**Rese** **Library**
**Medical**
**Education**

**BMA**

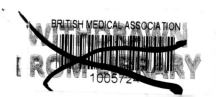

# Researching Medical Education

EDITED BY

## Jennifer Cleland

John Simpson Chair of Medical Education,
University of Aberdeen, UK; and
Chair of Council, Association for the Study of Medical Education (ASME)

## Steven J. Durning

Professor of Medicine,
Uniformed Services University,
Bethesda, Maryland, USA; and
Chair of the Association for Medical Education Europe (AMEE) Research Committee

## WILEY Blackwell

*Library of Congress Cataloging-in-Publication Data*

Researching medical education / edited by Jennifer Cleland, Steven Durning.

    p. ; cm.

  Includes bibliographical references and index.

  ISBN 978-1-118-83920-1 (pbk.)

  I. Cleland, Jennifer A., editor. II. Durning, Steven J., editor.

  [DNLM: 1. Education, Medical. 2. Biomedical Research. 3. Education, Dental. 4. Education, Nursing. 5. Learning. 6. Research Design. W 18]

  R735

  610.71–dc23

                                                       2015018491

A catalogue record for this book is available from the British Library.

Wiley also publishes its books in a variety of electronic formats. Some content that appears in print may not be available in electronic books.

Cover image: Definition "research" ©ineskoleva/istockphoto

Set in 9.5/11.5pt Palatino by SPi Global, Chennai, India

Printed in Singapore by C.O.S. Printers Pte Ltd

1  2015

# Contents

# Contributors

**Anthony R. Artino Jr.**
Associate Professor
Uniformed Services University of the Health Sciences
Bethesda,
Maryland, USA

**Juanita Bezuidenhout**
Educational advisor, Department of Interdisciplinary Health Sciences,
Faculty of Medicine and Health Sciences
Stellenbosch University
Cape Town and Consultant Histopathologist
JDW Pathology
Cape Town, South Africa

**Stephen Billet**
Professor of Adult and Vocational Education
School of Education and Professional Studies
Griffith University
Brisbane, Australia

**Alan Bleakley**
Professor of Medical Humanities
Falmouth University
Plymouth, UK

**Marise Ph. Born**
Professor of Personnel Psychology
Erasmus University,
Rotterdam
The Netherlands

**Ryan Brydges**
Assistant Professor
Department of Medicine
University of Toronto
Toronto, Canada

**Francois Cilliers**
Associate Professor
Education Development Unit
University of Cape Town
Cape Town, South Africa

**Jennifer Cleland**
John Simpson Chair of Medical Education
Division of Medical and Dental Education
University of Aberdeen
Aberdeen, UK

**Diana HJM Dolmans**
Professor
School of Health Professions Education
Maastricht University
The Netherlands

**Tim Dornan**
Professor of Medical Education
School of Medicine, Dentistry and Biomedical Sciences Queen's
University
Belfast, UK

**Erik Driessen**
Associate Professor of Medical Education
Maastricht University
Maastricht
The Netherlands

**Steven J. Durning**
Professor of Medicine
Uniformed Services University of the Health Sciences
Bethesda
Maryland, USA

**Kevin W. Eva**
Director and Professor of Educational Research and Scholarship,
Department of Medicine
University of British Columbia
Vancouver, Canada

**Tara Fenwick**
Professor of Professional Education
University of Stirling
Stirling, UK

**Trevor Gibbs**
Independent Consultant in Medical Education and Primary Care;
Development Officer
Association for Medical Education in Europe (AMEE)
Dundee, UK

**Tamara van Gog**
Professor of Educational Psychology
Erasmus University Rotterdam
Rotterdam
The Netherlands

**Larry D. Gruppen**
Professor
Department of Learning Health Sciences
University of Michigan Medical School
Ann Arbor, Michigan, USA

**Jenny Johnston**
Clinical Teaching Fellow
Queen's University Belfast
Belfast, UK

**Máire Kerrin**
Director,
Work Psychology Group
Derby, UK

**Theresa Kristopaitis**
Associate Professor,
Departments of Internal Medicine and Pathology
Loyola University Chicago
Stritch School of Medicine
Maywood, IL, USA

**Jimmie Leppink**
Postdoctoral Researcher in Education and Statistician
School of Health Professions Education
Maastricht University
The Netherlands

**Lorelei Lingard**
Director and Professor
Centre for Education Research & Innovation
Department of Medicine
Schulich School of Medicine and Dentistry
Western University, London
Ontario, Canada

**Anna MacLeod**
Associate Professor, Medical Education
Dalhousie University
Halifax, Canada

**Karen Mann**
Professor Emeritus, Medical Education
Dalhousie University
Halifax, Canada

**Maria Athina (Tina) Martimianakis**
Assistant Professor
Department of Paediatrics
University of Toronto
Toronto, Canada

**Meghan McConnell**
Assistant Professor
Clinical Epidemiology and Biostatistics
McMaster University
Hamilton, Canada

**William C. McGaghie**
Professor of Medical Education
Department of Medical Education
Northwestern University of Feinberg School of Medicine
Chicago, IL, USA

**Judy McKimm**
Professor of Medical Education and Director
of Strategic Educational Development
Swansea University
Swansea, UK

**Wendy McMillan**
Associate Professor in Dental Education
University of Western Cape
Cape Town, South Africa

**Jeroen J.G. van Merrienboer**
Professor
School of Health Professions Education
Maastricht University
The Netherlands

**Lynn V. Monrouxe**
Reader in Medical Education
Institute of Medical Education
Cardiff University
Cardiff, UK

**Maria Mylopoulos**
Assistant Professor
University of Toronto
Canada

**Sandra Nicholson**
Reader in Medical Education
Lead Community-Based Medical Education
Barts and The London
Queen Mary University of London
London, UK

**Graham R. Nimmo**
Consultant Physician in Intensive Care and Clinical Education
Western General Hospital
NHS Lothian
Edinburgh, UK

**Janneke K. Oostrom**
VU University,
Amsterdam,
The Netherlands

**Helen O'Sullivan**
Professor of Medical Education
Academic Lead for Online Learning
University of Liverpool
Liverpool, UK

**Fred Paas**
Professor of Educational Psychology
Institute of Psychology
Erasmus University Rotterdam
The Netherlands; and
Early Start Research Institute
University of Wollongong
Australia

**Fiona Patterson**
Professor, University of Cambridge
Director, Work Psychology Group
Derby, UK

**Linda Prescott-Clements**
Professor of Professional Education
University of Northumbria
Newcastle-upon-Tyne, UK

**Charlotte E. Rees**
Director and Professor Centre for Medical Education
University of Dundee
Dundee, UK

**Susan C. van Schalkwyk**
Deputy Director, Education;
Associate Professor in Health Professions Education
Stellenbosch University
Tygerberg, South Africa

**Lambert Schuwirth**
Professor of Medical Education
Flinders Innovation in Clinical Education
Flinders University
Adelaide, Australia

**R. Brent Stansfield**
Assistant Professor of Learning Health Sciences
Department of Medical Education
University of Michigan Medical School
Ann Arbor, Michigan, USA

**Linda Sweet**
Associate Professor
School of Nursing and Midwifery
Flinders University
Adelaide, Australia

**John Sweller**
Emeritus Professor of Education
University of New South Wales
Sydney, Australia

**David Taylor**
Reader in Medical Education
University of Liverpool
Liverpool, UK

**Dario Torre**
Associate Professor of Medicine
Drexel University College of Medicine
Philadelphia, USA

**Lara Varpio**
Associate Professor of Medicine
Uniformed Services University of the Health Sciences
Bethesda
Maryland, USA

**Cees van der Vleuten**
Scientific Director
School of Health Professions Education
Maastricht University
The Netherlands

**Geoff Wong**
Clinical Research Fellow
University of Oxford
Oxford, UK

# Foreword

Early in my career, a mentor enquired what sort of research I would undertake in my academic career. 'Education', I replied, triggering a perplexed look.

'Everyone in the university does education', he said patiently, 'but what will your *research* area be'?

'Education', I repeated.

Gazing at the floor he said searchingly, 'I'm looking for something more like … "I'm going to study the hypothalamic pituitary axis" or "I'm interested in thyroid function and depression"'.

'Education', I said once more, at which point I knew our time was up.

In just few decades, the field of medical and health professions education research has grown enormously, with new journals, international conferences, productive research centres and clear pathways for promotion at many universities. More importantly, the research itself is rapidly maturing in theoretical sophistication and methodological rigour. Long gone are the days when medical education was dominated by simple psychometric studies of examinations and a few descriptive curriculum reports. Today, when I tell a scholar (or a philanthropist) that I am researching health professions education, the look is more often one of interest than perplexity.

Perhaps the most interesting aspect of the marvelous new textbook you hold in your hands is that it provides a snapshot of how far we have come as a field. *Researching Medical Education* contains 24 chapters by authors from four continents and from many countries, representing a spectrum from well-known figures to emerging stars. Today our research family includes sociologists, historians, anthropologists, linguists, experimentalists, neurophysiologists, economists and clinicians of all kinds. Unlike many fields, we embrace theoretical and methodological diversities and have largely avoided the pointless disciplinary boundary skirmishes that sap energy and creativity from many academic areas. Medical and health professions education research is richer for its panoply of quantitative and qualitative methods and all manner of triangulation and integration.

Cleland and Durning's textbook is an indispensable resource for those new to the field of health professions education research. Using stories to introduce complex ideas, practice points to illustrate application and essential readings to guide further learning, the textbook provides the novice researcher with a place to begin and a program to advance. For those with more research experience, it provides a look at the current state of our field – illustrating in equal parts the journey we have taken and the challenges that lie ahead. Finally, this textbook will be invaluable for those responding to the growing demand for faculty development in education research: it will serve very well as a syllabus for a longitudinal masters or fellowship program. *Researching Medical Education* owes its existence to a wonderful organisation: The Association for the Study of Medical Education (ASME). Through its excellent journals and conferences, ASME is a leading light for high-quality research in education around the world. This textbook furthers ASME's reach and reputation. Furthermore, this textbook represents collaboration across ASME and the Association for Medical Education Europe (AMEE), thus illustrating the benefits of working together to share knowledge and networks.

Perhaps most importantly, *Researching Medical Education* is a guide to what Lingard so helpfully calls 'knowing which conversation we wish to join'. Decades ago I struggled to hear the faint voices of medical education research – today it has become a polyphonic conversation. *Researching Medical Education* comes at precisely the right time to capture this *zeitgeist*.

Brian D. Hodges, Toronto 2015

# Foreword from ASME

The idea for this exciting book came with the introduction of the Researching Medical Education (RME) conference of the Association for the Study of Medical Education (ASME), in its seventh year at the time of publication. From the outset, the RME was a great success, clearly tapping into the growing need to support those new to healthcare professions education research as well as providing continuing professional development for experienced researchers in the field.

*Researching Medical Education* remains true to its genesis by bringing together a wide range of medical education researchers to introduce, explain and illustrate, eruditely and enthusiastically, a breadth of topics and theories across healthcare profession research. It is wonderful to see this idea develop from its relatively humble beginnings to Jen and Steve's joint vision of creating an authoritative resource to inspire and support researchers to advance the science and scholarship of healthcare and medical education.

This is an exciting time in healthcare profession education. The number of masters programmes and doctorates in healthcare profession research is expanding rapidly worldwide. The field is moving forward in terms of rigorous and robust, cumulative and knowledge-building research. In short, the time is absolutely right for *Researching Medical Education*.

Dr Jane Stewart
*Chair of the Education Research Group (ERG) of the Association for the Study of Medical Education (ASME)*

# Foreword from AMEE

It has been said 'medicine used to be simple, ineffective and relatively safe; now it is complex, effective and potentially dangerous'.[1] If this is so how do we prepare students and trainees for independent practice? The expectation of evidence-based medicine, which was novel two decades ago, is now the norm. Hence, it is not so surprising that medical educationalists should be expected to research their discipline to help ensure that future doctors are trained and educated in evidenced-based ways. A new cadre of professionally trained medical educational researchers is emerging, this publication is timely to help and support their development. Not only is *Researching Medical Education* timely for individual researchers but also to support the intellectual development of the discipline as a whole. Linking theory to practice will allow the discipline to move from the previous 'show and tell' era into the mature academic discipline it needs to be for the effective and efficient education of future health care professionals and ultimately to improve patient care. We applaud the vision of the editors in commissioning this scholarly work and feel it will be of immense benefit to researchers in all stages of their careers.

**Trudie Roberts**
*President, Association of Medical Education in Europe*

**Ronald Harden**
*General Secretary, Association of Medical Education in Europe*

---

[1] C. Chantler. The role and education of doctors in the delivery of health care. Lancet 1999;353(9159):1178–1181.

# Preface

The intent of *Researching Medical Education* is to provide an authoritative guide to promote excellence in educational research in the healthcare professions (which includes medicine, nursing, dentistry and other fields).

Rigorous and original educational research in healthcare professions is critical to the future of healthcare education and, hence, ultimately, patient care. By encouraging thinking, discovery, evaluation, innovation, teaching, learning and improvement via research, the gaps between best practice and what actually happens in medical (and other healthcare professions) education can be addressed. In this way, knowledge can inform and advance education and practice, while education and practice can, in turn, inform and advance future research.

We have to ask the right questions, and answer them in the right way for a field of research to progress. To do so requires drawing on not just the existing education literature in healthcare professions but also the broader educational, sociological, cognitive and psychological literatures. These open our minds to different ways of thinking and working via different theories and methods, and different perspectives on the fundamental nature of research. To this end, our objectives in *Researching Medical Education* are to provide readers with the basic building blocks of research, introduce a range of theories and how to use a theory to underpin research, provide examples and illustrations of a diversity of methods and their use and, finally, give guidance on developing your practice as a researcher. By linking theory and design and methods across the context of educational research in healthcare professions, this book supports the improvement of quality, capacity building and knowledge generation within our field. This moves the focus of our work from local evaluation, assessment and audit to considering problems more generally, in terms of how they may contribute to new knowledge about learning, teaching and education.

There are many textbooks available that introduce theories, research designs and methodologies relevant to educational research in healthcare professions. However, most are not written specifically with this field of enquiry in mind and this can limit their impact. In contrast, this textbook is embedded with healthcare profession education and is illustrated throughout with examples from healthcare education and from selection to learning and teaching to professional development, drawn from international settings, using language and metaphors accessible to those working in, and wishing to work in, educational research. Reflecting our own backgrounds and the relationship of this book with the immensely successful *Understanding Medical Education*, the majority of examples are drawn from medical education. However, the aims and objectives of the book, and its key messages, are generalisable across any healthcare profession, or indeed any other profession, where learning knowledge, skills and attitudes are central to professional development.

*Researching Medical Education* provides a guide for Masters and PhD students in healthcare profession education and their supervisors; those who are new to the field, those who are generally inexperienced in research, those who are new to the field of educational research but have prior research experience in the clinical or biomedical domains and experienced researchers seeking to explore new ways of thinking and working. With this broad audience in mind, we have designed the book to be of value to degree programme students and faculty; those juggling a portfolio of clinical work, teaching and research; and those few whose sole focus is research. To achieve these objectives, our authors are a blend of clinicians and PhD researchers in healthcare profession education, representing a range of disciplines and backgrounds. Their contributions provide a blueprint of how to pose and address research questions, illustrated by practical examples – from the straightforward to the aspirational. Many examples are to illustrate how medical education and related research are currently progressing knowledge in the field. International examples help ensure that the messages in this textbook are relevant to all healthcare profession educators even though the structures, systems and processes of healthcare delivery and education vary across countries.

*Researching Medical Education* is presented in three sections. The first is labelled 'A primer of healthcare education research'. This section systematically introduces the initial steps in the research process. It starts with a broad overview of the two main research philosophies relevant to the educational research in healthcare professions and how these differ in terms of assumptions about the world, about how science should be conducted and about what constitutes legitimate problems, solutions and criteria from Cleland. McMillan then considers the influence of the individual researcher's preferences or 'worldview' on the research process, and introduces and explains the critical concepts of ontology, epistemology and reflexivity in research. Wong introduces the next step in the research process, of identifying, then critically examining, the quality, methodological and/or theoretical contribution of the existing literature on a particular topic, and explains the different purposes and approaches to producing a literature review. In the fourth chapter, Bezuidenhout and van Schalkwyk describe how to move from an idea or a problem to formulating a research question, using the analogy of distillation and concrete worked examples to illustrate the steps in this process. Following on from this, Stansfield and Gruppen discuss how to conduct a power analysis to help ensure your quantitative study has an adequate number of participants to find effects such as the impact of an intervention, an educational outcome or the relationship between variables.

The next section of *Researching Medical Education* introduces theory, of the utmost importance in terms of providing a solid foundation to any research. A good theory (one which is internally consistent and coherent) should describe, explain, enable explanations (not just the what, but the why and the how) and yield testable hypotheses or research questions. The use of theory should generate new routes for research – routes that are conceptually related to and build on prior research. Theories can be described in terms of their scope, with wider scopes reflecting generally higher levels of abstraction in the knowledge hierarchy. Mann and Macleod open this section with an introduction to a 'grand theory' (a very general theory that provides a framework for the nature and goals of a discipline), that of social constructivism. They promote alignment of worldview, theoretical frameworks and research approaches (methods) in relation to constructivism and its philosophical underpinnings.

This section then introduces a number of specific theories that are intended to guide empirical inquiry, action or practice. We first focus on theories that emphasise the collective, or social, where relationships between context, environment, people and things matter. Fenwick and Nimmo provide an overview of some main ideas shared across different sociomaterial theories and methods, those which foreground materials – bodies, objects, substances, settings, technologies, and so on – to examine how they act with and on the human activity and thought. Bleakley and Cleland focus on complexity theory as an overarching framework to inform and guide how healthcare profession researchers can meaningfully engage with highly complex contexts, such as clinical teams or educational systems, and where the outcomes of interactions are not always predictable. Johnson and Dornan then introduce activity theory, a socio-cultural perspective, which places a person's social and cultural surroundings, and history, as central to what they do. This system-level focus can be used to analyse situations and enable change beyond the individual. We continue with a chapter by Torre and Durning who discuss social cognitive theories, those that consider learning and performance as inherently social and where the uniqueness that each situation brings (in terms of environment, participants, interactions) can often lead to different learning and performance experiences and outcomes. We finish this section with Sweet and Billett who introduce the concept of participatory practices – what opportunities for learning are provided in healthcare workplace settings and how individuals elect to engage in and learn through those practices – for understanding, supporting and developing workplace-based learning.

The next chapters introduce rich families of theories where a number of different theories offer a particular perspective on the same phenomena. This is itself not unusual, but what is of interest is that each topic area encompasses theories that range from those that focus on the individual level (beliefs, processes and/or performance) to theories that offer a social or environmental lens through which to look at the same phenomena. Monrouxe and Rees consider the issues of professional identity and present a range of identity theories, from those that acknowledge that personal identities develop in a social world to individualist approaches that conceptualise identities as personal attributes. Cilliers and colleagues outline a number of different health behaviour theories and illustrate how these can be used as a means of illuminating, explaining and changing behaviour in teaching-learning settings, whether campus-based or practice-based. Artino and colleagues introduce theories of self-regulated learning (SRL), which describe the processes that individuals use to optimise their strategic pursuit of personal learning goals. These represent the continuum from largely social to largely cognitive descriptions of SRL. In these chapters, as with all chapters in this book, the chapter authors set out how these different theories may productively be used to plan studies, to analyse findings and, potentially, to relate findings from different studies.

We then move on to areas where the dominant theories are those that focus solely on individual-level beliefs, processes and/or performance. Patterson and colleagues introduce the concept of values in relation to selection, and invite us to consider the theoretical underpinnings of values and how values link to concepts such as personality, motivation and behaviours. McConnell and Eva provide an understanding of the role that emotions play in the training, assessment and development of clinicians and, using a cognitive psychology lens, introduce common theoretical constructs and key methodological issues inherent in studying emotion. van Merrienboer and Dolmans introduce the field of study of instructional design, a field that aims at developing evidence-informed guidelines and models for the design of instruction, ranging from the design of particular instructional materials, via lessons and courses, to complete curricula. Leppink and colleagues take this forward by setting out a comprehensive overview of the utility of cognitive load theory for effective instructional design that facilitates learning and problem solving in medical education and practice. McGaghie and Kristopaitis provide a critical-realist review of the state of knowledge on deliberate practice and clinical skill acquisition, including how clinical skills acquired in the medical education laboratory can transfer to patient care practices and patient outcomes.

We end with two chapters that examine the different ways of using theory. Nicholson and Cleland use the topic of widening access to medicine to illustrate how the use of different theoretical or conceptual frameworks can progress understanding and increase the sophistication of empirical work in a field. Varpio and colleagues focus on the necessity of acknowledging the differences within qualitative methodologies that make a difference, because these variations enable carefully directed research. They introduce and explain the concepts of methodological borrowing, shifting and importing in qualitative research.

In summary, theories are considered to be important aspects of the worldviews helping to generate a better understanding of the surrounding world. Each chapter includes examples of application of a theory but some emphasise explanation more than application, or vice-versa, depending on the topic and the nature of the research on that topic. Some of these theories are already used extensively in educational research in healthcare professions, whereas some are more novel but hold much promise. You will see when reading that different theoretical approaches align more with certain study designs and methodologies: in some chapters, the research studies are predominantly quantitative, to enable the measurement of cause-effect relationships, whereas in others, the methodologies and methods are typically qualitative, reflecting the nature of the phenomena and hence the research questions.

These are not the only theories, or ways of applying particular theories, which may be suitable for educational research in healthcare professions – others are not presented, for no other reason than that no one book can cover everything. What *Researching Medical Education* gives is an introduction to the breadth of theories from computing science, psychology, sociology, education and other fields, which may be used to help design a research question, guide the selection of relevant data, interpret the data and propose explanations of the underlying causes or influences of the observed phenomena in healthcare education research. Moreover, each chapter provides additional recommended references to help readers explore topics of interest in more detail. Most chapters also begin with a vignette and end with summary points, and we have placed emphasis on the practical aspects of the theories discussed in this book. Whatever be your question and natural inclination towards particular schools of theory, consider different theories and methods carefully. Do not jump too quickly, consciously or not, onto a single option without exploring others. The time spent in reflecting on which theory and methods are appropriate for your purposes early in the research process is time well spent.

The chapters so far have provided essential reading for planning and doing quality medical and healthcare profession research. Ensuring what we do is excellent is, however, only one part of educational research. The best research will have little impact if no-one knows of it or if it is not taken forward beyond a single study. Thus, the third section of *Researching Medical Education* provides guidance on developing your practice as an educational researcher. Driessen and Lingard focus on dissemination, taking a rhetorical approach to get writers and speakers thinking about how to tell a compelling story from their research work. McKimm and O'Sullivan look at a key element of educational research – how to lead and manage the research process – and how leadership and management theory can help your (and others') research run more smoothly. Finally, Taylor and Gibbs explain the importance of planning research in a way that ensures sustainability and long-term effectiveness.

We hope that *Researching Medical Education* stimulates fresh thinking and new ideas for educational research in medical and healthcare professions and encourages you to engage further with the many exciting theories, models, methodologies and analysis approaches introduced here, the use of which will progress our field of study.

Jennifer Cleland
Steven J. Durning

# Acknowledgements

Our thanks to the *Researching Medical Education* International Editorial Board members for their guidance on which theories, models and methods were included in this book. We also thank them for their help with reviewing submissions.

**Professor Peter Cantillon**, Chair of the Irish Network of Medical Educators (INMeD) and Primary Care, Department of General Practice, Clinical Science Institute, National University of Ireland, Galway, Ireland

**Professor Gudrun Edgren**, Director of the Centre for Teaching and Learning, Lund University, Lund, Sweden

**Professor Trevor Gibbs**, WHO Consultant in Medical Education, Adolescent Health and Primary Care and Association for the Study of Medical Education (AMEE) Development Officer, AMEE, Dundee, UK

**Professor Shipra Ginsberg**, Associate Professor and cross-appointed Scientist in the Wilson Centre, University of Toronto, Toronto, Canada

**Professor Judy McKimm**, Director of Strategic Educational Development, Swansea University, UK

**Professor Stewart Mennin**, Mennin Consulting and Associates, Sao Paulo, Brazil

**Professor Debra Nestal**, Professor of Simulation Education in Healthcare, Monash University, Melbourne, Australia

**Dr Mark Newman**, Reader in Evidence-informed Policy and Practice in Education and Social Policy, Institute of Education, University of London, London, UK

**Professor Patricia O'Sullivan**, Department of Medicine and Director of Research and Development in Medical Education, Office of Medical Education, University of California, San Francisco, USA

**Professor Daniel Pratt**, Professor Emeritus (Education) and Senior Scholar (Medicine), Department of Educational Studies, Faculty of Education, University of British Columbia, Canada

**Professor Jereon van Merrienboer**, Chair in Learning and Instruction and Research Program Director of the Graduate School of Health Professions Education, University of Maastricht, Maastricht, The Netherlands

**Professor Tim Wilkinson**, Director, MB ChB programme (Faculty of Medicine) and Deputy Dean (Christchurch), University of Otago, New Zealand

**Dr Kath Woolf**, Senior Lecturer in Medical Education, University College London, London, UK

**PART 1**

# A primer of healthcare education research

# 1 Exploring versus measuring: considering the fundamental differences between qualitative and quantitative research

*Jennifer Cleland*

*I overheard some of the trainees/residents talking about the things that are important to them in terms of career decision making. It struck me that things are a bit different from 'my day': for example, they seem much more concerned with work-life balance. After looking at the literature, a colleague and I decided that there were various gaps in terms of what is known about the factors that influence medical student and trainee careers decision making in our country, particularly since the training pathway changed about 10 years ago. We wanted to explore this further, so first carried out some telephone interviews to gather the views of students and trainees. The participants suggested a number of factors, which we had not thought of, as particularly important in careers decision making. We then wanted to find out which factors were most important to the majority of trainees and if there were differences across students and trainees at different stages of training. To achieve this, we used the data from our literature review and the interviews to design a questionnaire, which we sent out to all students and trainees nationally.*

## Introduction

This true scenario, one which has underpinned, to date, a 5-year programme of work,[1–3] highlights some of the differences between quantitative and qualitative research, but also how they can be used in a complementary manner in the same programme of research.

It is easy to assume that the differences between quantitative and qualitative research are solely about how data is collected – the randomised controlled trial (RCT) versus ethnographic fieldwork, the cohort study versus the semi-structured interview. These are, however, research methods (tools) rather than approaches (methodologies). There are very important consequences of choosing (implicitly or explicitly) a particular methodological stance or position to guide and inform your research

practice or an individual study. Quantitative and qualitative approaches make different assumptions about the world,[4,5] about how science should be conducted and about what constitutes legitimate problems, solutions and criteria of 'proof'.[6] They also use completely different languages (see Fig. 1.1).

*'When we speak of 'quantitative' or 'qualitative' methodologies we are in the final analysis speaking about an interrelated set of assumptions about the social world which are philosophical, ideological and epistemological. They encompass more than just data collection methodologies'* (Rist, 1977, p. 62[7])

In this chapter, drawing on Bryman,[8] I will talk about these assumptions and their implications for research practice. I will then compare and contrast the two approaches in terms of research design, methods are tools, analysis and interpretation. I will draw on examples from healthcare education research to illustrate these points. I will also discuss combined ('mixed-methods') approaches. The content of this chapter is more heavily 'weighted' towards quantitative research is but cross-referenced with corresponding key information about qualitative research, which is presented in other chapters in this volume.

## Philosophical differences

Research philosophies differ on the goals of the research and the way to achieve these goals. For example, is the purpose to test theories and discover general principles, or is it to describe and explain complex situations? Quantitative and qualitative research comes from different underlying assumptions of what is reality (ontology) and what is knowledge (epistemology) (see also chapters by McMillan, and Mann and Macleod in this book).

*Researching Medical Education*, First Edition. Edited by Jennifer Cleland and Steven J. Durning.
© 2015 John Wiley & Sons, Ltd. Published 2015 by John Wiley & Sons, Ltd.

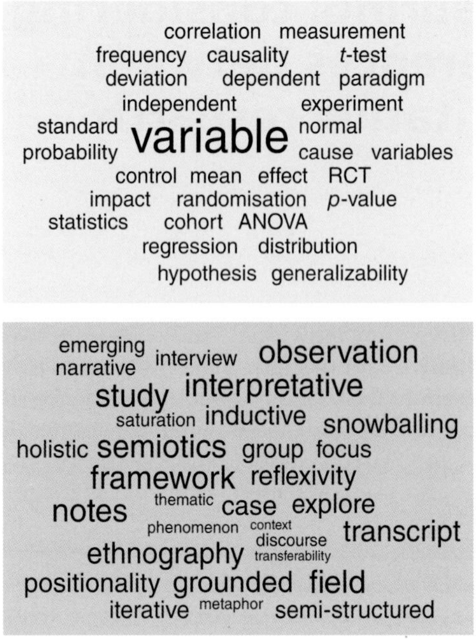

correlation  measurement
frequency  causality  *t*-test
deviation  dependent  paradigm
independent  experiment
standard  **variable**  normal
probability  cause  variables
control  mean  effect  RCT
impact  randomisation  *p*-value
statistics  cohort  ANOVA
regression  distribution
hypothesis  generalizability

emerging  narrative  interview  observation
study  interpretative
saturation  inductive  snowballing
holistic  semiotics  group  focus
framework  reflexivity
notes  thematic  case  explore
phenomenon  context
discourse
ethnography  transferability  transcript
positionality  grounded  field
iterative  metaphor  semi-structured

*Figure 1.1* Word clouds of quantitative and qualitative language.

## Quantitative research philosophies

Quantitative research draws originally from the positivist paradigm. The underlying premise of this paradigm (basic belief systems, or universally accepted models providing the context for understanding and decision making) is that the goal of knowledge is simply to describe the phenomena that we experience, and hence can observe and measure (i.e. objectivity). The researcher and the focus of the research are in this way independent of each other: the researcher has no influence on the research process. In a positivist view of the world, the goal of knowledge is to observe, measure and describe the phenomena experienced. The positivist perspective is founded on the idea that reality is tangible and measurable. Knowledge of anything beyond that (a positivist would hold) is impossible. In positivism, science was seen as the way to get at truth, to understand the world well enough so that we might predict and control it. This might seem a little extreme to us now, and it is fair to say that quantitative research has moved on from purely positivist views to post-positivism. Post-positivism does not reject the basic tenets of observation and measurement, but it recognises that all observation is fallible and that all theory is revisable. Post-positivitism is also characterised by an acceptance that the theories, background, knowledge and values of the researcher can influence what is observed.

In post-positivism, a variety of epistemologies underpin theory and practice in quantitative research[9]. One of the most common post-positivism stances is that of critical realism or criticality. A critical realist believes that there is a reality independent of our thinking about it that science can study, and questions (hence the 'critical' label) the infallibility of observation and theory. Moreover, they also believe that while everyone is influenced by their cultural experiences, world views, and so on, researchers can put aside their biases and beliefs to strive for objectivity. The differences between positivism and critical realism are discussed further in the chapter by MacMillan later in this book. For the purposes of the current chapter, however, it is sufficient to know that those working from a (post-) positivist position believe that the scientific method (i.e. the approaches and procedures of the natural sciences such as chemistry, biology and physics) is appropriate for the study of social phenomena (e.g. learning).

## Qualitative research philosophies

The premise of qualitative research is subjectivity[10]. Qualitative research is concerned with how the social world is interpreted, understood, experienced or produced. Reality cannot be measured directly. It exists as perceived by people and by the observer. Reality is relative and multiple, perceived through socially constructed and subjective interpretations[11]. There are many structured approaches to apprehending such realities and the methods and procedures of the natural sciences are not (generally) suitable for doing so (see later). The qualitative tradition is also underpinned by a number of different theories. These give researchers different 'conceptual lenses' through which to look at complicated problems and social issues, focusing their attention on different aspects of the data and providing a framework within which to conduct their analysis.[12] Many of these are described elsewhere in this book (for example, see chapters by Mann and McLeod, Monrouxe and Rees, Varpio and colleagues) and see also Reeves *et al.*[13] for a very useful overview.

## So what do these differences mean in practice?

Broadly speaking, quantitative research involves hypothesis testing and confirmation whereas qualitative research is concerned with hypothesis generation and understanding (see Table 1.1). Expanding on this, quantitative research tends to be deductive, seeking to validate an idea or theory by conducting an experiment and analysing the results numerically (see Table 1.1). Theory is often seen as something from which to derive a hypothesis, a tentative explanation that accounts for a set of facts and can be tested by further investigation. For example, one hypothesis we might want to test (the null hypothesis) is that there is a relationship between students' self-confidence in examination skills and the amount of time they spend on the wards. Hypotheses are often in the form of an if/then statement; for example, if we teach handwashing, then infection rates will reduce. A hypothesis is always provisional as data may emerge that cause us to reject it later on (i.e. the outcome might be to reject the null hypothesis if the data indicates no significant relationship between self-confidence and time on the wards).

In this way, in quantitative research, the theories determine the problems (the research moves deductively, from theory to the data), which generate the hypotheses, usually about causal connections. On the other hand, the use of theory in qualitative research tends to be inductive; that is, building explanations from the ground up, based on what is discovered (although more deductive qualitative studies are possible[14]). Inductive reasoning begins with specific observations and measures, for detecting patterns and regularities, formulating tentative hypotheses to explore, and, finally, ends by developing some general conclusions or theories.

Finally, it is useful to make one final point about how qualitative and quantitative research 'use' theory. Theory is often 'assumed' in quantitative research, while its use is much more explicit in the qualitative tradition. Because of this, you are unlikely to see statements of theoretical stance in quantitative studies whereas these are an expected feature of healthcare education qualitative studies[15].

## Comparing research design in quantitative and qualitative research

If quantitative research is concerned with establishing casual connections while qualitative research is concerned with describing phenomena in their natural setting, then different study designs are needed.

### Quantitative research design

There are four broad approaches to study design within quantitative research: descriptive, correlational, quasi-experimental and experimental. These are described briefly in Table 1.2 and illustrated

*Table 1.1* The hypothesis

To use the word hypothesis in qualitative research is incongruent (see Fig. 1.1). However, all studies have a research question. How these are decided, and written, differs depending on the philosophy of the study. For example, here is a reasonably typical example of a hypothesis from a quantitative study in medical education research: 'this study aimed to identify whether poor performance in degree assessments early in the medical degree course predicts poor performance in later MBChB assessments' ([16], p. 677). In this study, we wanted to know if x (early poor performance) predicted y (later poor performance). Compare that statement with this one from a qualitative study published in the same year: 'Our study aimed to answer the research question: why do assessors fail to report underperformance in medical students?' ([17], p. 802). This is a much more open and exploratory approach, as befits a study, which was concerned with exploring the views and beliefs underpinning assessor behaviour. See the chapter by Bezuidenhout and Schalkwyk in this book for a more in-depth discussion of the research question.

with hypothetical examples in the table. Published examples of each design are discussed in the text.

Descriptive research is used to describe characteristics of a population or phenomenon – for example, how many students failed a certain assessment, how positively trainees rate the teaching in a particular department, what factors are important in medical student career decision making. Descriptive studies do not answer how/when/why questions, just the 'what' question (What are the characteristics of the population or situation being studied?[18]).

Correlational research is used to identify trends and patterns in data. For example, Husbands *et al.*[19] examined the predictive validity of the UKCAT, an aptitude test used for selection into medical school in the UK, and compare this with traditional selection methods (e.g. performance in an individual interview), in terms of performance in the senior years of medical school. They examined the relationships between admissions variables, examination scores, gender and age group using statistical tests, and found that the UKCAT predicted performance in the later years of medical school better than other selection methods.

Quasi-experimental research is used frequently in healthcare education research as random assignment to study conditions is often difficult due to practical and ethical constraints (e.g. it would be unethical to withhold teaching from a 'control' group of students). However, this leaves quasi-experimental designs open to biases and confounders, (or 'threats to validity') of the conclusion about the relationship between the intervention and outcome studied.[20] For example, in the early days of problem-based learning (PBL), Distlehorst

*Table 1.2* Types of quantitative design

| | | | |
|---|---|---|---|
| *Descriptive research* seeks to describe the current status of the variable under study ('what is'). Designed to provide systematic information about a phenomenon. *Example*: a description of the alcohol use of medical and nursing students. | *Correlational research* explores relationships (associations) between study variables using statistical data. This type of research will recognise trends and patterns in data, but it does not go so far in its analysis as to prove causes for these observed patterns. *Example*: the relationship between early and later performance on degree assessments (see previous sections). | *Quasi-experimental research* attempts to establish cause–effect relationships among the variables. Groups are naturally formed or pre-existing rather than randomised. *Example*: the effect of attending extra clinical skills sessions on exam performance | *Experimental research* looks to establish the cause–effect relationship among a group of variables that make up a study. An independent variable is manipulated to determine the effects on the dependent variables. Subjects are randomly assigned to experimental treatments. *Example*: the effect of different types of curricula design on students' preparedness for practice |

and Robb[21] compared the academic performance (United States Medical Licensing Examination, clinical clerkship, and clinical practice examination) of students in a PBL curriculum with that of their counterparts in a standard curriculum, in the same medical school. They found that students in the PBL curriculum performed at least as well as, their counterparts and concluded that PBL students were not disadvantaged. This was on the face of it reassuring but the conclusion does not acknowledge the potential for this outcome to be due to confounders, such as the fact that a different type of learner may be attracted to PBL. If using a quasi-experimental design, it is thus critical to carefully consider threats to validity of the particular study and demonstrate that they can be ruled out. For example, if you think surgical experience will influence how students perform on a particular task make sure all participants do the task before their surgical rotation, if you are using a quasi-experimental design.

Finally, experimental research tests whether the independent variable(s) (controlled by the researcher) affects a dependent variable (the variable being measured for change) (see Table 1.3). An attempt may be made to control extraneous variables to ensure that the cause of change is, indeed, the independent variable – such as PBL in the aforementioned example. The RCT is an example of experimental research. A good illustration of an RCT in healthcare education research is provided by Watson *et al.*[22] who used an RCT design to investigate whether education in simulated learning environments (SLEs) could substitute for part of traditional clinical education for physiotherapy students. They designed two SLE models, and

*Table 1.3* Independent and dependent variables in quantitative research

An independent variable is exactly what it sounds like. It is not changed by the other variables you are trying to measure. Examples would include age or gender – other factors (such as diet, amount of time spent studying or exercising, ward attendance) are not going to change a person's age or gender. The point is to see if the independent variable causes some kind of change in the other, or dependent, variables. Dependent variables would include exam outcome, performance on a task, things that can be changed by other factors, such as how much you studied or practised. Thus, an independent variable causes a change in a dependent variable.

randomly assigned students (stratified by academic score) to either receiving SLE (intervention arm of the study) or 'traditional' (control arm of the study) teaching. The primary outcome measure (see later) was a blinded, structured assessment of student competency conducted over two clinical examinations. They found that students' achievement of clinical competencies was no worse in the SLE groups than in the traditional groups. Because of the design of the study (e.g. randomising students to SLE or traditional teaching, assessor not knowing what teaching the student had received), the authors could confidently say that they had provided evidence that clinical education in an SLE can in part replace clinical time with real patients without compromising students' attainment of the professional competencies required to practise. The chapter on Cognitive Load by Leppink and colleagues in this book is a good example of a topic area where most of the evidence is based on RCTs.

RCTs are a major undertaking but luckily, there is guidance on how to plan and report them. Sibbald and Roland[23] provide a useful summary of the important features of a 'gold standard' RCT, including randomisation and the 'double-blind' approach. CONSORT (Consolidated Standards of Reporting Trials) provides a set of recommendations, checklist and flow chart for reporting randomised trials, known as the Consort Statement (http://www.consort-statement.org/: see also[24]). Most journals and funding bodies require a CONSORT statement and flow diagram to be submitted alongside a paper reporting a randomised trial.

There is, arguably, less explicit guidance available for planning other quantitative designs – descriptive, correlational or quasi-experimental – but one useful source of guidance is critical appraisal tools. These provide guidance on the essential components of what should be included or considered in a study (for example, see the Critical Appraisal Skills Programme, or CASP (http://www.casp-uk.net/).

A critical feature of quantitative research design lies is pre-planning and prescriptiveness. All aspects of the study are carefully designed before data is collected. Each detail is worked out in advance – the study design, participants, data collection tools, data collection procedures (e.g. timing of follow-up) and the analysis plan. The aim of documenting quantitative research processes in detail, in advance, is to ensure that each step is performed in the same way each time. This also means that the study can be replicated or repeated using the same protocol at another time or by a different researcher, and the same findings will be the same. This document or 'protocol' is planned in great detail, and quantitative research protocols are publishable entities in their own right.

## Qualitative research designs

Compare the above with the description of research design in Becker et al.'s[25] classic qualitative study of medical students:

> *In one sense, our study had no design. That is, we had no well-worked-out set of hypotheses to be tested, no data-gathering instruments purposely designed to secure information relevant to these hypotheses, no set of analytic procedures specified in advance. Insofar as the term 'design' implies these features of elaborate prior planning, our study had none. If we take the idea of design in a larger and looser sense, using it to identify those elements of order, system, and consistency our procedures did exhibit, our study had a design. We can say what this was by describing our original view of the problem, our theoretical and methodological commitments, and the way these affected our research and were affected by it as we proceeded.* (p. 17)

In qualitative research, the design is predominantly determined by the research question and, as such, questioning and inquiring unfolds the process of understanding.[26] To do this requires scoping the project and considering what data is required in advance, with research design as 'a reflexive process operating through every stage of a project'.[27] Reflexive refers to being thoughtful, constantly examining what is affecting research decisions such as the wording of questions or how one interprets data. (A fuller explanation of reflexivity in the research process is provided by Mann and MacLeod in Chapter 6.) In the qualitative approach, the activities of collecting and analysing data, developing and modifying theory, elaborating or refocusing the research questions, are usually going on more or less simultaneously, each influencing all of the others (see Maxwell[28] for a useful model of qualitative research design (p. 216)). The researcher may need to reconsider or modify any design decision during the study in response to new developments. In this way, qualitative research design is less linear than quantitative research, which is much more step-wise and fixed.

These differences are a matter of degree, however. Most qualitative projects would have some pre-structuring at least in terms of the equivalent of a research protocol, setting out what you are doing (aims and objectives), why (why is this important) and how (theoretical underpinning, design, methods, analysis). Generally, however, a qualitative research plan would be less fixed than its quantitative equivalent, but it is still a critical component of the research process. There are several excellent textbooks that go into this in more detail[26,29–31] and you can read examples of different qualitative designs throughout this book.

## Data collection methods

There is no one best way of quantitative or qualitative data collection: the method depends on what you need to know. Only a broad overview of different types of method is provided here. For more detail, go to one of the major textbooks recommended at the end of this section.

## Quantitative data collection methods

Quantitative data collection methods involve objective measurements via structured data collection instruments that fit diverse experiences into predetermined response categories. The most common quantitative data collection tools are as follows:

- Surveys (e.g. questionnaires, structured interviews)
- Observations (e.g. number of students using the gym between 6 and 8 am)
- Measurements (e.g. ranking on graduation, number of doctors training in radiology)

Questionnaires or surveys (the terms are often used interchangeably) often look a relatively straightforward way to collect data. This is not the case. Designing a good questionnaire typically involves drawing on the literature, collecting some exploratory or consensus data, piloting a preliminary questionnaire for readability and acceptability, testing out the statistical qualities of the questionnaire, before actually using it in a study. Unless questionnaire design is the focus of your research, it is generally better to use a published questionnaire, ideally one which has been used previously with a similar population (group of participants) to the one you are studying.

Observations in quantitative research are structured in that the precise focus of the observations is decided in advance, and the method does not change as the study continues (compared to the more fluid research process in qualitative research). Collection of data by observations can be conducted on facts (e.g. the number of students in a classroom), events (e.g. the amount of collaborative work taking place between students in the classroom) or behaviours (e.g. the number of incidents of antisocial behaviour in a classroom), or skills (e.g. the number of attempts needed to put in a venflon correctly, checklist ratings of performance). Data collection is planned to allow for easy recording – for example, 'done' or 'not done'; 'excellent', 'good', 'borderline'. Workplace-based assessment tools such as the Mini-CEX are good examples of structured observation tools[32].

Remembering that analysis in quantitative research is about number 'crunching' and statistics, it is worth emphasising that simple word data can be transformed into number data for analysis. For example, 'Done' or 'not done' can be transposed into 0 and 1 for analysis, 'excellent', 'good' and 'borderline' can become 1, 2 and 3. This is particularly useful in surveys, where a popular technique is to ask respondents to choose between particular options or rate statements in different ways, such as 'agree strongly', 'agree', 'disagree' or 'disagree strongly', and give the answers a number (e.g. 1 for 'disagree strongly', 4 for 'agree strongly'). Note that questionnaires often use a mixed-methods design, incorporating both statement ratings and free text questions such as 'Please explain the reasons for your answer.' Mixed-methods approaches are discussed in more detail later in this chapter.

In terms of data collection procedures, quantitative studies tend to involve relatively large numbers compared with qualitative studies. Qualitative study samples need to be of sufficient size to enable statistical analysis and to demonstrate associative or causative relationships between variables (more about analysis later). As one of the ultimate aims of quantitative research is generalisability, representative sampling is critical. A representative sample should be an unbiased indication of what the population is like. For example, in Scotland at the time of writing, the medical student population is 60:40 female:male. A representative sample of Scottish medical students would, therefore, have female and male subjects in these proportions. Unfortunately, it would be fair to say that much quantitative research in healthcare education continues to be single-site, where all data is collected from one institution or one sub-group (e.g. surgical trainees/residents from one hospital, or even those from one surgical sub-specialty), which limits generalisability. See Table 1.4 for a comparison of sampling approaches in quantitative and qualitative research.

*Table 1.4* Sample sizes

The sample size for a quantitative study is calculated using formulas to determine how large a sample size will be needed from a given population in order to achieve findings with an acceptable degree of accuracy. Generally, researchers seek sample sizes, which yield findings with at least a 95% confidence interval (which means that if you repeat the survey 100 times, 95 times out of a hundred, you would get the same response), plus/minus a margin error of 5 percentage points. Please see Chapter 5 by Stansfield and Gruppen for guidance on sample size and power calculations.

Sampling of research participants in qualitative research is described as purposive, meaning there is far less emphasis on generalising from sample to population and greater attention to a sample 'purposely' selected for its potential to yield insight from its illuminative and rich information sources ([33], p. 40). See chapters by Mann and MacLead, Rees and Monrouxe, Varpio and colleagues in this book for more extensive descriptions of sampling in qualitative research.

## Qualitative data collection methods

The qualitative methods most commonly used for research purposes are mentioned very briefly in this chapter, as these are covered in more detail elsewhere in this book. They can be classified in three broad categories as follows:

- Interviews (individual or group)
- Observation methods
- Document review

The qualitative research interview seeks to describe and gain understanding of certain themes in the life world of the subjects. Interviews can be organised one-to-one or group (focus groups) depending on the topic under study and the cultural context, and the aims of the project. Observational data collection in qualitative research involves the detailed observation of people and events to learn about behaviours and interactions in natural settings.[34] Such study designs are useful when the study goal is to understand cultural aspects of a setting or phenomenon,[35] when the situation of interest is hidden, (tacit), or when subjects in the setting appear to have notably different views to other groups. Written materials or documents such as institutional records, personal diaries and historical public documents may also serve as a valuable source of secondary data, providing insight into the lives and experiences of the group under study. See Bowen[36] for an excellent introduction to the purpose and practicalities of document review within qualitative research.

See Dicicco-Bloom and Crabtree[37] for a useful summary of the content and process of the qualitative research interview, Creswell[31] for further discussion of the many different approaches in qualitative research and their common characteristics, and later in this book for examples of different approaches to qualitative interviewing and observation.

## Data management

Different research approaches generate different types of data. Quantitative research generates (quantifiable) numerical data, that is (if the sampling strategy is appropriate) generalisable to some larger population, for analysis. Aliaga and Gunderson[38] sum up quantitative research neatly as 'explaining phenomena by collecting numerical data that are analysed using mathematically based methods (in particular statistics) (p. 1). Qualitative research may use some form of quantification, but statistical forms of analysis are not seen as central ([39], p. 4). Instead, qualitative data analysis (QDA) aims to uncover emerging themes, patterns, concepts, insights, and understandings.[33] The data are allowed to 'speak for themselves' by the emergence of conceptual categories and descriptive themes. Trying to squeeze narratives into boxes (like '0' and '1') would result in the loss of contextualisation and narrative layering. The researcher must immerse themselves in the data in order to be able to see meaningful patterns and themes, making notes as they go through the processes of data collection and analysis, and then using these notes to guide the analysis strategy.

In both approaches, data has to be managed before it can be analysed. Statistical and qualitative data management and analysis software are pretty much essential at this stage unless you are working with a very small dataset. If you are working with numbers, or data, which can be sensibly coded into numerical form, you need a database that is designed to store and analyse numerical data. It is a good idea to enter your data directly into a statistical package to avoid problems transferring data from one package (e.g. a spreadsheet) to another for analysis[40]. SPSS is one of the most commonly used statistical software packages. On the other hand, if your study design is qualitative and hence your data takes the form of 'words' and text, or images and visual material, you may want to use a specialist qualitative database to facilitate data management and analysis. NVivo is a well-known QDA software package (note that qualitative software packages enable you to make and store notes, and explanations of your codes, so you do not need to juggle bits of paper and electronic data files). These and similar databases are available commercially (i.e. at a cost) and are used widely by universities. The choice of database may be dictated by the resources of your institution, your personal preference and/or what technical support is available locally.

A word of caution – data management software does not describe or analyse your data for you. You have to enter and manage data in such a way to facilitate the processes of description and analysis. Thinking about the analysis early on in the project plan can save a lot of time later in the process. See Cleland *et al.*[40] for comprehensive guidance on how to use quantitative and qualitative databases in education research.

## Data analysis

As mentioned earlier, different research methods generate different types of data and these different types of data require different analysis approaches.

### Quantitative data analysis

Quantitative analysis is the process of presenting and interpreting numerical data. Statistical analysis is inherent to quantitative research. Quantitative data analysis usually involves descriptive statistics and inferential statistics. Descriptive statistics give a 'picture' of the data in terms of, for example, number of male and female respondents, age of respondents, frequency of particular responses, as and describe the pattern of the data in terms of averages (mean, median and mode) and measures of variability about the average (range and standard deviation). A useful overview of descriptive data and how to present descriptive data can be found in Cleland *et al.*[40]

Inferential statistics are the outcomes of statistical tests, helping deductions to be made from the data collected, testing hypotheses and relating findings to the sample or population. In terms of selecting a statistical test, the most important question is 'what is the main study hypothesis and/or research question?' Are you looking for an association or relationship between x and y, or a difference between a and b? Different statistical tests are used for testing each type of question, and within each type of question, different statistical tests are used depending on the precise nature of your study design. The next question is 'what types of data are being measured?' Is your data in the form of frequencies or measured from a discrete scale (e.g. height)? Or is the data binary (e.g. pass/fail)? Is the data from two independent groups of subjects or from the same group before and after an intervention (such as training of some sort)? Is it from more than two groups? How many independent variables (see earlier) will be entered into the analysis, and how will you decide which ones to include?

Identifying the appropriate statistical test for quantitative analysis can be complicated but luckily most statistical analysis books provide handy decision trees to help with this. Some useful books for statistics in social science research are Foster *et al.*, Norman and Stryner, and Bryman and Cramer.[41–43] A useful article is McCrum-Gardner's 'Which statistical test to use?'.[44] The major statistical software packages all have paper and online manuals, which can be invaluable.

Last, but not least, do seek advice and support from a statistician, statistics-friendly supervisor or able colleague when planning your project. This will save you hours of frustration when you reach the point of data analysis. Indeed, this point is equally made in relation to qualitative research. It is common for novices to qualitative research to have their papers rejected because the different components of their study – theory, design, methods and analysis – do not align appropriately. Seek early advice and support from, and collaboration with, colleagues whose expertise lies in qualitative theory, research design and methods, and analysis.

### Qualitative data analysis

While bearing in mind that qualitative data collection and analysis are iterative rather than linear (see earlier), Miles and Huberman[45] explain the process of QDA as follows:

- data reduction (extracting the essence);
- data display (organising for meaning);
- drawing conclusions (explaining the findings)

While arguably, quantitative research follows these steps also, if one interprets data reduction as occurring through statistical analysis, the process of QDA is a little different. It usually follows an inductive approach where the data are allowed to 'speak for themselves' by the emergence of conceptual categories and descriptive themes. The researcher must be open to multiple possibilities or ways to think about a problem, engaging in 'mental excursions' using multiple stimuli, 'side-tracking' or 'zigzagging', changing patterns of thinking, making linkages between the 'seemingly unconnected' and 'playing at it', all with the intention of 'opening the world to us in some way' ([33], p. 544). The researcher must immerse themselves in the data in order to be able to see meaningful patterns and themes, making notes as they go through the processes of data collection and analysis, and then using these notes to guide the analysis strategy and the development of a coding framework.

In this way, good qualitative research has a logical chain of reasoning, multiple sources of converging evidence to support an explanation, and rules out rival hypotheses with convincing arguments and solid data. The wider literature and theory are used to derive analytical frameworks as the process of analysis develops and different interpretations of the data are likely to be considered before the final argument is built. For example, one of our own studies[15] aimed to explore how widening access policy is translated and implemented at the level of individual medical schools. Data was collected via individual interviews with key personnel. We initially conducted a primary level thematic analysis to determine themes. After the themes emerged, and following further team discussion, we explored the literature, identified and considered various theories, in some depth, before identifying the most appropriate framework for a secondary, theory-driven analysis.

There are some excellent text books that discuss QDA in detail.[9,31,46]

## Judging the quality of research

There are various criteria by which you can judge the quality of quantitative and qualitative research (see Table 1.5).

Validity refers to how well a measure captures what it is meant to measure. For example, how well does a questionnaire asking students to rate their satisfaction with a course assess satisfaction (rather than, for example, usefulness of the course, which is a different concept). Credibility, on the other hand, is about whether the study has been conducted well and the findings seem reasonable. External validity is the extent to which the results of a study can be generalised to other situations and to other people. For example, if peer-based learning in first year anatomy is found to be effective, will it also be effective in the clinical years or with students from another institution where the curriculum differs (this is where sampling is critical, see earlier)? Similarly, the transferability criterion asks if the findings of a study can be useful in other, similar contexts. Reliability refers to a measure's precision and stability extent to which the same result would be obtained with repeated trials. Judgements of the dependability of research findings consider the extent to which the research process was carried out in a manner, which may be reviewed or audited by another. Finally, in quantitative research, objectivity refers to freedom from bias. According to Lodico,[47] objectivity is possible when the researcher has little opportunity to interact with participants, as is the case when using quantitative methods to test hypothesis using statistical tests. The qualitative equivalent of confirmability refers to researchers providing sufficient detail of data collection and analysis that readers can see how their conclusions were reached. The criteria for judging qualitative research[4] are discussed further in chapter six.

*Table 1.5* Criteria for judging research

| Criteria for Judging Quantitative Research | Criteria for Judging Qualitative Research[4] |
| --- | --- |
| Internal validity | Credibility |
| External validity | Transferability |
| Reliability | Dependability |
| Objectivity | Confirmability |

## Mixed methods

Despite some traditionalists' reservations, it is now widely accepted that quantitative and qualitative approaches, designs and methods are compatible in the same programme of research. While most researchers have a preference for one camp over the other, depending on their own personal philosophy, many take a pragmatist approach to research, using different methods depending on the research question they are trying to answer[46] and combine different methods in the same research programme. This may seem in direct opposition to the quote at the start of this chapter but pragmatism is a philosophy in itself.[47–50]

Pragmatism contents that the key question is not 'is it true?', or 'is it right?', but 'does it work?' John Dewey, for example, believed that when we first face a problem, our first task is to understand our problem through describing its elements and identifying their relations. Identifying a concrete question that we need to answer is a sign that we are already making progress. Much has been written on Dewey – a good starting point is Dewey: A Beginner's Guide.[51]

If we take a pragmatic approach to research methods, the main question is 'what kind of question is best answered by what methods?' The pragmatic philosophical stance is perfect for mixed-methods design, which incorporates both quantitative and qualitative methods. Mixed-methods research is a flexible approach, where the research design is determined by what we want to find out rather than by any predetermined epistemological position. Lingard *et al.*[52] set out some useful considerations when mixing methods within one study or across several studies in a research programme. They stress that central to the effectiveness of a mixed methods study is a clear relationship among the methods in order to ensure that the data converge or triangulate to produce greater insight than a single method could. Good mixed methods research negotiates the differences between qualitative and quantitative approaches (in terms of philosophy, design, methods and analysis) by articulating how and why both are integrated. See Creswell and

*Table 1.6* Key characteristics of quantitative and qualitative research.

| Approach or philosophy | Quantitative | Qualitative |
|---|---|---|
| Assumptions | • Positivism/post-positivism<br>• Social phenomena and events have an objective reality<br>• Variables can be identified and measured<br>The researcher is objective and 'outside' the research | • Constructivism/interpretivism<br>• Reality is socially constructive<br>• Variables are complex and intertwined<br>The researcher is part of the process |
| **Purpose** | • Generalisability<br>• Prediction<br>• Explanation | • Contextualisation<br>• Interpretation<br>• Understanding |
| **Approach** | • • Hypothesis testing<br>• Deductive, confirmatory, inferential – from theory to data<br>• Manipulation and control of variables<br>• Sample represents the whole population so results can be generalised<br>• Data is numerical or transformed into numbers<br>• Counting/reductionist<br>• Statistical analysis | • Hypothesis generation<br>• Inductive and exploratory – from data to theory<br>• Emergence and portrayal of data<br>• The focus of interest is the sample (uniqueness)<br>• Data is words or language, minimal use of numbers<br>• Probing/holistic<br>• Analysis draws out patterns and meaning |

Plano Clark[53] for an excellent guide to designing and conducting mixed methods research.

So, returning to the example with which we opened this chapter, we started the programme of research into medical careers by seeking to extend understanding of the factors, which were important to medical students and trainees/learners in their careers decision making. Interviewees were selected on the basis of the degree to which they represented the diversity of background characteristics among the population under study. We analysed this data using framework analysis, and used the findings to inform the questions included in an initial survey of medical students across Scotland. These surveys included forced-choice and open questions. Data from the surveys and the interviews were triangulated in the analysis process in order to produce greater insight than would be gained by a single method. For instance, while the interview results emphasised the importance of location, the survey results illustrated that work-life balance, or quality of life, was the over-arching factor in careers decision making, and the importance of specific quality-of-life-related factors differed by stage of training.

## Conclusion

In this chapter, I have set out the fundamental differences between qualitative and quantitative research approaches, which are summarised in Table 1.6. It may be clear from how I have done so that my personal stance is that both have a place in healthcare education research, reflecting the agenda in education (in the United Kingdom at least), where both qualitative and quantitative research are used to produce generalisable/transferable knowledge, which informs theory, practice and policy, and contributes to methodological and theoretical developments in the field.

---

### Practice points

- All research requires a philosophical stance, a research question, study design, data collection methods and data analysis.
- Quantitative and qualitative research differ fundamentally at each of these steps in the research process.
- Incongruence across the different stages of any research project is very obvious to those reading and judging research.
- All designs and methods have their strengths and weaknesses, and it is critical to be aware of these when thinking about how best to address a particular research goal.

---

## Further reading

Miles, M.B., Huberman, M. & Saldana, J. (2013) *Qualitative Data Analysis: A Methods Sourcebook*, 3rd edn. Sage Publications, Thousand Oaks. This update of Miles & Huberman's classic research methods text presents the fundamentals of research design and data management, followed by five distinct methods of analysis: exploring, describing, ordering, explaining and predicting.

Creswell, J.W. (2013) *Educational Research: Planning, Conducting, and Evaluating Quantitative and Qualitative Research*, 4th edn. Pearson, Boston, a very practical and helpful book which is a recommended text for many courses.

## References

1 Cleland, J.A., Johnston, P., French, F.H. & Needham, G. (2012a) Associations between medical school and career preferences in Year 1 medical students in Scotland. *Medical Education*, **46**, 473–484.

2 Cleland, J.A., Johnston, P.W., Walker, L. & Needham, G. (2012b) Attracting healthcare professionals to remote and rural medicine: learning from doctors in training in the north of Scotland. *Medical Teacher*, **34**, e476–e482.

3 Cleland, J.A., Johnston, P.W., Michael, A., Khan, N. & Scott, N.W. (2014) A survey of factors influencing career preference in new-entrant and exiting medical students from four UK medical schools. *BMC Medical Education*, **14**, 151. doi:10.1186/1472-6920-14-151

4 Guba, E. & Lincoln, Y. (1981) *Effective Evaluation*. Jossey-Bass, San Francisco.

5 Guba, E.G. (1978) *Toward a Methodology of Naturalistic Inquiry in Educational Evaluation. Monograph 8.* UCLA Center for the Study of Evaluation, Los Angeles.

6 Kuhn, T. (1970) *The structure of scientific revolution*, 2nd edn. University of Chicago Press, Chicago.

7 Rist, R. (1977) On the relation among educational research paradigms: from disdain to détente. *Anthropology and Education Quarterly*, **8**, 42–69.

8 Bryman, A. (1988) *Quantity and Quality in Social Research (Contemporary Social Research)*. Routledge.

9 Savin-Baden, M. & Major, C. (2013) *Qualitative Research: The Essential Guide to Theory and Practice*. Routledge, London.

10 Carson, D., Gilmore, A., Perry, C., & Gronhaug, K. (Eds.). (2001). *Qualitative Marketing Research*. London, England: SAGE Publications, Ltd.

11 Carson, D., Gilmore, A., Perry, C. & Gronhaug, K. (2001) *Qualitative Marketing Research*. Sage Publications, London.

12 Bordage, G. (2009) Conceptual frameworks to illuminate and magnify. *Medical Education*, **43**, 312–319.

13 Reeves, S., Mathieu, A., Kupar, A. & Hodges, B.D. (2008) Why use theories in qualitative research? *BMJ;*, **337**, e949.

14 Yin, R.K. (2009) *Case Study Research: Design and Methods*. Sage Publications, Thousand Oaks, CA.

15 Cleland, J.A., Nicholson, S., Kelly, N. & Moffat, M. (in press) Taking context seriously: explaining widening access policy enactments in UK medical schools. *Medical Education* 2015, **49**: 25–35.

16 Cleland, J.A., Milne, A., Sinclair, H. & Lee, A.J. (2008a) Cohort study on predicting grades: is performance on early MBChB assessments predictive of later undergraduate grades? *Medical Education*, **42**, 676–683.

17 Cleland, J.A., Knight, L.V., Rees, C.E., Tracey, S. & Bond, C.M. (2008b) Is it me or is it them? Factors that influence the passing of underperforming students. *Medical Education*, **42**, 800–809.

18 Brickman, L. & Roy, D.J. (eds) (1998) *Handbook of Applied Social Research Methods.* Sage Publications, Thousand Oaks, CA.

19 Husbands, A., Mathieson, A., Dowell, J., Cleland, J.A. & MacKenzie, R. (2014) Predictive validity of the UK Clinical Aptitude Test in the final years of medical school: a prospective cohort study. *BMC Medical Education*, **14**, 88 http://www.biomed central.com/1472-6920/14/88.

20 Cook, T.D. & Campbell, D.T. (1979) *Quasi-Experimentation: Design and Analysis Issues for Field Settings.* Rand McNally, Chicago.

21 Distlehorst, L.H. & Robbs, R.S. (1998) A comparison of problem-based learning and standard curriculum students: Three years of retrospective data. *Teaching and Learning in Medicine*, **10**, 131–137.

22 Watson, K., Wright, A., Morris, N. *et al.* (2012) Can simulation replace part of clinical time? Two parallel randomised controlled trials. *Medical Education*, **46**, 657–667.

23 Sibbald, B. & Roland, M. (1998) Understanding controlled trials: Why are randomised controlled trials important? *BMJ*, **316**, 201 doi: http://dx.doi.org/10.1136/bmj.316.7126.201.

24 Togerson, D. & Togerson, C. (2008) *Designing Randomised Trials in Health, Education and the Social Sciences.* Palgrave MacMillan, Basingstoke.

25 Becker, H.S., Greer, B. & Hughes, E.C. (1961) *Boys in White: Student Culture in Medical School.* Transaction Publishers, London.

26 Denzin, N.K. & Lincoln, Y.S. (2011) *The SAGE Handbook of Qualitative Research*, 4th edn. Sage Publications, Thousand Oaks.

27 Hammersley, M. & Atkinson, P. (1995) *Ethnography: Principles in Practice*, 2nd edn. Routledge, London.

28 Maxwell, J. (2008) Designing a qualitative study. In: Bickman, L. & Rog, D.J. (eds), *The Handbook of Applied Social Research Methods*, 2nd edn. Sage Publications, Thousand Oaks, CA.

29 O'Brien, B., Harris, I., Beckman, T., Reed, D. & Cook, D. (2014) Standards for Reporting Qualitative Research: A Synthesis of Recommendations. *Academic Medicine*, **89**, 1245–1251.

30 Silverman, D. (2012) *Interpreting Qualitative Data*, 4th edn. Sage Publications, Thousand Oaks, CA.

31 Creswell, J.W. (2013) *Educational Research: Planning, Conducting, and Evaluating Quantitative and Qualitative Research*, 4th edn. Pearson, Boston.

32 Norcini, J.J., Blank, L.L., Arnold, G.K. & Kimball, H.R. (1995) The Mini-CEX (Clinical Evaluation Exercise): a preliminary investigation. *Ann Intern Med*, **123**, 795–799.

33 Patten, M.Q. (2002) *Qualitative Research and Evaluation Methods.* Sage Publications, Thousand Oaks, CA.

34 Pope, C. & Mays, N. (1995) Reaching the parts other methods cannot reach: an introduction to qualitative methods in health and health services research. *BMJ*, **311**, 42–45.

35  Lambert, H. & McKevitt, C. (2002) Anthropology in health research: from qualitative methods to multidisciplinarity. *BMJ*, **325**, 210–213.

36  Bowen, G.A. (2009) Document analysis as a qualitative research method. *Qualitative Research Journal*, **9**, 27–40.

37  Dicicco-Bloom, B. & Crabtree, B.F. (2006) The qualitative research interview. *Medical Education*, **40**, 314–21.

38  Aliaga, M. & Gunderson, B. (2000) *Interactive Statistics*. Prentice Hall, Upper Saddle River, NJ.

39  Mason, J. (1996) *Qualitative Researching*. Sage Publications, Thousand Oaks, CA.

40  Cleland, J.A., Scott, H., Harrild, K. & Moffat, M. (2013) Using databases in medical education research. AMEE Guide 77. *Medical Teacher*, **25**, e1100–e1122.

41  Foster, L., Diamond, I. & Jefferies, J. (2014) *Beginning Statistics: An Introduction for Social Scientists*, 2nd edn. Sage Publications, Thousand Oaks, CA.

42  Norman, G.R. & Streiner, D.L. (2008) *Biostatistics: The Bare Essentials*, 3rd edn. BC Decker, Hamilton, Ontario.

43  Bryman, A. & Cramer, D. (2012) *Quantitative Data Analysis with IBM SPSS 17, 18 & 19: A Guide for Social Scientists*. Routledge.

44  McCrum-Gardner, E. (2008) Which is the correct statistical test to use? *British Journal of Oral and Maxillofacial Surgery;*, **46**, 38–41.

45  Miles, M.B. & Huberman, M. (1994) *Qualitative Data Analysis: An Expanded Source Book*, 2nd edn. Sage Publications, Thousand Oaks, CA.

46  Higgs, J., Cherry, N., Macklin, R. & Ajjawi, R. (2010) *Researching Practice: A Discourse on Qualitative Methodologies*. Sense Publishers, Rotterdam, The Netherlands.

47  Lodico, M., Spaulding, D. & Voegtle, K. (2010) *Methods in Educational Research: From Theory to Practice*. John Wiley & Sons, San Francisco.

48  Dewey, J. (1910) *How We Think*. Heath, Lexington, MA. Reprinted, Prometheus Books, Buffalo, NY, 1991

49  James, W. (1907) *Pragmatism, A New Name for Some Old Ways of Thinking, Popular Lectures on Philosophy*. Longmans, Green, and Company, New York, NY.

50  Peirce, C.S. (1958). In: Hartshorne, C. & Weiss, P. (eds),, vols. 7–8, Arthur W. Burks (ed.) *Collected Papers of Charles Sanders Peirce*, vols. 1–6. Harvard University Press, Cambridge, 1931–1935.

51  Hildebrand, D. (2008) *Dewey: A Beginner's Guide*. One World Publications, London.

52  Lingard, L., Albert, M. & Levison, W. (2008) Grounded theory, mixed methods, and action research. *BMJ*, **337**, a567.

53  Creswell, J.W. & Plano Clark, V.L. (2010) *Designing and Conducting Mixed Methods Research*. Sage Publications, Thousand Oaks, CA.

# 2 Theory in healthcare education research: the importance of worldview

*Wendy McMillan*

*Geoff teaches third-year dentistry students. He is puzzled that students frequently ask whether what he is teaching will be assessed in the final examination – because he carefully matches what he teaches with course outcomes and makes these connections explicit to the students. He decided to research the source of this question so that he can help his students to learn better. A colleague from his Faculty's Education Unit said that he should clarify what he believes about assessment before he starts the research. Geoff had not really thought about assessment – it is just something which you do to see whether students understood what you have taught. When Geoff started to read what other people thought about assessment, he was puzzled because different people had different understandings of assessment. He noticed that these understandings even affected study design. Some researchers said that students experience assessment as reward or punishment. This research studied how students' experiences of assessment as reward and punishment influenced their learning practices. Other research said that students are active participants in their own learning and constantly trying to make sense of what they learn. This research studied how students used assessment opportunities to help them make meaning. Geoff noticed that researchers seemed to take their own assumptions about assessment for granted and usually neglected to specify these assumptions to the reader.*

## Introduction

This vignette about assessment highlights the important role that assumptions play in education research. Our assumptions are influenced by our worldview – in other words, by how we understand the world to be. Worldview influences how we interpret what goes on around us. This chapter is going to unpack how these assumptions work, and how they influence education research design, analysis and reporting. By the end of this chapter, the reader should be able to explain

- the purpose of education research;
- the role that theory plays in research study design, method, analysis, and how theory

informs the kinds of conclusions that might be drawn;
- the way in which research is shaped by the researcher's worldview;
- how worldviews are shaped by ontological and epistemological assumptions;
- the importance of reflexivity in research;
- how a summary of existing literature is different from a worldview or theory;
- different ways in which theory might be used to contribute to knowledge generation.

## The purpose of education research

Why would one want to engage in education research? Geoff was clear that he wanted to understand how his dental students experienced assessment, in order to help his students to learn better and so to become 'good' dentists. Improved patient outcomes are the ultimate goal of medical education and medical education research.[1] The purpose of education research, thus, is to generate the kinds of information that healthcare educators need in order to understand, and thereafter to improve, teaching and learning – with the ultimate purpose of improving healthcare practice, patient care and patient outcomes.[1] Description alone is inadequate if the purpose of research is to generate insight.[2] Without an in-depth understanding, for example, of how students interpret assessment, such planning would be based on teachers' assumptions and conjecture.[2] By understanding the students' experiences and how these shape students' learning, the planning of assessment as part of the teaching and learning process can be evidence-based.[2] Understanding requires not just a description of what is happening, but some ideas about why it is happening – in other words, an explanation of what is happening. So, it would not be helpful for Geoff to know how many students passed (or failed) particular assessment activities in which performance categories. To understand why students want to know whether something will be

*Researching Medical Education*, First Edition. Edited by Jennifer Cleland and Steven J. Durning.
© 2015 John Wiley & Sons, Ltd. Published 2015 by John Wiley & Sons, Ltd.

assessed in the final examination, Geoff is going to need to find out about the motives, experiences, feelings, opinions, perceptions and choices of his students.[3] Qualitative research is most suited to getting answers for questions about people's behaviour.[3]

Qualitative research aims to generate an 'interpreted understanding' (p. xii) of people's social world through learning about people's experiences and their interpretations of these experiences.[4] Whitley[5] suggests that there are three basic differences between qualitative and quantitative research. First, qualitative research is designed to provide data which explores a topic of interest framed as a research question, rather than to test a hypothesis.[5] Thus Geoff's study would probably set out to collect data to help him answer the research question, 'How do students' understandings of assessment shape their learning behaviour' rather than to test the hypothesis, 'Perceptions of reward and punishment influence what students learn'. Second, sample size for qualitative research is usually quite small – often between 20 and 40 participants[5] – because the emphasis in qualitative research is on collecting detailed data so as to be able to create in-depth understandings of the lived experiences of a carefully selected representative sample of people. Thus Geoff would probably select students in his third-year dentistry class as participants, rather than studying dental students across a variety of institutions. If his dentistry class was very large, he might select a sample of 20 – 40 students within the class, from across the performance groupings, to serve as his cohort. Third, the study design for qualitative research is more fluid than for quantitative research. It is common and accepted practice for the study design to be modified as findings emerge.[5] Thus Geoff might find in his study that students learn only what they think will be immediately relevant in the clinical context. This finding might result in him deciding to administer an open-ended questionnaire to all 120 of his third-year students to find out what they believe are the aspects of his module, which are important for clinical application. This information will be helpful to him because he can use it to plan how to highlight the clinical relevance of the things which he teaches which the students do not necessarily see as clinically relevant. These differences are discussed in further detail in Chapter 1.

## The importance of worldview to study design

Qualitative research, therefore, has the potential to provide the kinds of information that are really useful in understanding aspects of teaching and learning. However, much healthcare education research fails to actually generate these understandings because it stops short at description.[2] Analysis remains as a surface description of what people said and did.[3] Merely describing what his students think about assessment will not help Geoff to plan a teaching environment, which better supports dental students' learning and professional development. In order to create that sort of environment, Geoff will need to know what the meaning is of all the data that he collects – in other words, he will need to understand what all the data tells him as a teacher about what motivates students to learn and how different kinds of teaching strategies, learning activities, and assessment tasks cause students to make different decisions about how and what they learn.

However, in order to generate this kind of understanding, Geoff will need to be clear what he believes about learning and assessment. He will need a theory of learning and assessment in order to conduct his analysis.[6] Geoff has already encountered two theories of assessment, which draw on two different worldviews (see Table 2.1[7–24]) – that students experience assessment in terms of reward and punishment (which draws on the worldview of positivism[12] and its associated theory of behaviourism[12] to understand assessment), and that students are active participants in their own learning and constantly trying to make sense of their learning experiences (which draws on the worldview of interpretivism[10,11,25] and its associated constructivist[13,14] theory of learning to understand assessment). There are many more theories and, as Geoff discovered, each theory is shaped by a particular set of assumptions about how the world is. In other words, worldview (and the theories which are generated by it) determines what gets studied, how it gets studied, how the data gets interpreted, and what counts as valid findings (see also Chapter 1).[7]

Two examples illustrate this relationship. If Geoff believes that students experience assessment as reward and punishment, his research will focus on this aspect of assessment. He might decide to use focus group interviews because talking with others helps people to think about and clarify their own beliefs and assumptions more easily than in a one-on-one interview.[26] He could ask students to explore what it is about assessment

*Table 2.1* Summary of three worldviews[7–11]

| | Positivism | Interpretivism | Criticalism |
|---|---|---|---|
| **Ontology** *(assumptions about the nature of reality)* | • There is a reality 'out there', and it can be known.<br>• Laws and mechanisms govern the workings of that reality.<br>• Research can (in principle) find out the true state of that reality. | • There are multiple realities because meaning is grounded in experience.<br>• Knowledge can be derived from sources other than the senses.<br>• Reality is complex, and context-dependent. | • Reality may be objective or subjective, but truth is continually contested by competing groups. |
| **Epistemology** *(assumptions about the nature of knowledge)* | • The investigator and the object under investigation are two independent entities.<br>• It should be possible to study something without influencing it.<br>• Part of good research is employing strategies to reduce or eliminate any influence.<br>• What is found – if replicable – it true.<br>• The investigator might acknowledge 'true for now', but the assumption is that 'true' can indeed be found with the correct techniques, information or research question. | • Knowledge is derived from people's experiences – both those of the researcher and the research participants.<br>• Perceptions and experiences of both the researcher and the research participants affect what is seen and conceptualised.<br>• There are multiple ways of knowing. | • Power relations determine what (and whose) knowledge counts.<br>• Power is implicated in the relationship between the researcher and the researched.<br>• What can be known is inextricably intertwined with the interaction between the researcher and the researched. |
| **Related theories** | • Behaviourism[12]<br>• See also Chapter 20 | • Social constructivism/social constructionist theory (emphasis on construction of meaning)[13,14]<br>• Socio-cultural theory (emphasis on context of complex social environments)[15]<br>• Socio-materialism, including actor-network theory[16] and complexity theory[17] (emphasis on inter-relatedness of all aspects within a system) | • Critical theory[18]<br>• Critical realism[19,20]<br>• Race[21]/class[22] theory[23] |
| **Example of research question** | Positivist research usually tests a hypothesis and does not ask a research question:<br>• 'Perceptions of reward and punishment influence what students learn' | • 'How do students' understandings of assessment shape their learning behaviour?' | • 'What is the influence of diversity and the educational climate in shaping clinical competence of oral health students'[24] |

activities, and how they are conducted, that is experienced as positive or negative. However, while he might probe how assessment-as-reward or assessment-as-punishment affects what students choose to study and how they study it, he is unlikely to explore whether students perceive a relationship between preparing for assessment and learning to be a competent healthcare professional, and if they do, how students understand this relationship. If, on the other hand, Geoff believes that students are active participants in their own learning and that students use assessment opportunities to assist themselves to make meaning, he will make use of different interview questions and will conduct his data-collecting interviews differently. He might interview individual students about how they learn and how they use assessment to support and direct their learning. He might ask the students to share examples of their study notes, and he may even try to analyse the annotations that they make on these notes. He might seek out groups of students who study together, and conduct focus group interviews with them about how they construct and share knowledge together and about the role which assessment plays in this process. In other words, Geoff's research focus will determine how he collects the data and what data he collects.

And, it is not only the means and nature of data collection that will be different for these two studies. The analysis and the interpretation of the data will also be influenced by what Geoff believes about learning and assessment. A study of assessment through the lens of reward and punishment draws on the behaviourist theory of learning. Behaviourism assumes that learning is achieved through stimulus-response.[12] Analysis of the data would set out to find evidence of how assessment services as a stimulus, and how positive or negative assumptions about this stimulus influence students' response behaviour. Conclusions from this study would be framed in terms of what kinds of assessment stimuli lead to what kinds of student learning responses. Recommendations might suggest ways in which assessment stimuli could be adapted to ensure a positive response.

A study of assessment that explores how students use assessment activities as part of the construction of knowledge, in contrast, draws on constructivist theories of learning. Constructivism assumes that students are active participants in their own learning and constantly trying to make meaning of their learning experiences.[13,14] Analysis of the data would set out to find evidence of the kinds of actions and activities which students engage in as part of their learning and the ways in which they engage with assessment activities as part of this process. Conclusions from this study would be framed in terms of the kinds of assessment activities that best encourage students to engage with the knowledge, skills, and dispositions of the subject and to construct their own personal meaning from that engagement. Recommendations might suggest ways in which the teacher could facilitate this kind of active engagement, and would include suggestions about assessment as a part of the entire teaching and learning environment.

It is clear that studies based on different worldviews – while even studying the same topic and trying to find solutions to the same classroom challenge – have different study designs, and will come up with different interpretations and different recommendations.

## Personal assumptions and worldview

Before he can design his study, Geoff is now faced with the challenge of having to be explicit about what he believes about learning and assessment. We all have beliefs and assumptions about how the world is. Usually, we are unaware of these beliefs and assumptions until someone else appears to be thinking or behaving in an 'odd' way – or as happened with Geoff, when he was faced with apparently contradictory understandings of his research concept.

There are basically two kinds of assumptions about the world, which we tend to take for granted and seldom make explicit or examine.[25] We have assumptions about the nature of reality and what can be known about the world – that is, what counts as 'true'[25] and what we believe is 'real'.[27] For example, researchers who conducted research to test the hypothesis 'Perceptions of reward and punishment influence what students learn' would probably assume that the 'truth' was out there for them to find. In other words, they would be assuming that reality is static, fixed and ordered in accordance with a supreme and impartial 'truth'[25] – they would hold a positivist worldview (see Table 2.1). In contrast, someone who asked 'How do students' understandings of assessment shape their learning behaviour' would assume that different students understand learning differently and that that question could not be answered without getting an insight into what the students themselves thought. For this person, who holds an interpretivist worldview, reality is subjective and changing, and there is no ultimate truth – only people's differing experiences of it. These assumptions about what counts as truth are referred to as ontological assumptions.[25]

In educational research, ontological assumptions will shape what a researcher accepts as evidence of the nature of teaching and learning and will determine the kinds of questions that the researcher believes can be asked about the teaching and learning reality and what the researcher will accept as valid answers to them.[25] These assumptions about the nature of knowledge are referred to as epistemological assumptions.[7,26,12,25,8–10,28] For example, if the researcher adopts a worldview that assumes that reality is ordered according to a supreme truth (i.e. a positivist worldview), then the purpose of research will be to generate a theory that accurately describes that reality – and only knowledge about reality that can be proved to be objective and neutral will count as valid.[25] Thus the researcher of the hypothesis, 'Perceptions of reward and punishment influence what students learn', would try to study student learning without influencing it and would conscientiously employ strategies to reduce or eliminate any influence by the researcher on the research topic, including on the students who would be the subjects of the study.[25,8–11] Validity of the study would depend on whether it could be replicated.[25,8–11] In contrast, the researcher of the question, 'How do students' understandings of assessment shape their learning behaviour', would assume that knowledge is derived from people's experiences and would therefore expect there to be multiple of ways of understanding assessment and they would treat each as equally valid.[25,10,11]

Three broad worldviews can be identified – positivism, interpretivism and criticalism.[25,8–11] Each worldview is determined by particular beliefs, which in turn shape the research questions that can be asked, what counts as valid information about the research context, and what kinds of conclusions can be drawn. Table 2.1 summarises the three worldviews, their associated ontologies, epistemologies and educational theories. It also suggests the kinds of research questions that would emerge from each worldview.

## Positivism

Healthcare practitioners will be familiar with the assumptions about reality and knowledge of what is referred to as positivism or the positivist worldview[7–10,25] (see Chapter 1). The study by Hodges and McIlroy[28] of the validity of global ratings for scoring Objective Structured Clinical Examinations (OSCEs) is an example of an education study designed within the ontological and epistemological assumptions of positivism.

However, it is hard to find out the truth about some aspects of reality – especially, about things related to people such as their motives, experiences, feelings, and reasons for doing or not doing things. Since insight into teaching and learning is usually about understanding the behaviour and motivations of students and their teachers, positivism may not be a very effective or suitable framework for understanding these aspects. Other worldviews might better help education researchers to understand the world of students and university teachers, their experiences and their assumptions.

## Interpretivism

Interpretivism, as a worldview, argues that reality is subjective, and therefore that there can be no ultimate truth.[10,11,25] It is sometimes difficult for researchers who have worked in the positivist worldview to understand the assumptions that are embedded in the interpretivist worldview. The article by Frost and Regehr,[14] which draws on social constructionist theory, is helpful in this regard. Social constructivism is an interpretivist theory, which assumes that the people whose experiences are being researched each have a unique experience and a unique and subjective interpretation of that experience (see also the chapter in this book by Mann and MacLeod). In their study, Frost and Regehr[14] highlight how identity as a doctor is constructed in a variety of ways, resulting in many different identities within a single research cohort. The authors examine these different constructs and conclude that an interpretivist worldview allows for an examination of the construction of diverse identities that would be impossible through a worldview such as positivism, which assumes that there is only one truth. Similarly, Govaerts and Van der Vleuten[15] use socio-cultural theory to understand how students and their assessors perceive learning and competence in the work-based environment. In two separate articles, Bleakley[16,17] suggests ways in which social materialism theories (such as actor-network theory[16] and complexity theory[17]) might be used to understand aspects of medical education.

## Criticalism

Interpretivism allows for individual perspectives to be heard and for education researchers to examine understandings from the perspective of those involved in a particular teaching and learning activity or environment. Criticalism[9,25], however, while also assuming that individual perspectives are important, argues that not all experiences can be treated as equal because some experiences are the consequence of prejudice, discrimination and exploitation on the part of more powerful others. Experiences of access to healthcare in apartheid South Africa would be an example of the way in which experience is determined by more powerful others.

Studies drawing on the assumptions of criticalism focus on power and the way in which power operates to marginalise some participants in social interactions. Criticalism has been used to study both patient care[18–21] and the experiences of healthcare students.[22,23] Drawing on qualitative interviews with first-year oral hygiene students, McMillan[23] uses race and class theory to examine the relationship between students' experiences of the transition to university, their first-year academic performance and the expectations that universities have of first-year students. She shows how university expectations serve to discriminate against those who come from homes with little or no prior experience of university. Her study shows how, while each individual student has a personal and subjective experience of university, race and social class shape common experiences for students. Beagan[22] uses class theory to reveal experiences of exclusion and marginalisation of working class medical students.

### Being 'up front' about worldview

Whether researchers are explicit about it or not, ontological and epistemological assumptions will underpin the worldview which they use as a lens to study aspects of teaching and learning. Differences in these assumptions shape not only study design, but also what emerges as data, how this data can be analysed and even the conclusions that can be drawn and recommendations that can be made from the study. However, what researchers frequently neglect to do is to make explicit the worldview and assumptions upon which their studies are based.[3,29]

In order for a research study to be evaluated for significance and validity and reliability – as well as to ensure that the reader understands 'where a study comes from' – the researcher needs to 'own up' to his/her worldview and its associated assumptions. Geoff's puzzlement when he was faced with different perspectives on assessment was exactly because the authors had not indicated the assumptions and worldviews that they took for granted and which had shaped the lenses which they used to look at assessment.

The demand to be upfront can be challenging to healthcare practitioners who have usually been educated and trained – and continue to work and research within – a positivist (or what is frequently referred to as a 'scientific') worldview. As a consequence, the positivist worldview takes on the semblance of being the only possible way to view the world. However, the preceding discussion about ontology and epistemology has highlighted that worldviews vary. It has been argued that different understandings of what questions might be asked of reality and what counts as convincing evidence of answers to these questions are appropriate for different research contexts and for different views about how the world actually is.

How then might a researcher be transparent in reporting healthcare education research? One way would be for researchers to actually reflect on their assumptions about knowledge and reality, and to consider what worldview would provide the most suitable lens and tools for understanding the particular healthcare education issue under investigation. Reflexivity[30] is one mechanism for ensuring this kind of disciplined inquiry.[31] Reflexivity involves thoughtful analysis or disciplined self-reflection.[31] It involves continuous evaluation by researchers of what they are assuming, and a continuous checking that the assumptions are aligned with and appropriate for the research situation, the research question, and the methodologies and methods adopted. Thus, Geoff is going to need to ask himself what he believes about assessment. Does he believe that assessment comes after learning; that it is something separate from learning – in which case behaviourist understandings of reward and punishment will probably underpin his research question and study design. Or, does he believe that assessment is an integral part of learning and that students are active participants in their own learning – in which case constructivist understandings of 'making sense' will probably shape his research question and study design. Geoff will need to be alert to the worldviews that underpin each of these theories.

Geoff might ensure the rigor of this process – the on-going self-evaluation and alignment of all aspects of the research process – through a number of mechanisms. An audit trail, tracking decisions made during the research process, is one such mechanism.[32] This audit trail of the thinking processes, which were integral to the study design and its implementation and subsequent analysis and reporting, might be kept in the format of a reflective journal.[32] Journalling allows researchers to think about what they are doing and why and about their assumptions and how these shape what they do and why they do these things. It is also an excellent mechanism for capturing personal inconsistencies, biases and even prejudices.[32,33] These reflections will be important for later claims regarding validity and reliability.[33,34]

It may now be evident that acknowledging a worldview or taking on a theory is not the same as reviewing the literature (See chapter 3 later in this book for more on literature reviewing). A researcher may include articles from a number of different worldviews into a review of the literature. This indeed would be appropriate as the purpose of a literature review is to show what people are currently saying and researching about in a particular subject. However, when the time comes to design the study, the researcher will need to be clear about his or her assumptions of how the world operates. This awareness of worldview will form the foundation for deciding on a suitable theory for the study – one that will allow the research issue to be adequately studied and reported.

## The relationship between theory and research

The point was made at the beginning of this chapter that the purpose of healthcare education research is to generate the kinds of information that healthcare educators need in order to understand, and thereafter to improve, teaching and learning so as to improve the quality of healthcare delivery. The discussion so far has highlighted the importance of understanding how ontological and epistemological assumptions shape research study design. Table 2.1 indicates that a relationship exists between ontological and epistemological assumptions and the kinds of theories that a researcher might select. In this section, attention turns to how theory contributes to the knowledge generation required to understand, and thereby, improve teaching and learning. The issue being studied, the ontological and epistemological assumptions of the researcher, and the research question usually determine how theory is used to generate knowledge.

Theory in research contributes to knowledge generation in two different ways. Inductive inquiry uses theory to inform study design and analysis. A specific theory is taken up before the study is designed. All aspects of the study design – including the framing of the research question – are informed by the theory. Most importantly, the concepts identified in the theory as central are used in the analysis. Locating a study within an existing theory allows the researcher to draw on existing concepts, to justify the focus of and techniques used to conduct the study and to organise, analyse and

interpret the data that is collected.[35] Theory used in this way provides an organisational framework for interpreting the data and for representing the data after analysis.[29] For example, McMillan[36] drew on self-regulated learning theory to study the learning strategies of academically successful dentistry students. She used the core concepts of this theory – cognitive strategies, metacognitive strategies, motivation – to interpret the data. From her findings, she made recommendations of how the ways in which academically successful students manifest these concepts might be developed in less academically successful students.

On the other hand, deductive inquiry contributes to the development of theory.[37,38] While ontological and epistemological positions are identified before these studies are conducted, a specific theory is not usually identified. The researcher waits for the concepts to emerge from the data. Grounded theory adopts this approach.[39–41] Some grounded theory studies explicitly develop theory – such as the study by Pratt[38], which set out to theorise the professional identity development of surgeons. Others use findings to generate models or frameworks for understanding particular aspects of a discipline – such as the study by Sbaraini *et al.*[37], which used grounded theory to develop a model of the process of adapting a preventive protocol into dental practice.

## Conclusion

This chapter has highlighted the way that worldview – and associated ontological and epistemological assumptions – shapes how researchers understand the world, what kinds of questions they believe can be asked of that world, and what kinds of information count as answers to these questions. The point has also been made that this worldview influences the actual study design, from the formulation of the research question to the collection and analysis of the data. The importance of reflection as part of research methodology has also been emphasised. Increasingly, in the writing up of research proposals and articles, researchers are being asked to 'own up' to their worldviews and theoretical positions. Frost and Regehr,[14] for example, state their theoretical position up front as part of their description of the structure of their article, 'We then survey the social science literature to describe the tenets of a social constructivist theory of identity. We draw on this theory to explore what the tension between the discourses of diversity and standardisation might mean for medical students and the ways in which they are constructing their professional identities'. Similarly, Clarke[42] describes how she used a reflective journal to understand her research process when studying the experiences of patients with chronic pain, 'My learning was clearly outlined as I realised the importance of suspending judgement and the influence of my beliefs and values. This was difficult on occasion and sometimes the diary was used to help me understand a situation from my viewpoint and then it allowed me to focus on the same situation from the patient's viewpoint'. The first step that Geoff will need to take in his study of assessment will be to define his own ontological and epistemological assumptions – for it is only once these have been made overt that he will be able to design a study that will allow him to address his concern and so help his students to better focus their attention when they learn.

## Practice points

- The purpose of education research is to generate explanations of teaching and learning.

- Research design, data collection and analysis, and explanations generated from research are dependent on the researcher's assumptions about the nature of reality. These assumptions determine the kinds of questions that can be asked and what counts as an acceptable answer.

- Education researchers need to recognise and 'own up' to their assumptions, and make their assumptions clear when reporting on research.

- Worldview, study design, data collection and analysis need to be aligned in order to generate authentic and useful explanations of teaching and learning – which in turn will contribute to improved healthcare.

## References

1 McGaghie, W.C. (2010) Medical education research as translational science. *Science Translational Medicine*, **2**, 19cm8. Available: http://www.newzet.com/d/16508/content/2/19/19cm8. full (Accessed 1 July 2014).

2 McMillan, W. (2010) Moving beyond description: research that helps improve teaching and learning. *African Journal of Health Professions Education*, **1**, 3–7.

3 Kelly, M. (2010) The role of theory in qualitative health research. *Family Practice*, **27**, 285–290.

4 Ritchie, J. & Lewis, J. (2003) *Qualitative Research in Practice*. Sage, London.

5 Whitley, R. (2009) Introducing psychiatrists to qualitative research: a guide for instructors. *Academic Psychiatry*, **33**, 252–255.

6 Reeves, S., Albert, M., Kuper, A. & Hodges, B.D. (2008) Why use theories in qualitative research? *British Medical Journal*, **337**, 631–634.

7 Carter, S.M. & Little, M. (2007) Justifying knowledge, justifying method, taking action: epistemologies, methodologies, and methods in qualitative research. *Qualitative Health Research*, **17**, 1316–1328.

8 Weaver, K. & Olson, J.K. (2006) Understanding paradigms used for nursing research. *Journal of Advanced Nursing*, **53**, 459–469.

9 Guba, E.G. & Lincoln, Y.S. (1994) Competing paradigms in qualitative research. In: Denzin, N.K. & Lincoln, Y.S. (eds), *Handbook of Qualitative Research*. Thousand Oaks, California, pp. 105–117.

10 Tavakol, M. & Zeinaloo, A.A. (2004) Medical research paradigms: positivistic inquiry paradigm versus naturalistic inquiry paradigm. *Journal of Medical Education*, **5**, 75–80.

11 Monti, E.J. & Tingen, M.S. (1992) Multiple paradigms of nursing science. *Advances in Nursing Science*, **21**, 64–80.

12 Conole, G., Dyke, M., Olivier, M. & Seale, J. (2004) Mapping pedagogy and tools for effective learning design. *Computers and Education*, **43**, 17–33.

13 Appleton, J.V. & King, L. (1997) Constructivism: a naturalistic methodology for nursing inquiry. *Advances in Nursing Science*, **20**, 13–22.

14 Frost, H.D. & Regehr, G. (2013) "I AM a doctor": negotiating the discourses of standardisation and diversity in professional identity construction. *Academic Medicine*, **88**, 1–8.

15 Govaerts, M. & Van der Vleuten, C.P.M. (2013) Validity in work-based assessment: expanding our horizons. *Medical Education*, **47**, 1164–1174.

16 Bleakley, A. (2012) The proof is in the pudding: putting actor-network-theory to work in medical education. *Medical Teacher*, **34**, 462–467.

17 Bleakley, A. (2010) Blunting Occam's Razor: aligning medical education with studies in complexity. *Journal of Evaluation in Clinical Practice*, **16**, 849–855.

18 Waitzkin, H. (1989) A critical theory of medical discourse: ideology, social control, and the processing of social context in medical encounters. *Journal of Health and Social Behaviour*, **30**, 220–239.

19 Connelly, J. (2001) Critical realism and health promotion: effective practice needs an effective theory. *Health Education Research*, **16**, 115–120.

20 Kontos, P.C. & Poland, B.D. (2009) Mapping new theoretical and methodological terrain for knowledge translation: contributions from critical realism and the arts. *Implementation Science*, **4**, 1. Available: http://www.implementationscience.com/content/4/1/1 (Accessed 20 December 2013).

21 Brown, T.N. (2003) Critical race theory speaks to the sociology of mental health: mental health problems produced by racial stratification. *Journal of Health and Social Behaviour*, **44**, 292–301.

22 Beagan, B. (2005) Everyday classism in medical school: experiencing marginality and resistance. *Medical Education*, **39**, 777–784.

23 McMillan, W. (2007) Understanding diversity as a framework for improving student throughput. *Education for Health*, **20**, 71–81. Available http://www.educationforhealth.net/ (Accessed 10 November 2007).

24 Brijlal P. (2014) *The influence of diversity and the educational climate in shaping clinical competence of oral health students*. Unpublished doctoral dissertation. Cape Town: University of the Western Cape.

25 Bunniss, S. & Kelly, D.R. (2010) Research paradigms in medical education research. *Medical Education*, **44**, 358–366.

26 Kitzinger, J. (1995) Introducing focus groups. *British Medical Journal*, **311**, 299–302.

27 Tuffin, K. (2005) *Understanding Critical Social Psychology*. Sage, London.

28 Hodges, B. & McIlroy, J.H. (2003) Analytic global OSCE ratings are sensitive to level of training. *Medical Education*, **37**, 1012–1016.

29 Sandelowski, M. (1993) Theory unmasked: the uses and guises of theory in qualitative research. *Research in Nursing and Health*, **16**, 213–218.

30 Finlay, L. (1998) Reflexivity: an essential component for all research. *British Journal of Occupational Therapy*, **61**, 453–456.

31 Jensen, G.M. (1989) Qualitative methods in physical therapy research: a form of disciplined inquiry. *Physical Therapy*, **6**, 492–500.

32 Bradbury-Jones, C. (2007) Enhancing rigour in qualitative health research: exploring subjectivity through Peshkin's I's. *Journal of Advanced Nursing*, **59**, 290–298.

33 Fischer, C.T. (2009) Bracketing in qualitative research: conceptual and practical matters. *Psychotherapy Research*, **19**, 583–590.

34 Williams, E.N. & Morrow, S.L. (2009) Achieving trustworthiness in qualitative research: a pan-paradigmatic perspective. *Psychotherapy Research*, **19**, 576–582.

35 Charmaz, K. (1990) 'Discovering' chronic illness: using grounded theory. *Social Science and Medicine*, **30**, 1161–1172.

36 McMillan, W. (2010) "Your thrust is to understand" – how academically successful students learn. *Teaching in Higher Education*, **15**, 1–13.

37 Sbaraini, A., Carter, S.M., Evans, R.W. & Blinkhorn, A. (2011) How to do a grounded theory study: a worked example of a study of dental practices. *BMC Medical Research Methodology*, **11**, 28. doi: 10.1186/1471-2288-11-128. Available http://www.biomedcentral.com/content/pdf/1471-2288-11-128.pdf Accessed 20 January 2014.

38 Pratt, M.G., Rockmann, K.W. & Kaufmann, J.B. (2006) Constructing professional identity: the role of work and identity learning cycles in the customization of identity among medical residents. *Academy of Management Journal*, **49**, 235–262.

39 McMillan, W.J. (2009) Finding a method to analyse qualitative data: using a system of conceptual learning. *Journal of Dental Education*, **73**, 53–64.

40 Boychuk Duchscher, J.E. (2004) Grounded theory: reflections on the emergence vs. forcing debate. *Journal of Advanced Nursing*, **48**, 605–612.

41 Kennedy, T.T. & Lingard, L.A. (2006) Making sense of grounded theory in medical education. *Medical Education*, **40**, 101–108.

42 Clarke, K. (2009) Uses of a reflective diary: learning reflectively, developing understanding and establishing transparency. *Nurse Researcher*, **17**, 68–76.

# 3 Literature reviews: who is the audience?

*Geoff Wong*

*Dr Scarlet thinks he has a great idea – to use smart phones to teach heart sound auscultation. He wants to do some research to show that it is not only as good as current teaching approaches, but better. He approaches one of his colleagues in his department, who he knows had experience and expertise in educational research to discuss his idea. He is rather surprised to find that his colleague seems less enthusiastic than he is about this idea. During their discussion Dr Scarlet's colleague suggests that it may be worth his while to first undertake a literature review – to find out what is known about this topic area. This, the colleague suggests, might help him further develop the focus of his research idea (i.e. what is known and not known about this topic and so identify where the research gaps are). He explained that doing a literature review may take time, but might ultimately save him wasting his time if he were to find that this topic had already been well researched. Several questions immediately spring to Dr Scarlet's mind. Do I really need to do a literature review? What type of review do I need to do? Where can I learn how to do one? How will I know if it will be good enough?*

## Introduction

At some point in their career, most healthcare professionals will read or carry out a literature review. Indeed, in any type of research, including medical education, it is nearly impossible to avoid literature reviews. Once you start looking at literature reviews, it does not take long to notice that there is a number of different approaches to literature reviews. This chapter explores the range of review approaches and provides guidance on how to decide which one is best for your purpose.

## What is a literature review?

There are many definitions on what a literature review is and thus is not.[1] These range from a discussion about, or account of, the published works on a topic area; to summaries of existing knowledge; right through to a piece of work that critically examines the quality, methodological and/or theoretical contribution of the existing literature. In other words, literature reviews are undertaken for a range of different purposes – as a means of introducing the background around a topic; to summarising what is know about a topic area; to examine, analyse and make sense of data that relates to a specific topic and to answer specific research questions. Along with this variation in the purpose of a literature review, there are multiple differences in the processes, or approach, needed to produce a review. Examples of commonly used review approaches are used in this chapter to illustrate this variation.

Furthermore, the type of documents that may be legitimately included in a literature review varies. Some will only include studies of a particular type, others published and unpublished documents. The "quality" of the documents may or may not be vetted before they are considered worthy of inclusion in the review.

Another aspect of literature reviewing that differs across approaches is the extent to which searching is undertaken for potentially relevant documents. For example, does the review include only research studies of a particular design, research papers published within a certain timeframe, or does it encompass unpublished and 'grey' literature? (Grey literature is published written material, such as governmental and other reports, that has not been published in a conventional way, and can be difficult to identify and obtain through the usual channels of abstract and citation databases of peer-reviewed literature. Grey literature has been broadly defined to include everything except peer-reviewed books and journals accepted by Medline.) The rationale for different ways of carrying out literature reviews, and what kind of papers are included in the review, depends the purpose of the review, which is, in turn, linked to the research question (for more on the research question, see Bezuidenhout and Schalkwyk later in this book).

The corollary is that a literature review means different things to different people *and* that approaches to literature reviewing differ. This chapter will help

*Researching Medical Education*, First Edition. Edited by Jennifer Cleland and Steven J. Durning.
© 2015 John Wiley & Sons, Ltd. Published 2015 by John Wiley & Sons, Ltd.

make sense of this variation through the use of some simple rules of thumb. By the end of this chapter, the reader will be able to do the following:

- Explain the importance of the audience's perspective in literature reviews
- Begin the task of undertaking a literature review through the application of five rules of thumb.

## The importance of purpose and audience

Literature reviews are done for a specific purpose. For example, as part of a thesis, for a competitive grant application, as background for a research study or as a research project in its own right. Within a research study, thesis and a competitive grant, the role of a literature review is to demonstrate a detailed awareness of what the current knowledge is in a topic area and make the case for why the chosen research is needed. When a literature review is undertaken in its own right, the purpose is more often to produce evidence for decision making – for example, by clinicians on choice of medications or educators on which standard setting procedure is best for their clinical (OSCE, Objective Structured Clinical Examination) exam.

This variation in the reasons or purpose of doing a literature review is the first clue to why there is such a plethora of approaches to reviewing. Different literature review approaches have been developed for different purposes. The key decision for any researcher wishing to undertake a literature review is to ensure that the approach chosen is suitable for the purpose of the review. The suggestion within this chapter is that this choice should be driven by the consideration of who the audience is for the literature review.

Consider Dr Scarlet, unless he plans to undertake his literature review and then never show the fruits of his labours to anyone, his review will be read by others. When making his choice of literature review approach, he should be asking to whom his review is targeted. In other words, who is going to read the review? Who is the audience? Why, because it is a literature review's audience that decides whether he made the right choice of literature approach to use. It is they who will decide if his choice of approach was 'right' or 'wrong'. In addition they will decide on how well the approach has been applied – that is if his review is 'good', 'bad', 'rigorous', 'high quality', worthy of funding or publication, down right 'sloppy' and so on. His audience will be his judge, jury and executioner – both on his choice of literature approach and the quality of the work done when in the literature review. In other words, the audience judges whether or not the right literature review approach was chosen for the stated purpose and if the processes used were appropriate.

To illustrate the point on literature review processes, consider PhD theses. The purpose for needing to provide a literature review in a thesis may be the same for a historian and doctor in training – to give a critical assessment of the relevant literature. But the approach (and by implication the processes undertaken within the review) will not necessarily be the same. Just to take one process difference, what might be considered a legitimate document to include within a literature review will vary. To an audience of historians, a contemporaneously written document on an area relevant to the thesis written by a single person might be invaluable. However, to an audience of medical researchers applying a widely used level of evidence in biomedical research (see Box 3.1), such a piece would constitute the very lowest type of evidence available – on the same level as a expert opinion, thus potentially not warranting inclusion.

---

**BOX 3.1   Levels of evidence used in biomedical research**

| Level | Description of nature of evidence |
|---|---|
| 1++ | High-quality meta-analyses, systematic reviews of randomised controlled trails (RCTs), or RCTs with a very low risk of bias |
| 1+ | Well-conducted meta-analyses, systematic reviews, or RCTs with a low risk of bias |
| 1- | Meta-analyses, systematic reviews, or RCTs with a high risk of bias |
| 2++ | High-quality systematic reviews of case control or cohort or studies High-quality case–control or cohort studies with a very low risk of confounding or bias and a high probability that the relationship is causal |
| 2+ | Well-conducted case control or cohort studies with a low risk of confounding or bias and a moderate probability that the relationship is causal |
| 2- | Case control or cohort studies with a high risk of confounding or bias and a significant risk that the relationship is not causal |
| 3 | Nonanalytic studies, for example, case reports, case series |
| 4 | Expert opinion |

Source: http://www.sign.ac.uk/guidelines/fulltext/50/annexoldb.html.

The expectations of the different audiences for literature reviews are often set out publicly (e.g. in publications or training manuals) or taught at relevant courses. It is to these standards and norms an audience will judge a literature review. Later on in this chapter this point is illustrated using examples based on some of the more commonly used review approaches.

There are, however, two caveats to be aware of when using the audience's perspective to choose review approaches. Firstly, a literature review may have more than one audience. For example, a literature review might be undertaken as part of a grant application, but is then written up for publication. The two audiences would be peer-reviewers, but one set would be applying standards from a funder's perspective and the other, the standards of experts in the field. The funder's reviewers would be likely to have to judge if a literature review supports the argument that the proposed study represents value for money, something that is not of great concern to a journal's peer-reviewers. Secondly, it can be a challenge to identify what the standards and expectations are that the audience will apply when reading the review. These two conundrums may seem insoluble, but possible solutions are (again) discussed in the following section.

## Choosing between literature review approaches using the audience perspective

There are many different 'brands' or approaches to literature reviews, some of the more mainstream approaches are covered in this section. Note that, by including or excluding a literature review approach, there is no judgement on any one approach being better or worse than another. Rather, the criterion for inclusion and discussion is more pragmatic – the approaches listed below are the ones that you are likely to come across in your work in healthcare education research. These approaches are also the ones that have undergone most methodological development, so it is easier to work out for what purpose the approach is more suitable, and what constitutes high quality. Later on, some guidance is provided on approaches that have not been mentioned in this chapter.

So far, the use of the term 'systematic review' has been avoided as it is one that may potentially cause a great deal of confusion. For some, systematic review conjures up in their minds a certain review approach – most frequently a Cochrane systematic review (an approach discussed in more detail later). For others the term more closely follows the dictionary definition of systematic – namely a review that is structured, methodical, orderly, organised and so on. As such, any review might be considered systematic, but whether the audience considers it to be so is the important consideration. When 'systematic review' is used in this chapter, we say what 'brand' of review it is.

## Cochrane and other related systematic review approaches

Cochrane reviews are probably one of the most widely recognised literature review approaches and so warrant early mention. In the space of just over two decades, this approach has grown to become a synonymous with high quality and trustworthiness in healthcare reviews.[2]

Cochrane reviews attempt to identify, appraise and synthesise all the empirical evidence that meets pre-specified eligibility criteria to answer a given research question. The researchers use explicit methods aimed at minimising bias, to produce their findings. There are three types of Cochrane review:
- Intervention reviews assess the benefits and harms of interventions
- Diagnostic test accuracy reviews
- Methodology reviews

Cochrane reviews base their findings on the results of trials which meet certain quality standards. Within Cochrane reviews processes are applied which aim to reduce the impact of bias across different parts of the review process. These processes include exhaustive searching for relevant studies from a number of different sources; the use of explicit predefined criteria to select and judge the quality of studies for inclusion; the systematic collection of data and; appropriate synthesis of data.

The researchers in this approach have through national and international collaboration (often on a voluntary basis) via the Cochrane Collaboration, developed training courses and materials, a journal for Cochrane reviews and transparent processes for producing reviews. Producing a Cochrane systematic review is a 'start to finish' process that runs all the way through from (for example) submitting a protocol for a review topic, to getting peer review feedback on the protocol, to final peer review of the completed review prior to (hopefully) publication in the Cochrane library.

This collaboration has produced an impressive range of resources for those interested in using its approach. For example, newcomers can access an informative overview (http://www.cochrane.org /about-us/newcomers-guide), the highly detailed training manual – The Cochrane Handbook (http://handbook.cochrane.org/) and a range of training courses in different languages and countries of the world (http://www.cochrane.org/training). In addition there is an active community of researchers that those interested in this approach may contact (http://www.cochrane.org/about-us/get-involved).

Using the audience perspective, there is no doubt as to what is to be expected of a researcher who wishes to undertake a Cochrane review. The whole process is clearly spelt out by the Cochrane Collaboration. For a Cochrane review, the 'first' and 'last' audience will be the individuals who will peer-review your protocol (and very helpfully) provide feedback on it and finally decide on whether to publish it in the Cochrane Library (http://www.thecochranelibrary.com). The expectations of this audience also extend to the purpose to which Cochrane reviews may be used (i.e. intervention reviews, diagnostic test accuracy reviews and methodology reviews). For example, when it comes to the suitability of the research question to the review approach, The Cochrane Handbook provides clear guidance which should enable any researcher to work out if the question to be addressed will be suited to a Cochrane approach. The Handbook points out that 'It is not helpful to include evidence for which there is a high risk of bias in a review, even if there is no better evidence.' If a topic area is known to have studies of 'poor' quality (and by implication probably at high risk of bias), then this approach may not be suitable. For example, in a Cochrane review examining 'Community wide interventions for increasing physical activity' (http://onlinelibrary.wiley.com/doi/10.1002/14651858.CD008366.pub2/full) the majority of the studies identified and included in the review were of low or unclear quality. The authors concluded that 'It could be postulated that, given the conflicting findings, community wide interventions lack efficacy, however we believe such a conclusion would be premature given the poor quality of studies.' In other words, while it is possible to conduct a rigorous Cochrane review when the evidence is of low quality, only limited conclusions can be drawn due to the nature of the studies available for inclusion into the review. This scenario thus raises the issue of whether the time and effort devoted to undertaking the review was justifiable.

In addition, the Cochrane Handbook advises that the research question should be of a certain format PICO (*P*articipants, *I*nterventions, *C*omparisons and *O*utcomes). So if your question cannot be expressed in this format, a different literature review approach may be more suitable (see later for different ways of carrying out literature reviews). An example of a PICO type question would be as follows: In medical students [*P*articipants] what is the effect of an Internet based learning module [*I*ntervention] compared to face to face lectures [*C*omparison] on knowledge gains [*O*utcome]? A non-PICO type question would be: Why do some medical students prefer not to use Internet based learning modules?

It is rarely possible to carry out a Cochrane review if you are single researcher, working in isolation because of their prescribed format and process. From the materials on the Cochrane website and published Cochrane reviews, it should become apparent that a review of this type is not to be undertaken lightly – these are a significant piece of work. Box 3.2 outlines two 'best case scenarios' of how to approach undertaking a Cochrane review, one drawn from healthcare delivery, the second from healthcare education.

Four rules of thumb can be gleaned from the example of Cochrane systematic reviews:

1 Read the instructions. If a literature review approach provides guidance and documentation, then make sure you are familiar with the relevant contents. In other words, make sure you read the 'instructions' provided.

2 Do your homework. For a review approach that has a library of quality-vetted published reviews then, if you are in any doubt as to what constitutes a 'high-quality' review, you should read and learn from the published reviews. These illustrate very clearly the expectations of the review approach.

3 Get training. If a funder recommends specific approaches or endorse certain literature review approaches, then if you need to, go on a training workshop for that approach. Training may have a cost attached, and of course attending training means time away from your 'day job', but an investment in training upfront can save you a lot of wasted time, and stress, further down the line.

4 Seek collaboration and support. There are many researchers who have experience in undertaking certain review approaches (e.g. Cochrane reviews). If you need help, you may be able to find someone locally whom you can turn to for help. If there is no-one local, try looking for potential advisors you have identified as working on similar reviews in the literature, or search for contacts via online medical education communities such as MedEdWorld (http://www.mededworld.org/Home.aspx).

**BOX 3.2 Two hypothetical case studies of how to approach undertaking a Cochrane review**

Dr Green regularly treats patients who are overweight. She is aware that a new medication, *zipese* has just come onto the market that claims to help patients lose weight. She is interested to know if this medication is as good as it claims to be. She spends some time looking online (including in the Cochrane Library) to see if a review already exists on this new drug – she was not able to find one. She did however notice that there were at least half a dozen published RCTs on it.

She approaches one of her colleagues whom she knows has undertaken research before to ask her about how she might start the process of undertaking a review.

Within a few months they have formed a small team of people interested in reviewing the efficacy of *zipese*. They start off by formulating a PICO question – In patients with obesity, what is the efficacy of *zipese* compared to usual care on weight loss? They explore and discuss the issues of; which review approach; team expertise in reviews; seeking funding; individuals' roles in the review and; the published literature on *zipese*.

A member of the team suggests that they might want to undertake a Cochrane review. He is familiar with this approach and explains to the rest of the team that the purpose of their review would fit in with would be expected by the Cochrane Collaboration's peer-reviewers. For example, he explains that they are able to identify a clear PICO question, are undertaking a review on a defined intervention and that published trials exist. He further suggests that if the rest of the team would like to check for themselves if his suggestion fits with the expectations required of a Cochrane review, they can access the Cochrane Collaboration's online resources.

Having checked themselves, the team agree on the approach. However they find that they need the input of an expert librarian and that one of them needs to undertake further training in Cochrane reviews.

The team then set about assigning tasks and use the detailed freely available resources from the Cochrane Collaboration to help them understand what is required of them.

In healthcare education, Dr Green regularly teaches students using standardised patients (SPs). She wonders if using SPs is as good as using real patients in terms of students' learning outcomes. She spends some time looking online (including in the Cochrane Library) to see if a review already exists. She was not able to find one but did notice that there were trial data on this topic area.

She approaches one of her colleagues whom she knows has research experience to ask how she might start the process of undertaking a review.

This colleague is enthusiastic and supportive of the proposal to review the literature on use of SPs in medical education. Within a few months they have formed a small team of people interested in working together on this review. They start off by formulating a PICO question – When teaching medical students, what is the efficacy of simulated patients compared to real patients on learning outcomes? They explore and discuss the issues of; which review approach; team expertise in reviews; seeking funding; individuals' roles in the review and; the published literature on simulated patients.

A member of the team suggests that they might want to undertake a Cochrane review. He is familiar with this approach and explains to the rest of the team that the purpose of their review would fit in with would be expected by the Cochrane Collaboration's peer-reviewers. For example, he explains that they have already identified a clear PICO question, are undertaking a review on a defined intervention and that published trials exist on the topic. Having checked the expectations required of a Cochrane review via the Cochrane website, the team agree on this approach. They identify that they need to supplement the existing skills set of the team with the input of an expert librarian and that one of them needs to undertake further training in Cochrane reviews.

The team then set about assigning tasks and use the detailed freely available resources from the Cochrane Collaboration to help them understand what is required of them in terms of the process of a Cochrane review.

These four rules of thumb should enable any researcher to work out whether or not the purpose of their review will fit in with a particular review approach. In addition, it should be possible to work out what will be expected when undertaking a Cochrane or any other systematic review approach. The main thrust of these rules are to encourage any researcher intending to undertake a literature review to look to the most up-to-date methodological literature for answers – rather than to rely on the opinion of any one author. For some review approaches, such as the Cochrane Collaboration, the Campbell Collaboration and BEME (see Box 3.3), continuing methodological work by different researchers around the globe has resulted in a regularly peer-reviewed and updated range of resources that are made freely available online. The work on such resources is never ending, but at any point in time, they represent the collective wisdom and consensus of what is expected of a Cochrane, Campbell or BEME review, respectively (i.e. the expectations of the audience).

---

### BOX 3.3   Organisations that draw on and adapt the Cochrane Collaboration's approach

Some of the literature review processes and standards set by the Cochrane collaboration have been adapted by other organisations.

The Campbell collaboration's (http://www.campbellcollaboration.org/) goal is to provide systematic reviews in education, crime and justice, social welfare and international development. Many of their review processes are similar to those of the Cochrane Collaboration. As with the Cochrane Collaboration, they offer guidance on what is expected of a researcher undertaking a Campbell review (http://www.campbellcollaboration.org/resources/research/the_production.php) and provide training courses and resources (http://www.campbellcollaboration.org/resources/training.php).

In medical education, the BEME Collaboration (http://www.bemecollaboration.org) sets out to develop evidence informed education in the medical and health professions through amongst other things, systematic reviews. Many of this collaboration's review processes are informed by the work of the Cochrane Collaboration and other scholars in literature reviews. Clear guidance is provided to researchers who wish to produce BEME reviews (http://www.bemecollaboration.org/BEME+Reviews+General+Information/), ensuring that there will be no doubt about what the expectations are from this audience.

To recap, it is important to appreciate that:
- Opinions vary between literature review methodologists. The implication of this is that it is important for any researcher hoping to use a literature review method to seek out where current consensus stands on (for example) the various processes with a review.
- Each review approach is constantly evolving, what might be accepted as the norm now may change in a year's time. Thus, regularly updated, trusted online resources may well prove to be the most up to date.

Researchers may seek funding for their literature reviews. The audience in these situations are the funding agencies' reviewers and various decision making committees. Some have decided to adopt the literature review standards set out by the Cochrane Collaboration – see for example the resource webpage of the United Kingdom's National Institute of Health Research (http://www.nets.nihr.ac.uk/resources/systematic-reviews). The principle set out in the four simple rules of thumb above can be adapted to help increase the chances of getting funded – bearing in mind that the audience has now changed to that of the funder.

## Realist syntheses and meta-narrative reviews

Realist synthesis[3] and meta-narrative reviews[4] are two relatively newer literature review approaches compared to Cochrane and other related literature review approaches. Meta-narrative reviews and realist reviews both differ in many ways to Cochrane reviews. The most important difference is arguably the way they make sense of the published (and unpublished) research. Brief overviews of these two review types are provided in Box 3.4.

---

### BOX 3.4   Brief overviews of meta-narrative reviews and realist reviews

Meta-narrative reviews are designed to be used for reviews of topics which have been *differently conceptualised and studied* by different groups of researchers. For example many groups have studied inter-professional learning in different countries and with different professional groups. Some have conceptualised this as when two or more professions learn with, from and about each other to improve collaboration and the quality of care; others have conceptualised it as a means of breaking down the barriers between professional silos; others as a threat to professional identities, and so on. If we were to summarise this topic area in a way that was faithful to what each different group set out to do, we would have to start by asking how each of them approached the topic, what aspect of 'inter-professional learning' they chose to study and how. In order to understand the many approaches, we would have to consciously and reflexively *step out of* our own world-view (see chapter by MacMillan earlier in this book), learn some new vocabulary and methods, and try to view the topic of 'inter-professional learning' through multiple different sets of eyes. When we had begun to understand the different perspectives, we could summarise them in an over-arching narrative, highlighting what the different research teams might learn from one another's approaches.

Realist reviews, on the other hand, seek to makes sense of research by unpacking and understanding what the influence is of context on observed outcomes. This approach to sense making is succinctly summarised by the research question 'What works for whom under what circumstances, how and why?' Realist inquiry considers the interaction between context, mechanism and outcome. In a realist world, intervention X is not thought of as having effect size Y with confidence interval Z. Rather, intervention X (e.g. a programme introduced by postgraduate training policymakers who seek to create a particular outcome, such as improving surgical trainee laparoscopic skills) alters context (e.g. by making new resources available – such as funding a laparoscopic simulator for each training centre), which then triggers mechanism(s) which produce both intended and unintended outcomes (such as trainees doing more simulated practice [an intended outcome] but simulator resources being stretched so trainees complain about unequal access to simulators [an unintended outcome]). X may work very will in one context but poorly or not at all in another context. Realist inquiry seeks to unpack the context-mechanism-outcome relationship, thereby explaining examples of success, failure, and various eventualities between. Theoretical explanations of this kind are referred to as 'middle-range theories' (i.e. ones which involve abstraction but are close enough to observed data to be incorporated in propositions that may be permit empirical tested).

These two review approaches serve to illustrate an important point on the use of the audience perspective. Review approaches that have been developed and used for longer (like the Cochrane approach) tend to have greater consensus on many aspects – from what purpose they may be more suited for, right through to the methodological developments. In effect, it is clearer what the audiences will expect – as illustrated in the section above on the Cochrane approach.

When a review approach has been recently developed (e.g. meta-narrative in 2004 review) or introduced form one discipline into another (realist synthesis in 2006), then there is much less certainty as to what the approach is good for – that is its purpose. For example, some have argued that sub-group analyses in a Cochrane review already enables researchers to answer the 'for whom' question. As such if the purpose of a review is focussed on this specific narrow question, realist reviews are not as suitable as an approach. The common counter argument is that the 'for whom' question is only part of what a realist review seeks to answer when it is used to make sense of interventions.

Such issues around what type of purpose a review approach can address and what the (at any point in time) consensus may be will continue to evolve as different literature approaches are used more and more. Where there are uncertainties (in purpose and/or review processes) the 'response' from the audience will not be unified and will often focus on areas where 'controversies' continue to exist between literature review approaches and the processes within a review. Rule of thumb 2 (Do your homework) is particularly important – read and learn from published reviews using this approach – but there is an additional point:

5 Expect to be challenged. If you use a newer or less used literature review approach, then you should expect that you will be called upon more often to justify and defend aspects of your review – from the fit between purpose and review approach to the processes used within it.

One way for the proponents of new or less used literature review approaches to make life easier for their fellow researchers is to start to develop quality and publication standards and training materials and courses. This has been case with realist synthesis and meta-narrative reviews with the creation of the RAMESES project website (http://www.ramesesproject.org/) in 2013. While it must be recognised that more developmental work will likely be needed when any new initiative develops such resources, they act as an important anchor point from which to build and serve as a resource for researchers. Box 3.5 provides hypothetical examples on when it might be appropriate to use a meta-narrative review or a realist review.

---

> **BOX 3.5   Two hypothetical case study of when to undertake a meta-narrative review or a realist review.**
>
> **Meta-narrative review**
>
> Dr Black is interested in teaching medical students about the topic of medically unexplained symptoms. He is however aware that different schools of research have conceptualised this topic differently. For example he is aware that some researchers believe that the symptoms are not medically unexplained but merely waiting for medical science to explain them – that is more research is needed to better understand the illness. For others, the diagnosis is viewed as a 'dustbin' diagnosis which regularly attending patients are saddled with. To make sure his teaching takes into account these differing perspectives he decides that he needs to undertake a literature review. As this topic has been differently conceptualised and studied by different groups of researchers, it would be suitable for a meta-narrative approach.
>
> **Realist review**
>
> Dr White is interested in educational interventions designed to get doctors to change their prescribing behaviour. He has been reading the literature on this topic and found that there have been a large number of trials undertaken. In addition he has also noticed that a number of literature reviews exist. His overall conclusion is that some educational interventions seem to work some of the time on some doctors. In other words, the educational interventions used to try to change the prescribing behaviour of doctors seem to be context sensitive and probably individual specific in their effects. He wonders what review approach might be suitable. As Dr White wants to understand the influence of (amongst other things) context on outcomes (in this case prescribing behaviour), a realist review approach would be a suitable option.

## Meta-ethnography and mixed-method approaches

There is no standard method for conducting literature reviews of qualitative research.[5] The most recognised and widely used in health services

research is meta-ethnography.[6] In this literature review approach, induction and interpretation of the qualitative data within included studies is used. During synthesis sense making comes from the translation of studies into one another – ideas, concepts and metaphors are understood and transferred across the different studies. Box 3.6 provides an indication on when it might be appropriate to use a meta-ethnography.

Other approaches exist and it is beyond the scope of this chapter to discuss these in any more detail. However a useful summary that lists and then briefly describes each approach may be found in the University of York's Centre for Reviews and Dissemination (CRD) guidance for undertaking reviews in health care (https://www.york.ac.uk/inst/crd/SysRev/!SSL!/WebHelp/6_5_SYNTHESIS_OF_QUALITATIVE_RESEARCH.htm)

---

> **BOX 3.6   A hypothetical case study of when to undertake a meta-ethnography review**
>
> Dr Ochre is part of a research team investigating the experiences of medical students from disadvantaged backgrounds as they settle into their first year in medical school. The research team want to undertake a review of the literature to understand what the experiences are for this group of medical students. The final goal is to use their review findings to develop specific services for them.
>
> The nature of the data the research team has to deal with in their review will be qualitative. The question that Dr Ochre asks is what review approach should they use. Her colleagues have suggested meta-ethnography as this is one well developed approach for synthesising data from qualitative studies.
>
> Dr Ochre is set the task to find out more about this approach and she consults both the published methodological literature and example reviews and seeks out a course she might be able to go on.

---

The implication is that when undertaking a literature review of qualitative data, there is a choice of approaches. However, with choice comes the challenge of justifying the choice of approach. Rule of thumb 5 (above) comes into play in a more prominent way. If, for example, meta-ethnography is chosen as an approach to synthesise qualitative data as part of a higher degree, then it should be expected that a peer-reviewer or examiner (the audience) will ask why this review approach, as opposed to any, other was chosen. There are not (as yet) published 'quality' standards for meta-ethnography reviews, so a researcher would have to refer back to a selection of the original published methodological works and examples of use of this approach to construct an argument in favour of the choice of approach. The consequence is more work is needed to justify the use of an approach to the audience, but this may be work that is worth doing if this approach is more likely to address the purpose of a review.

Another example of where literature review processes and purpose vary is the emerging field of mixed-methods review. Broadly these review approaches seek to understand a body of literature through the use of both quantitative and qualitative data.[7] The use of mixed methods in literature reviews is a rapidly developing field and so it is difficult to provide much advice. However, rules of thumb 2, 3, 4 and 5 may help those wishing to use such approaches to coherently and plausibly argue the case for using such approaches.

A resource that provides a reasonably comprehensive overview of the range of literature review approaches is the Canadian Institutes of Health Research Synthesis Resources webpage (http://www.cihr-irsc.gc.ca/e/36331.html). This webpage provides a list of the more commonly used literature review approaches and for each a key list of methodological resources.

### What about the research question?

Researchers are often asked what their research question is and told that developing a 'good' research question is an important skill for researchers ([8]; and see Bezuidenhout and Schalk-wyk in this book). Literature reviews can be used to answer research questions, but this is just one of the many purposes they can be put to. In relation to the perspective advocated in this chapter it is the audience who judge whether a research question is 'good' or not, and if it can be suitably answered using a specific chosen review approach. In other words, a researcher may develop a research question and choose a literature review approach to address it, but the judgement of whether the choice of approach is capable of answering the research question is not only the researcher's to make. For example, a research question may be to estimate the effects size of an educational intervention on a specific learning outcome and a research grant proposal is developed. To answer the question the researchers decided to use the Cochrane systematic review approach and to undertake, if possible, a numerical summation (meta-analysis) of the data. The audience – the funding body the proposal is submitted to, will judge if the literature review approach is capable of answering the research question using. The standards used for these judgements are often public available and should be sought out.

### Future developments

The future challenge in this area lies in reviewing the literature on interventions that are either more 'messy' or (some might term) complex,[9] to produce review findings that inform the implementation of interventions[10] or when developing and designing complex interventions.[11] It is the research communities' desires to rise up to the challenge posed by complex interventions and/or the implementation agenda that has, and continues to, drive methodological development in existing literature review methods and the birth of new approaches. Methodological development in literature reviews is an exciting frontier and for those interested in this field of research, there are many opportunities to get involved – mainly by contacting the various organisations engaged in methodological development.

### Conclusion

Literature reviews are an important research approach. It can be difficult to decide on which approach to use. The solution to this conundrum may lie by considering who the audience is for a review's findings. A review may have different audiences at different points in its production so consider this in your decision making process. By using the audience's perspective it may be possible not only to decide whether they would agree that the literature review approach chosen is the most appropriate for the research question, but also what processes are needed to undertake a rigorous review.

---

**Practice points**

- There are many types of literature review approaches.
- Methodological development is well advanced for some approaches leading to a degree of consensus about the suitability of an approach for a particular purpose.
- For other approaches, less consensus exists on when the approach should be used and what constitutes rigour in a review's processes.
- Taking the perspective of who the audience(s) might be for a review is one possible way to address the issue of the suitability of purpose and processes within a review.
- Where consensus is high on the appropriate use of and processes within a review, working out what an audience expects is easier. Where there is less agreement, more time and effort will be needed for justification of approach selection and review processes.

# References

1 Gough, D., Oliver, S. & Thomas, J. (2012) *An Introduction to Systematic Reviews*. Sage, London.

2 Stern, C. (2014) In honour of Archie Cochrane: Twenty years of providing high-quality information based on the evidence [online]. *Journal of Stomal Therapy Australia*, 34.

3 Pawson, R. (2006) *Evidence-Based Policy: A Realist Perspective*. Sage, London.

4 Greenhalgh, T., Robert, G., Macfarlane, F., Bate, P., Kyriakidou, O. & Peacock, R. (2005) Storylines of research in diffusion of innovation: a meta-narrative approach to systematic review. *Social Science and Medicine*, **61**, 417–430.

5 Britten, N., Campbell, R., Pope, C., Donovan, J., Morgan, M. & Pill, R. (2002) Using meta ethnography to synthesis qualitative research: a worked example. *Journal of Health Services Research & Policy*, **7**, 209–15.

6 Noblit, G. & Hare, R. (1988) *Meta-Ethnography: Synthesizing Qualitative Studies*. Sage, Newbury Park.

7 Harden, A. & Thomas, J. (2010) Mixed methods and systematic reviews: examples and emerging issues. In: Tashakkori, A. & Teddie, C. (eds), *Handbook of Mixed Methods in the Social and Behavioral Sciences*. Sage, Thousand Oaks, pp. 749–774.

8 Greenhalgh, T. (2010) *How to read a paper: the basics of evidence-based medicine*, 4th edn. Wiley-Blackwell/BMJ Books, Oxford.

9 Wong, G. (2013) Is complexity just too complex? *Journal of Clinical Epidemiology*, **66**, 1199–201.

10 Eccles, M., Armstrong, D., Baker, R. *et al.* (2009) An implementation research agenda. *Implementation Science*, **4**, 18.

11 Craig, P., Dieppe, P., Macintyre, S., Michie, S., Nazareth, I. & Petticrew, M. (2008) Developing and evaluating complex interventions: the new Medical Research Council guidance. *BMJ*, **337**, a1655.

# 4 Developing the research question: setting the course for your research travels

*Juanita Bezuidenhout and Susan van Schalkwyk*

*How often have you walked out of a class, left a tutorial or completed a ward round with a group of students and wondered about the extent to which the students had actually grasped what it was that you were hoping to share with them? Or what about having marked an assignment or exam, observed a student during an OSCE and then been perplexed because the responses given bear no resemblance to what you had discussed with them previously. This type of reflective thinking, prompted by our natural curiosity, is what moves us to start asking questions about our teaching and our students' learning. When we approach these issues in a scholarly manner, we embark on educational research. The key driver in such research activity is the research question which is the focus of this chapter.*

## Introduction

In the previous chapter, you explored the role of theory in educational research and the development of theoretical and conceptual frameworks. We now move to the heart of the research process, namely the research question. Once you have decided that your curiosity regarding an interesting phenomenon warrants further investigation, i.e. research, you will embark on an iterative process that leads to the development of a research question. In the first part of this chapter, we unpack the characteristics of the research question as it evolves, including its role and function. Thereafter, we take you through a process of developing a research question of your own.

Developing the research question can be characterised as going through a process of triple distillation. Distillation is defined as 'The action of purifying a liquid by a process of heating and cooling' or 'The extraction of the essential meaning or most important aspects of something'.[1] Through repeated distillation, a distillate becomes more pure and concentrated. Often the liquid is distilled twice, but in rare instances it is distilled thrice, resulting in increased purity and concentration. In each instance, the distillation process ultimately leads to a refined product from which all extraneous and unnecessary information has been removed. Each distillation requires the researcher to work iteratively until the final product emerges. Given our focus in this chapter, we review the distillation process (Fig. 4.1) as a metaphor to guide our discussion. In addition, we refer to an actual healthcare profession education (HPE) research project (see Box 4.1) to provide specific and practical examples.

> **BOX 4.1  Scenario of an actual health professions education research project that will be used as background to provide specific and practical examples of research questions.**
>
> A medical faculty in South Africa establishes a rural clinical school (RCS), taking medical students away from the academic hospital to spend their entire final year at a district or regional hospital (year-long longitudinal rural clerkship). This intervention requires changes to the curriculum and results in different teaching and learning experiences for students and clinicians. Numerous questions immediately come to mind. Has the intervention been effective? How have the students experienced the rural platform? What have been the outcomes in terms of student learning? And so forth. These are the sorts of questions that serve as catalysts for educational research.

By the end of this chapter you will be able to do the following:

- Identify the principles of a 'good' research question.
- Describe the different types of questions and their implications for and impact on the research process.
- Explain the process of developing a research question.
- Develop your own research question.

---

*Researching Medical Education*, First Edition. Edited by Jennifer Cleland and Steven J. Durning.
© 2015 John Wiley & Sons, Ltd. Published 2015 by John Wiley & Sons, Ltd.

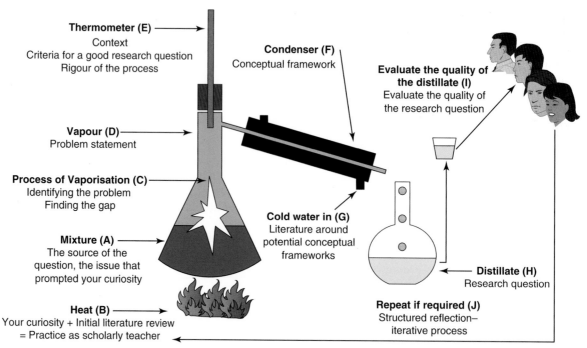

**Thermometer (E)**
Context
Criteria for a good research question
Rigour of the process

**Condenser (F)**
Conceptual framework

**Evaluate the quality of the distillate (I)**
Evaluate the quality of the research question

**Vapour (D)**
Problem statement

**Process of Vaporisation (C)**
Identifying the problem
Finding the gap

**Cold water in (G)**
Literature around potential conceptual frameworks

**Mixture (A)**
The source of the question, the issue that prompted your curiosity

**Distillate (H)**
Research question

**Heat (B)**
Your curiosity + Initial literature review = Practice as scholarly teacher

**Repeat if required (J)**
Structured reflection– iterative process

*Figure 4.1* The purpose of distillation is to separate a specific liquid, the distillate (H), from a mixture (A) of liquids/s and other ingredients. This mixture is heated (B), resulting in series of reactions (C) that will produce a vapour (D). The exact temperature (E) of the process is important, to ensure that only those molecules that must form part of the distillate will vaporise. Impurities and superfluous elements are left behind in the container. The vapour is then guided through a condenser (F) in which cold water is circulated (G). This condenses the vapour, and the distillate (H) can be collected. The distillate then has to be evaluated to ensure its quality (I). If necessary, the process has to be repeated (J). In this illustration, the components of developing a research question are equated to the steps in the distillation process.

## Why a research question?

Why is it necessary to have a research question? Is it not sufficient to have a topic or an idea and to develop aims and objectives accordingly? The research question is, however, pivotal to any educational research project and has a particular purpose in the research endeavour – that of providing direction, both in terms of reading relevant literature and in the selection of data collection methods.[2,3] In essence, the research question becomes your guide that directs all other activities during the research process and against which decisions with regard to research design, the presentation of results and the way in which the results are interpreted and discussed will be measured.[4,5] The quality of the research question (Fig. 4.1H) determines the quality of the research.

Irrespective of the nature of your research, it is critical that you are interested in the topic.[3,6] Your enthusiasm, particularly when it is aligned with your practice, can spark an interest amongst other potential collaborators. In addition, as you enhance your expertise and understanding of the topic, your stature as someone who sufficiently understands the topic in order to effectively explore it will become established.[6]

## The research question under the microscope

As suggested in the opening narrative of this chapter, an important source of questions (Fig. 4.1A) in HPE research resides in our practice/activity as teachers, whether it be in the clinical context or focusing on a theoretical issue.[7,8] Your reading of the literature can also prompt a research question. For example, you may have a particular interest in problem-based learning (PBL) and have recently implemented it in your programme. However, as you read about this approach, you become aware of the challenges that others have documented when applying PBL and you may question how these challenges manifest in your own context.[7] A third important source of research questions comes from a desire for teachers to determine the extent to which a particular educational approach has been effective, usually in terms of enhancing student learning. HPE is currently being challenged to adopt innovative approaches that will facilitate transformative learning experiences of our students.[9] Implementing such innovative approaches brings with it a responsibility to be accountable and to produce evidence of the usefulness, or not, of these approaches, and to respond accordingly. When the RCS was implemented, part of the planning made provision for a 5-year longitudinal cohort study that would investigate the impact of this unique intervention. Thus your curiosity to find out more is what generates the heat that initiates the distillation process (Fig. 4.1B).

Research questions come in many different guises and can have many different objectives (Table 4.1). When starting out in HPE research, one typically will focus on less-complex research questions. However, studies in this field are seldom one dimensional and often address a matrix of 'layered problems'[10] with sub-questions being developed to support an overarching question (see the first example in Table 4.1).

## The 'good' research question

What is a 'good' research question? Critically, a research question should have significance and relevance.[11] When the RCS was established, it was the first of its kind in South Africa. In addition, it represented a considerable financial and human resource investment on the part of the university. Determining the impact of such an intervention, therefore, had relevance at both institutional and national levels. Educational research questions should also advance educational theory and practice.[7] They should pre-empt any discussion around methods, be focused and offer the potential to uncover the real issues. Good questions are concise, focussed and direct, devoid of ambiguity, self-explanatory, unbiased, appropriate, elegant and simple, timely and theoretically rich.[2,7,8] They should be clear and examinable – in other words they need to be answerable.[7] Addressing a gap in the literature is also a fundamental criterion of a good research question.[7] Ultimately, as mentioned earlier, a good research question is one that piques the interest of the researcher. Together, these criteria serve as the thermometer for the distillation process, carefully measuring the quality of the question being defined (Fig. 4.1E).

The structure of the research question thus carries the hallmark of the principles mentioned above.

*Table 4.1* The guises and objectives of research questions: In relation to a particular phenomenon or event, the research question is typically used to interrogate an intervention through one of the actions described here

| Objective | Example |
| --- | --- |
| Describe | *What does the curriculum for the final year medical students at the RCS look like?* |
| Sub-questions | *What content is included in the curriculum? How often do students attend tutorials? What is the mode of engagement between students and lecturers/supervisors? How is the assessment conducted?* |
| Explain | *'Why do students elect to attend the RCS in their final year?'* |
| Explore | *'How do final year medical students experience the year-long placement?'* |
| Investigate | *'What is the potential of the RCS to enhance retention of rural health care practitioners?'* |
| Predict the outcome | *'Will final year medical students attending the RCS practice their profession in rural areas?'* |
| Compare/Justify | *'How does the performance of final year medical students at the RCS compare to that of the final year medical students at the academic hospital?'* |

It contains a minimum of three parts and should identify the variables that you, as a researcher, are investigating: an intervention or a specific situation (an independent variable); the outcome, such as the performance, attitudes or behaviour (a dependent variable) and who you are going to study (the population).[12,13] In the case of the RCS study, the implementation of the RCS is the independent variable, the impact of the intervention is the dependent variable and the students and clinicians are the population. When you want to compare two or more interventions, your question will contain four parts, namely the Population; the Intervention; the Control or alternative intervention and the Outcome (PICO Participants, Interventions, Comparisons and Outcomes).[14] In a complex environment, such as education, there are often additional variables that are important, including the moderator and mediator variables. Moderator variables determine what effect the intervention has on different groups, for instance in the RCS study, the intervention might have had a different impact on students from a rural background than on students from an urban background.[15] A mediator variable explains how the intervention works and describes the process by which the intervention achieves its effect. In the case of the RCS, the students started developing a professional identity because they became part of the local community of practice. Moderator and mediator variables are more commonly present in quantitative than qualitative research.[15]

## Developing the research question

Despite all the information available on the research question, and notwithstanding what has been written above, many who are new to HPE research find it challenging to develop a research question. We hope your reading thus far has nevertheless sown the seeds of a research question in your mind. In the next few sections, we focus on the evolution of your preliminary question. In this instance, Morrison's notion of the development of research questions in HPE, as being both a science and an art, will be central to our thinking.[16]

### Identifying a 'problem'

The issue that has prompted your curiosity (Fig. 4.1A) is often labelled the 'problem'.[8] A research problem can, for example, emerge from an investigable hunch; an aspect warranting further investigation, a teaching and learning practice that can be improved, a concern with published research findings that appear at odds with one's lived experience, the translational nature of existing findings and conceptual or theoretical foci.[17] Clearly identifying the problem will highlight the gap that your study may fill. You will then formulate what is known as a problem statement to guide the construction of your research question.

Identifying a problem (Fig. 4.1B+C) can be steered by a series of questions, starting with what is significant to know. This relates to the prevalence and/or seriousness of the issue and the likelihood that the results will be of benefit to a wider audience. Significance also relates to what the research can add to the literature by, for example, investigating a timely, less-studied topic, challenging existing dogma, improving methodologies or exploring a key issue in a different context, such as was the case in the RCS study.[18,19]

To identify the problem, you must engage with the current literature relating to the topic, especially as your next task is to determine whether there is a gap in the knowledge and what the gap is.[13] How

does one identify a gap? Clearly, immersion in the body of knowledge will help define your field of enquiry. If this reviewing of the literature, the detail of which will be covered in a next chapter, does not provide answers to your envisaged research question, you have identified a gap. At this stage, it may be prudent to revisit the previous chapter, specifically the section regarding your worldview. You have to be aware of how your assumptions about the nature of reality (ontology) and the nature of knowledge (epistemology) will influence how you perform your review of the literature and therefore how you will justify why you believe the gap exists. This will inform the formulation of your research question and the subsequent research design.[20] The RCS study was unique given that the concept of a longitudinal rural clerkship was studied for the first time in an African context. The research therefore sought to address this gap by determining the mechanisms at play in this particular context.

The last question to answer in this section is why the gap in the knowledge has not yet been filled. This often speaks to feasibility and can relate to aspects of research design, such as setting realistic goals and objectives. Challenges in relation to the time frame, resources available, ethical matters and data collection and analysis are further issues that can influence feasibility.[6]

With the 'heat' you have generated (Fig.4.1B), you should be able to formulate a problem statement. Your statement will typically be structured by describing the study's context, for example 'Increasingly medical students are being trained at distributed rural sites...', followed by an introduction to the statement of intent, often using a transition such as 'however' or one of its synonyms[19]: '... however little is known of how this is implemented in the African context and how it influences the students' clinical learning experiences. This problem statement is the 'vapour' of your distillation process.

### Establishing a conceptual framework

Following on the problem statement, the conceptual framework (Fig. 4.1F) sets the stage for the research question that will drive your study and provides the lens through which the study will be investigated.[4] A conceptual framework is your own interpretation of a system of concepts, assumptions, expectations, beliefs and theories that supports and informs your research[21] and it may include a theory, an approach or a model that represents a way of thinking about a problem and helps to explain how complex things work.[20] It will therefore help you frame your problem. A conceptual framework can be constructed in either narrative or graphical form and may include the key elements, concepts, theories and variables that inform your research and the potential relationships between them.[22] It can even include your ideas and beliefs about the research. The conceptual framework is therefore a very personal articulation of how you view the phenomena you are studying.[21]

As you have seen in the previous chapter, your research will usually be situated in a specific paradigm, for example, positivism, interpretivism or criticalism, although you could combine, with caution and care, aspects of different paradigms.[21] This positioning will help guide the construction of your conceptual framework, the formulation of your research question, and the design of your research.

There are four main sources you could draw from when developing your conceptual framework. These include your experiential knowledge, the existing literature (theory and research), exploratory or pilot studies and thought experiments.[21] A conceptual framework will therefore clarify and position your research question within a specific theoretical context and guide you in formulating the question, choosing the variables and interpreting the results. The process of constructing a conceptual framework requires that one consider

multiple perspectives before it can be finalised.[23] This can add depth to your study and encourage you to engage with your research on a different level, for example, moving from descriptive or justification studies to more clarificatory work.[24] A strong conceptual framework will also allow future researchers to draw on your study.

In the case of the RCS study (Fig. 4.2), the research is positioned within an interpretivist paradigm. The design of the intervention was informed by the philosophical positions of social accountability and patient-centredness and published research on the impact of similar interventions in other contexts. Theories that played a major role in the development included transformative learning,[25] communities of practice and situated learning[26] and professional identity development[27] – all theories that inform the potential impact of the intervention on the populations studied. Figure 4.2 provides an example of a framework that is based on these different perspectives.

## Refining the research question

Let us get back to the research question. As you have seen, the process of delineating a problem

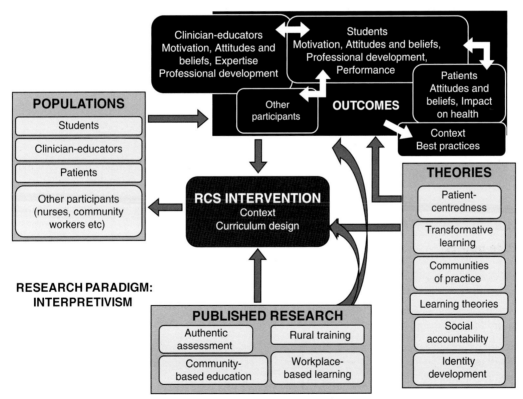

*Figure 4.2* A graphic representation of conceptual framework affords the researcher the opportunity to visualise the various components that contribute to the development of the research question. This example represents a potential conceptual framework for the RCS intervention. The research paradigm, the theories and published research that informed the conceptualisation, the context and the various populations and variables are all represented in this framework.

statement, developing a conceptual framework and formulating a research question is iterative in nature. Each phase contributes to the distillation process towards refining the research question (Fig. 4.1H). In the case of the RCS research, our initial research question was very broad, simply asking whether the intervention had been successful. As we worked through the process of refinement, however, our question became more focused as we came to discern the key issues that needed to be investigated.

At this point, therefore, it is time to examine the quality of the choices you have made in developing your question (Fig. 4.1I). We previously discussed a range of criteria for good research questions. Examine your question and decide whether it meets these criteria. Engage with others informally, or at conferences and seminars to obtain input as to the value and appropriateness of your research question. Revisit the literature and confirm that your question addresses the gap you initially identified (Fig. 4.1J).

## Conclusion

At the beginning of this chapter, we argued that the research question is the cornerstone of any research endeavour. We also suggested that the development of a research question is both a science and an art. The science is mirrored in the triple distillation process with each step and each component emphasising the action of refinement until the final product emerges. The art is seen in the iterative application of review, revision and critical reflection that influence the decision making towards scholarship. In the chapters that follow, the focus will be on putting the research question into play and designing a study that will offer a valid response.

### Practice points

- Find research questions in aspects of your own practice that are of genuine interest to you.
- Develop a problem statement.
- Identify a conceptual framework.
- Embrace the iterative nature of formulating a research question.
- Critically consider the criteria for good research questions.

## Essential readings

Beckman, T.J. & Cook, D.A. (2007) Developing scholarly projects in education: a primer for medical teachers. *Medical Teacher*, **29**, 210–218.

Boet, S., Sharma, S., Goldman, J. & Reeves, S. (2012) Review article: medical education research: an overview of methods. *Canadian Journal of Anesthesia*, **59**, 159–170.

Bordage, G. (2009) Conceptual frameworks to illuminate and magnify. *Medical Education*, **43**, 312–319.

Cook, D.A. (2010) Getting started in medical education scholarship. *Keio Journal of Medicine*, **59**, 96–103.

Coverdale, J.H., Roberts, L.W., Balon, R. & Beresin, E.V. (2013) Writing for academia: getting your research into print: AMEE Guide No. 74. *Medical Teacher*, **35**, e926–e934.

## Recommended readings

Cohen, L., Manion, L. & Morrison, K. (2011) *Research methods in education*, 7th edn. Routledge, Oxon.

Cook, D.A., Bordage, G. & Schmidt, H.G. (2008) Description, justification and clarification: a framework for classifying the purposes of research in medical education. *Medical Education*, **42**, 128–33.

Ringsted, C., Hodges, B. & Scherpbier, A. (2011) The research compass': an introduction to research in medical education: AMEE Guide no. 56. *Medical Teacher*, **33**, 695–709.

Bickman, L. & Rog, D.J. (2009) *The SAGE Handbook of Applied Social Research Methods*. SAGE Publications, Inc., Thousand Oaks, CA.

Miles, M.B. & Huberman, A.M. (1994) *Qualitative data analysis: an expanded sourcebook*. SAGE Publications, Inc., Thousand Oaks, CA.

## References

1  Oxford Dictionaries. (2014) http://www.oxforddictionaries.com/definition/english/distillation?q=distillation. (Accessed 7 July 2014).

2  Maree, K. (2007) *First Steps in Research*. Van Schaik, Pretoria.

3  Shea, J.A., Arnold, L. & Mann, K.V. (2004) A RIME perspective on the quality and relevance of current and future medical education research. *Academic Medicine*, **79**, 931–938.

4  McGaghie, W.C., Bordage, G. & Shea, J.A. (2001) Review Criteria. Problem statement, conceptual framework, and research question. *Academic Medicine*, **76**, 923–924.

5  Regehr G. (2010) It's NOT rocket science: rethinking our metaphors for research in health professions education. *Medical Education*, **44**, 31–39.

6  Coverdale, J., Louie, A. & Roberts, L.W. (2005) Getting started in educational research. *Academic Psychiatry*, **29**, 14–21.

7 Boet, S., Sharma, S., Goldman, J. & Reeves, S. (2012) Review article: medical education research: an overview of methods. *Canadian Journal of Anesthesia*, **59**, 159–170.

8 Ringsted, C., Hodges, B. & Scherpbier, A. (2011) 'The research compass': an introduction to research in medical education: AMEE Guide no. 56. *Medical Teacher*, **33**, 695–709.

9 Frenk, J., Chen, L., Bhutta, Z.A. *et al.* (2010) Health professionals for a new century: transforming education to strengthen health systems in an interdependent world. *Lancet*, **376**, 1923–1958.

10 Lavelle, E., Vuk, J. & Barber, C. (2013) Twelve tips for getting started using mixed methods in medical education research. *Medical Teacher*, **35**, 272–276.

11 Coverdale, J.H., Roberts, L.W., Balon, R. & Beresin, E.V. (2013) Writing for academia: Getting your research into print: AMEE Guide No. 74. *Medical Teacher*, **35**, e926–e934.

12 Bordage, G. & Dawson, B. (2003) Experimental study design and grant writing in eight steps and 28 questions. *Medical Education*, **37**, 376–385.

13 Cook, D.A. (2010) Getting started in medical education scholarship. *Keio Journal of Medicine*, **59**, 96–103.

14 Glasziou, P., Irwig, L., Bain, C. & Colditz, G. (2001) *Systematic Reviews in Health Care: A Practical Guide*. Cambridge University Press, Cambridge, UK.

15 MacKinnon, P. (2011) Integrating mediators and moderators in research design. *Research on Social Work Practice*, **21**, 675–681.

16 Morrison, J. (2002) Developing research questions in medical education: the science and the art. *Medical Education*, **36**, 596–597.

17 Cohen, L., Manion, L. & Morrison, K. (2011) *Research methods in education*, 7th edn. Routledge, Oxon.

18 Van Schalkwyk, S.C., Bezuidenhout, J., Conradie, H.H. *et al.* (2014) 'Going rural': driving change through a rural medical education innovation. *Rural and Remote Health*, **14**, 2493. (Online). Available: http://www.rrh.org.au

19 Blitz, J., Bezuidenhout, J., Conradie, H., de Villiers, M. & van Schalkwyk, S. (2014) 'I felt colonised': emerging clinical teachers on a new rural teaching platform. *Rural and Remote Health*, **14**, 2511. (Online). Available: http://www.rrh.org.au

20 Beckman, T.J. & Cook, D.A. (2007) Developing scholarly projects in education: a primer for medical teachers. *Medical Teacher*, **29**, 210–218.

21 Bickman, L. & Rog, D.J. (2009) *The SAGE Handbook of Applied Social Research Methods*. SAGE Publications, Inc., Thousand Oaks, CA.

22 Miles, M.B. & Huberman, A.M. (1994) *Qualitative Data Analysis: An Expanded Sourcebook*. SAGE Publications, Inc, Thousand Oaks, CA.

23 Bordage, G. (2009) Conceptual frameworks to illuminate and magnify. *Medical Education*, **43**, 312–319.

24 Cook, D.A., Bordage, G. & Schmidt, H.G. (2008) Description, justification and clarification: a framework for classifying the purposes of research in medical education. *Medical Education*, **42**, 128–133.

25 Mezirow, J. (2003) Transformative learning as discourse. *Journal of Transformative Education*, **1**, 58–63.

26 Wenger E. 2000. Communities of practice and social learning systems. *Organisation*, **7**, 225–246.

27 Dall'Alba, G. & Barnacle, R. (2007) An ontological turn for higher education. *Studies in Higher Education*, **32**, 679–691.

# 5 Power analyses: planning, conducting and evaluating education research

*R. Brent Stansfield and Larry Gruppen*

*Steve taught a course for several years and his students have found the course material to be difficult. Last summer, he developed a new learning module – readings, exercises and intermittent quizzes – to help his students. He thinks the module is having a positive effect: his current crop of students is performing better than his previous cohorts and he would like to publish a paper demonstrating its effectiveness. He has 35 students' exam performance from last year (without the module) and the current 35 students' exam performance (with the module). He knows he will need to perform an independent samples t-test, but he does not know if he has enough data to publish the results. If it is not enough, he can gather more: he can ask the school administrators for prior years of no-module student performance and he can collect more with-module data in the coming years, but he would rather not delay his publication unnecessarily. How many student records will Steve need for those statistical tests to give him reliable answers?*

## Introduction

As discussed in this book (Chapter 1), quantitative research inherently involves statistical analysis of numerical data. Power analysis is an important step in deciding how many subjects or data points are needed in a quantitative study. Power analysis helps ensure your study is planned adequately to find effects such as the impact of an intervention, an educational outcome or the relationship between variables. You may remember from Chapter One that quantitative research is planned in detail in advance of a study commencing, and power calculation (for instance, determining the necessary number of subjects) is a critical step in the methodology of any quantitative study. If you are applying for funding for a study, power calculation will be one of the specific methodological points looked for by grant committees, as it will be at the other end of the research process when you write up your study and it is peer-reviewed for publication.

Therefore, why is it important to calculate power? The purpose of power analysis is to focus on the size of your effect, which helps you understand and communicate its practical significance.[1] If a study is 'under-powered', and the results are negative (for example, a randomised control trial that found no difference between the treatment and control groups), then the question will always remain whether the lack of effect was due to insufficient numbers rather than anything to do with the ineffectiveness of the intervention.

Hopefully, this example makes clear the importance of conducting power analyses before you collect or analyse statistical data, then compute and report effect sizes with confidence intervals when publishing your results. Thus the aims of this chapter are to familiarise you with the basic concepts that underlie power calculation so that you can improve the effectiveness of your own educational research and communicate more clearly the strength of the effects you find.

Going back to the example given at the beginning of this chapter, a *power analysis* gives you the answer by *estimating the number of measurements necessary in order for a statistical test to have a particular chance of finding a study effect of a particular size*. There are four components of a power analysis:

1 The effect size
2 The probability of Type I error
3 The probability of Type II error
4 The sample size.

1 The *effect size* is the strength of the relationship or effect that you are examining in your study measured in statistical units (standard deviations or percentage of total variance). For Steve's learning module study, the effect he is interested in is the difference in exam scores between the intervention group (with-module) and the non-intervention group (no-module). There are several estimates of effect size, and we describe the most common in the following sections.

*Researching Medical Education*, First Edition. Edited by Jennifer Cleland and Steven J. Durning.
© 2015 John Wiley & Sons, Ltd. Published 2015 by John Wiley & Sons, Ltd.

Smaller effect sizes are harder to detect and require more measurements in order to be seen.

2 The *probability of a Type I error* is conventionally set at 5% (0.05). This is the probability of (incorrectly) finding a statistically significant effect if, in reality, there is no effect. This probability is named *alpha* ($\alpha$) and it is what we compare the *p*-value of our statistical test to when determining statistical significance. If Steve's learning module is not effective, any *t*-test he uses to test its effectiveness has a 5% chance of giving him a statistically significant finding anyway; this finding would be a false positive, which is called a Type I error.

3 The *probability of a Type II error* is the probability of NOT finding a statistically significant result when the effect you are testing actually DOES exist. This probability is named *beta* ($\beta$), and it is the complement of what we call *power* ($1-\beta$). Beta is conventionally set at 20%, which means 80% is considered adequate power. An experiment with $\beta = 20\%$ (0.20) for a given effect size has 80% power for that effect size and therefore an 80% chance of yielding a statistically significant statistical test for that effect if it exists. If Steve's learning module actually improves student performance with a medium effect size (around 0.5 standard deviations) then his *t*-test with 35 students per group gives him 80% power for that effect size. That means that he has a 20% chance of NOT finding a statistically significant effect despite the effectiveness of the module; this finding would be a false negative, which is called a Type II error. The effect is there, but Steve did not find it: if he claims the effect is not there, he has erred.

4 The *sample size* is the number of participants in your study. More participants give you more power. The smaller the effect size, the larger the necessary sample size must be to have adequate power to detect the effect.

These parameters are all related mathematically. Once you define three of these parameters, a power analysis will calculate the value of the fourth. Since the first two of these parameters are typically set by convention ($\alpha = 0.05$ and $\beta = 0.20$), you will usually need to determine or estimate one of the last two yourself. For your learning module study, you already know the sample size: you have 35 students per group. Therefore, you can take that sample size, set power at 0.80 and alpha at 0.05 and do a power analysis to estimate the smallest effect size you could detect.

Because Steve has a two-group design and wants to run a *t*-test, he can use Cohen's *d* as his effect size estimate. Cohen's *d* is the effect size of the difference between two samples. It is the ratio of the difference

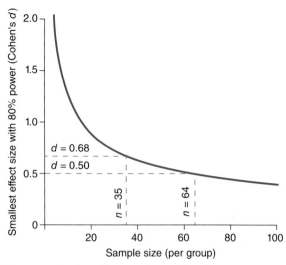

**Figure 5.1** Smallest effect size detectable with 80% power for sample sizes up to 100 per group.

between the group means to the within-group standard deviation. Cohen assigned a rule of thumb for interpreting this effect size: a small effect is around $d = 0.20$, a medium effect is around $d = 0.50$ and a large effect is around $d = 0.80$.[2]

The curve in Figure 5.1 shows the smallest effect Steve has 80% power to detect (with $\alpha = 0.05$) as a function of his sample size (number of students per group). Larger samples allow him to detect smaller effects with that given level of power. Steve can use that chart to see that his sample size of 35 gives him 80% power to detect an effect of $d = 0.68$.

If he suspects that the real effect size of the impact of his learning module is smaller than that, he can set alpha and power at the same levels (5% and 80%, respectively) and define the smallest effect size he is interested in detecting and then do a power analysis to calculate the minimum number of students in each group he will need: his required *sample size*. Let us say he thinks the real effect size is medium (closer to $d = 0.50$). He can trace the curve in Figure 5.1 and find he will need 64 students in each group to achieve 80% power. In that case, he should wait another year and test another 35 students with the module and ask his administrators for another year of old non-module test scores.

Let us say that Steve's learning module in reality has a medium-size positive impact on student learning; it improves a class' mean exam score by half of a standard deviation ($d = 0.50$). If Steve neglects to conduct a power analysis and simply runs his *t*-test on the easily available data ($n = 35$ students per group), he will only have 54% power: there will be a 46% chance that his test would be non-significant despite the actual efficacy of his intervention. This Type II error would be tragic: a non-significant result is likely doomed to never be published and Steve may conclude (falsely) that his learning module is ineffective. The power analysis would show Steve that doubling his sample size will greatly reduce the chances of making error.

## Compute and Report Effect Sizes with Confidence Intervals

Let us fast-forward a year. Steve wisely conducted his power analysis and decided to double his sample size. He now has 70 students in each group. He conducts his *t*-test and finds that students with the learning module score statistically significantly higher than those without ($p < 0.05$). He looks at the means and standard deviations of the groups and calculates his observed effect size: $d = 0.60$. There is a true effect size – if he could run an infinite number of students with and without his learning module, he would find precisely how much the module improves students' test scores. The results of his study, with only 70 students per group (much smaller than infinity), yields an estimate of that precise amount: his observed effect size has some uncertainty associated with it. This uncertainty comes from numerous factors (age, gender, educational background of the students, random variation in their mood and attention on the day of the test and myriad other factors too many to account for), and if he were to rerun the same analysis using different groups of students, he would certainly get somewhat different effect size estimates. The true effect size is probably not 0.60, but some value somewhat higher or lower than what he observed. Because of this, when reporting effect sizes, we should always report *confidence intervals* around them. Confidence intervals are essential to any report of observed study results.[3] Confidence intervals tell you just how precise is the estimate of a given statistical parameter obtained from a study.

The confidence interval provides us with the range of values of *d* that are likely to reflect the true effect size. Specifically, the 95% confidence interval around $d = 0.6$ may be as low as 0.4 and as high as 0.8. In other words, any value of the true effect size inside the confidence interval would be more than 5% likely to yield the effect size we observed. It is important to remember that the confidence interval is NOT a region where the true effect size is 95% likely to be. It is instead a range of true effect sizes that make our observed data reasonably plausible. A 95% confidence interval ranging from 0.3 to 0.5 indicates that if the true effect size were anywhere outside that range, there would be less than a 5% chance of a dataset yielding the effect size estimate it did.

This example also illustrates the connection between confidence intervals and *p*-values in statistical testing. In the logic of Null-Hypothesis Significance Testing (NHST), we determine whether observing a *d* of 0.60 is sufficiently unlikely (probability of 5%) given that the true effect of the intervention is zero (the null hypothesis). If so, we can reject the null hypothesis that the true effect is zero. The confidence interval lets you make that very same judgment by examining whether the null hypothesis (no relationship, difference between two means = 0.0, etc.) is included in the confidence interval. In the case of the 95% confidence interval from −0.1 to 0.7, the null result (0.0) is included in that interval, then a true effect size of zero could plausibly yield our observed results and so you should NOT reject the possibility that the true correlation is zero: your statistical test is not 'statistically significant'. In contrast, the 95% confidence interval of 0.1–0.5 does not contain 0.0; hence, this study would let you conclude that the observed results are unlikely to have occurred ($p < 0.05$) if the true effect size was zero.

Reporting an effect size with a confidence interval in your published research allows your readers to compare your results directly with those of others. Steve's estimated effect size of $d = 0.60$ (95% CI 0.40–0.80) might be larger than his colleague's result, who tried a similar learning module without intermittent quizzes: his colleague may have found $d = 0.45$ (95% CI 0.30–0.60). This information helps researchers generate new hypotheses (for instance, that intermittent quizzes are an important component for learning modules). If Steve and his colleague had merely reported their *t*-tests and statistical significance, no such comparison could be made and they might not think up the hypothesis of the importance of intermittent quizzes.

Cohen's *d* is standard for two-group designs like Steve's. It is directly comparable to other effect size measures that are in units of standard deviation. For instance, Steve's colleague might have asked her students how many hours they spent using the learning module and computed Pearson's *r* to measure the effect. Since *r* is a standardized, unitless measure, it can be converted into *d*, so that Steve and his colleague might compare results directly. The conversion is direct: $d = 2r/\mathrm{sqrt}(1 - r^2)$.

More complicated study designs require a different type of effect size measure, one that measures the percentage of variance explained by your model. Eta-squared ($\eta^2$) is the most common of these. Others you might encounter include omega-squared, *f*-squared and *R*-squared. These are all computed a bit differently, but they are all estimates of effect size that range from 0 (the model explains none of the variance) to 1 (the model explains all of the variance) and all of these can be reported with confidence intervals.

Therefore, how does one report the results of a study that provides more information than the traditional $p < 0.05$? The fundamental recommendation is to report each of the elements identified earlier. Note that:

- Alpha, sample size and power are often provided in the Methods section.
- The effect sizes and confidence intervals are typically reported in the Results section.

The more visible consequence of following these guidelines will be the demise of reporting the observed $p$-values (e.g. $p < 0.0035$ or $p < 0.0001$) and instead, simply reporting the criterion $p$-value (typically $p < 0.05$ or $0.01$) and signify which of the observed results meet that criterion. The second consequence will be the inclusion of effect size measures and associated confidence intervals. By including this information, the reader has a better understanding of the clinical significance and therefore the real-world implications of the effect.

Table 5.1[4] illustrates these practices. The overall $p$-criterion is 0.05. The observed mean values for the outcome measures (types of errors) are reported along with variance measures (standard deviations) and the observed differences in means. The effect sizes are reported as the proportion of variance accounted for in each outcome measure.

Confidence intervals provide information on the precision of each of these estimates. The criterion $p$-value (0.05) is provided as a footnote and applies to all the variables in the table.

As an example of how power analysis and confidence intervals help us understand the results of a study, we can look at a published research article, such as the vast majority of published articles, that contains neither. A published study described the efficacy of training physicians in patient-centred communication.[5] They used a short form of the training with which they successfully trained 15 physicians and measured another 15 as a control group. They also used a long form of the training with which they trained 20 physicians with no control group. Each physician was measured twice: shortly before the training (or lack of training for the control group) and a month later. The primary measure was a coding of the patient-centredness of their communication derived from audio tapes of five real patient interactions; the coding generated several scores for the incidence of various patient-centred communication behaviours (asking open-ended questions, psychosocial talk, etc.).

One of their planned comparisons was of the change from pre- to post-training communication scores between the 15 short-training physicians and the 15 control physicians. They used an independent samples $t$-test to compare the pre- to post-training change in various communication scores of

*Table 5.1* An example of reporting effect sizes with 95% confidence intervals

| Error | Mean (SD) frequency per student | | | |
| | Intervention group ($n = 30$) | Control group ($n = 53$) | Mean difference (95% CI) | % variance accounted for (95% CI) |
| --- | --- | --- | --- | --- |
| Lack of Medical Subject Headings (MeSH) explosion | 0.7 (0.8) | 1.3 (1.0) | −0.6 (−1.0, −0.2)* | 7.7 (0.9, 18.8) |
| Missing MeSH terms | 0.7 (0.8) | 1.2 (0.9) | −0.5 (−0.9, −0.1)* | 6.8 (0.3, 18.8) |
| Lack of appropriate limits | 0.8 (0.7) | 0.9 (0.5) | −0.1 (−0.4, 0.2) | —† |
| Inappropriate Boolean operator/failure to combine all relevant search concepts appropriately | 0.7 (0.7) | 0.6 (0.5) | 0.1 (−0.2, 0.4) | —† |
| Failure to search for best evidence | 0.4 (0.5) | 0.7 (0.5) | −0.3 (−0.5, −0.1)* | 7.7 (0.9, 18.8) |
| Missing one or more concepts | 0.6 (0.6) | 0.7 (0.5) | −0.1 (−0.3, 0.1) | —† |
| Inappropriate limits | 0.2 (0.4) | 0.3 (0.5) | −0.1 (−0.3, 0.1) | —† |
| Search inefficiency | 0.1 (0.4) | 0.3 (0.3) | −0.2 (−0.4, −0.1)* | 5.5 (0.9, 18.8) |
| Incorrect search terms | 0.1 (0.3) | 0.3 (0.4) | −0.2 (−0.4, −0.0)* | 3.6 (0.1, 12.90) |
| Total search errors | 4.4 (3.3) | 6.2 (2.8) | −1.8 (−0.4, −3.2)* | 7.6 (0.4, 20.6) |

Types and Frequencies of Search Errors in the Post-Elective Searches of 83 Fourth-Year Medical Students in an Evidence-Based Medicine Elective. University of Michigan Medical School. Ann Arbor, Michigan, 2001–2003.
*$p < 0.05$, independent $t$-test.
†Percent variance and confidence intervals are not computed for differences that are not statistically significant.
*Source*: Gruppen *et al.*[4] Reproduced with permission of Wolters Kluwer Health.

intervention and control group physicians and reported no statistically significant results. While they did not report a power analysis, their power can be computed: an independent samples *t*-test with 15 subjects per group has 80% power to detect an effect of $d = 1.06$ or greater. This is a very large effect size, and so we would not expect statistically significant results if the training had only a small or even moderate effect on physicians' communication behaviour. Thus, the negative finding is not surprising and contains little information about what the true effect size might be, other than the fact that it is probably smaller than one standard deviation.

Another of their planned comparisons was to compare all three groups (control, short-training and long-training) on various aspects of patient-centred communication. One of these comparisons found that the 20 long-trained physicians increased their use of open-ended questions (the mean pre- to post-training difference was 4.5) more than the 15 short-trained physicians (mean difference was 3.0) and controls (mean difference was 3.2). This effect, tested by one-way analysis of variance (ANOVA) had a *p*-value above but close to alpha ($F = 2.8$, $p = 0.068$) and hence was declared non-significant. Using the group means and the sample size, we are able to reverse-engineer the statistic[1] and find that their observed effect size was around eta-squared $= 0.106$. For percentage-explained effect size measures, this is a moderate-to-large effect and could have been reported as such. Instead, the authors reported the non-significant difference and that 'there was some indication that long-program physicians engaged in more asking of [open-ended] questions'.

The aforementioned patient communication article describes a possibly powerful communications-skills training tool, but a power analysis would have informed them that their sample size was too small to find statistical significance for all but very large effect sizes. In light of their low power, they could have reported their observed effect size estimates with their wide confidence intervals in addition to (or instead of) their significance tests to better demonstrate the potential efficacy of the tool. However, they are only able to report very unstable estimates of their tool because of their paucity of data and the 95% confidence intervals for many of their observed estimates include zero – a complete lack of efficacy of their training tool – as a plausible true effect size.

## Practicalities and pitfalls

Hopefully, the aforementioned paragraph has demonstrated the importance of power analysis and sample size calculations in any type of quantitative healthcare education research (see Gruppen *et al.*,[4] for an example from medical education). One question new researchers often ask is whether or not they should or could go ahead with a study without the necessary sample size to be likely to detect an effect. For example, if you need data from 100 people in each arm of a trial to detect an effect but there are only 50 people per arm available to you, is the study still feasible? We would strongly advise against going ahead with such a project. Your results are likely to be inconclusive and uninformative. Moreover, it is unethical to trouble subjects and waste limited resources in the service of collecting insufficient data; this work will very likely not yield fundable projects or publishable results. In such cases, go back to your research question and consider if another type of study design will provide more statistical power with the same sample restrictions.

One way to improve statistical power is to choose a more reliable outcome measure. Remember that the denominator of the effect size is the unexplained variance in the model. A more reliable measure will have less variance, making the denominator smaller and therefore the effect size larger. This will increase your observed effect size and thus your statistical power for detecting this larger effect. For instance, if the authors of the patient communications article cited earlier had pooled their various measures of different types of patient-centred communication into one more stable estimate of overall patient-centredness, they might have reduced their measurement error and thus increased their observed effect sizes. If they had reduced their residual variance of the one-way ANOVA cited earlier by 10%, their observed effect size would have jumped to eta-squared $= 0.116$ and would likely have been statistically significant.

If you are comparing across sites (e.g. comparing the impact of tutor training, where the tutors under study work across a number of different campuses), then you may use a particular

---

[1] To do this, we need to determine the degrees of freedom of the *F*-test, which are 2 df for the model (the number of groups minus 1) and 47 for the residual (50 subjects minus 1 minus the number of model df). We then determine the mean-square term of the model as a variance of the model parameter estimates (group means iterated by group sample sizes) and use that to determine the mean-square of the residual (since *F* is the ratio of the model mean-square to the residual mean-square). These mean-square terms are multiplied by the degrees of freedom to determine the sums-of-squares for the model and the residual. Eta-squared is the proportion of the model sum-of-squares to the total sum-of-squares.

type of randomised controlled trial to do so: the cluster-randomised trial.[6] These are very common in healthcare research. In this type of quantitative design, the power calculation has to take into account the possible influence of site as well as the qualities of the primary outcome measure.

## Conclusion

Finally, you may be relieved to hear that there is plenty of guidance available as to how to plan power analysis. Cohen[2] is the seminal reference. The Internet is a good source of resources and there are many online tools that allow you to choose a statistical test, plug in parameters and solve for the one you want (the necessary number of subjects or the statistical power of a given sample size for a given effect size). As stated by Cleland earlier in this book, statisticians are key colleagues when planning and analysing quantitative research. Seek statistical advice on power calculations and analysis and indeed on all aspects of the research planning early on: this will save much time and angst later in the research process.

---

### Practice points

- Estimating effect size and computing power are important aspects of study design and help avoid Type II error.

- Whether determining an adequate sample size for an estimated effect size or determining the smallest detectable effect size for a given sample size, power analysis informs the researcher about the likelihood of finding statistical significance.

- Reporting the size and confidence interval of an observed effect communicates the strength of the observed effect in a way that is easily comparable with results from other studies.

- Together, power analysis and effect size reporting improve the efficacy of research and the usefulness of the literature for understanding the clinical significance of findings and of comparing findings between studies.

---

## References and resources

1  Kirk, R.E. (1996) Practical significance: a concept whose time has come. *Educational and Psychological Measurement*, **56**, 746–759.
2  Cohen, J. (1988) *Statistical power analysis for the behavioral sciences*, 2nd edn. Erlbaum, Hillsdale, NJ.
3  Kirk, R.E. (2001) Promoting good statistical practices: some suggestions. *Educational and Psychological Measurement.*, **61**, 213–218.
4  Gruppen, L.D., Rana, G.K. & Arndt, T.S. (2005) A controlled comparison study of the efficacy of training medical students in evidence-based medicine literature searching skills. *Academic Medicine*, **80**, 940–944.
5  Levinson, W. & Roter, D. (1993) The effects of two continuing medical education programs on communication skills of practicing primary care physicians. *The Journal of General Internal Medicine*, **8**, 318–324.
6  Fayers, P.M., Jordhøy, M.S. & Kaasa, S. (2002) Cluster-randomized trials. *Palliative Medicine*, **16**, 69–70.

# PART 2
## Theory informing educational research

# 6 Constructivism: learning theories and approaches to research

*Karen Mann and Anna MacLeod*

*Your School of Medicine and Health Professions Education has begun to implement a program of interprofessional education for your pre-licensure students. An early initiative has involved bringing together second year students from the different professional schools for discussions about their professional roles and about current healthcare issues. Following the experience, students complete a standardised questionnaire surveying their attitudes, knowledge and feedback on the program. The student evaluations of the program have been mixed; a significant proportion of the class has expressed both dissatisfaction with and low interest in the experience.*

*You decide that it is important to understand why these results are occurring. You have questions such as: 'How do students understand "interprofessional education" and its goals? Do students from different professional schools hold different views? What is their experience, and what meaning do they make of it?' A colleague suggests that perhaps you need an approach that might help you to understand the evaluation results. She suggests 'constructivism' as an approach. You decide to learn something about it …*

## Introduction

Constructivism forms the basis of one of the major ways in which we can view the world (see also MacMillan earlier in this book). Creswell[1] describes a worldview as 'a general orientation about the world and the nature of research that a researcher holds' (p. 6). Like other paradigms, a worldview is the foundation of a group of beliefs about the nature of knowledge and how we come to know the world.

The term 'constructivism' has several meanings, all of which relate in some way to the idea of meaning-making, of making sense, both collectively and socially, of the world in which we live. This focus on meaning is integral to our work as healthcare profession educators and researchers. First, it underpins our understanding of how people learn and forms the basis for what are called constructivist theories of learning. These theories, in turn, lead to particular approaches to teaching and learning; they also provide a framework for our questions about learning and teaching, as we try to improve our understanding and our educational practice. Second, the focus on meaning calls for approaches to research that help us to understand the ways that people make meaning of their experience.

In this chapter, our goal is to promote alignment of worldview, theoretical frameworks and research approaches in relation to constructivism and its philosophical underpinnings. We then turn to an overview of constructivist theories of learning. In the third part of the chapter, we focus on constructivist approaches to research: its traditions and methods. Throughout the chapter, we provide examples from various disciplines including clinical medicine, healthcare profession education and nursing.

By the end of this chapter, you should be able to understand or to explore further:

- The philosophy of constructivism
- How it gives rise to certain theories of learning which we rely on in our daily practice
- Constructivist approaches to research and within them, five major research traditions
- The role of the researcher in constructivist research
- How research is conducted within this paradigm and the methods used in research
- Approaches to ensure quality and rigor; how they relate to such criteria in other paradigms
- Some important considerations and common pitfalls.

Constructivism has arisen as an alternative to positivism as a way of understanding the world. In that sense, it differs from positivism in important and fundamental ways. These include ontology, epistemology and methodology.[2] We will explain each briefly, in the following sections.

*Ontology* asks: 'What is the nature of reality? What is there to know? What can be known?' The positivist view holds that there is a real world

*Researching Medical Education*, First Edition. Edited by Jennifer Cleland and Steven J. Durning.
© 2015 John Wiley & Sons, Ltd. Published 2015 by John Wiley & Sons, Ltd.

and a single reality. While some uncertainty is acknowledged, the nature of that world can be understood through careful testing and measurement of a defined set of ideas. In contrast, constructivism holds that there are multiple realities or a 'relativist' view. In this view, each of these realities arises from the 'construction' of meaning and understanding, based on the individual's context, previous experience and knowledge, attitudes and beliefs.

*Epistemology* asks: 'What is the nature of the relationship between the knower and the known[2]?' The positivist worldview takes an 'objectivist' approach, that, as researchers, we can separate ourselves from the process or event we are describing and therefore discover its true form or process. By contrast, in the relativist or 'subjectivist' view of constructivists, the researcher and the researched are inseparable. The researcher brings to the exploration his or her beliefs, prejudices, experiences and values. These influence both what is studied and how the observations are seen.

The two approaches are summarised in Table 6.1.

*Methodology* asks 'How can we know what can be known?' The constructivist approach differs from the positivist approach in the methodology regarded as appropriate to answer the questions raised. Constructivist approaches to understanding are mainly qualitative, including questions such as why and how events and processes occur and how individuals and groups make meaning of them. While quantitative approaches are not excluded, they complement the qualitative methods. Positivist researchers rely mainly on quantitative approaches to mitigate and minimise subjectivity, with the goal of uncovering true knowledge of the real world, to explain and predict causal connections.

An example may be helpful to illustrate these different ways of viewing the world. Let's assume that we are interested in understanding how empathy is learned. Using a positivist approach, we might search the literature to determine approaches to measuring empathy. Having selected a validated scale, we might then choose to measure empathy in a group of learners at critical points during their education, for example, at entry to a program, at the transition to predominantly clinical learning, and at completion of the program. We could measure any changes across these times, and try to understand what they mean through the scores obtained and the constructs, which the scale purports to measure. We might compare these scores to scores obtained on other scales that are thought to measure concepts related to empathy, to see if relationships exist. In contrast, using a constructivist approach, we might want to understand more about how learners understand empathy, what meanings they make of it and how it is enacted in their experience. This might involve interviewing learners at different levels to gather their understandings of empathy and their personal experiences and perspectives on how it is learned. We would be interested perhaps in understanding how learners relate empathy to other concepts in their experience, or whether some new understanding of empathy and how it is learned might emerge from our analysis. (Of course, positivists may look at this also, but from the worldview that there is only one truth.)

As can be seen from the aforementioned comparisons, these worldviews or paradigms influence choices and actions made as a teacher, as a researcher and as an individual or group. We now turn first to a brief introduction to constructivist theories of learning. (These will be addressed in more depth in other sections of this book.) Following that, we turn to constructivist approaches to research.

*Table 6.1* A comparison of constructivist and positivist worldviews: ontology, epistemology and methodology

| Element | Constructivism | Positivism |
|---|---|---|
| Ontology | There are multiple realities. Individuals construct different understandings based on their past experiences and knowledge. | There is a single reality. The nature of reality can be understood through careful measurement and testing. |
| Epistemology | The researcher and the researched are inseparable. The researcher's beliefs and experiences influence the questions asked and how the findings are understood. | The researcher is separate from the phenomenon, event or process under study. Measures can be taken to eliminate bias and minimise subjectivity. |
| Methodology | Approaches are mainly qualitative. The goal is to understand how and why events occur and how individuals make meaning of them. | Approaches are mainly quantitative. The goal is to uncover the nature of the real world, in order to explain and predict causal connections and associations. |

## Constructivist theories of learning

The constructivist worldview has given rise to theories of learning which are increasingly relevant in healthcare profession education.[3-7] In approaching these theories of learning, it is helpful to see how they reflect the constructivist ontology (views of the nature of reality) and epistemology (the nature of the relationship between the knower and the known).[1] In the constructivist view, learning occurs as learners actively construct the meaning of new knowledge in the light of their previous experience, knowledge, attitudes and values. In this process, while there is general agreement about many things that are 'known', it is also recognised that individuals construct or represent their knowledge in different ways. Rather than being independent of context, meaning is closely related to context. Theories of learning based on constructivism generally fall into two main categories: personal or individual, and social. The personal constructivist aspect is generally included in cognitivist theories of learning, while social constructivism has generally been included among the social theories of learning. Each is explained briefly in the following sections.

*Personal constructivism* began in the first quarter of the 20th century with Piaget.[8] According to Piaget's theory of cognitive development, cognitive schemata or mental structures are developed as persons make meaning of their environment. These schemata become increasingly complex as people learn, through actively thinking and problem-solving about activities. Individuals build their knowledge and construct and expand their schemata by testing them against their current knowledge, readjusting and expanding the schemata, and integrating the new knowledge into their existing structures. We see this in medical education as students gradually build their clinical knowledge, adding to it with new knowledge and experience. A knowledge schema organised and encapsulated around a particular diagnosis is called an 'illness script'.[9]

Much of our knowledge of problem-solving, building knowledge, the effects of practice, development of expertise and other aspects of learning in medicine, is based in this framework of cognitive constructivism. The field of medical education research was opened up significantly by the work of several researchers working in this area.[10-13] Indeed, the resulting understandings of the processes by which medical learners acquired and processed knowledge contributed beyond medical education to the general field of cognitive psychology. This cognitivist–constructivist approach and the principles that underlie and derive from it have become established as a major theoretical foundation for problem-based learning.[13] These principles include the importance of prior knowledge; activation of prior knowledge; elaboration of knowledge; learning in context; and transfer of knowledge. Principles of adult learning build on constructivist foundations of drawing on past experience and knowledge, motivation to learn, and ability to be self-directed in learning.

Reflection, self-assessment and the development of clinical reasoning are also approaches to learning and development informed by constructivism. Each of these outlooks on learning presents issues of interest to researchers in healthcare profession education, as they are regarded as essential capabilities of professionals. They have proved to be extremely complex issues, and many questions remain to be answered. For example, studies of reflection have defined it as a cognitive and affective process through which learning occurs as a result of reflection on experience. However, questions of how this reflection affects action, learning and decision making are still being actively explored. Studies addressing these questions have been conducted using both qualitative and quantitative approaches, independently and in concert, in mixed methods studies. Readers wishing to read more will find a large literature to draw upon; two review papers may provide a useful start.[14,15]

The theories described earlier emphasise the individual learner and internal processes: the knowledge, skills and attitudes that are acquired in the process of active learning, experience and meaning making. In recent years, contemporary notions of constructivism have expanded to include a social aspect of learning, called 'social constructivism', in which the importance of social, cultural and environmental influences is emphasised. In this approach, learning occurs through dynamic interactions between the individual, the environment and the persons, objects and activities occurring there.

*Social constructivism* underlies and incorporates several important aspects of our current understandings of learning. Social cognitive theory[16] and other social theories of learning emphasise how learning occurs in (see chapter by Torre and Durning in this book) interaction with others and with the environment. Socio-cultural theories of learning, originating in the fields of sociology and anthropology have also helped us to understand learning as a social process. These have been further developed by scholars such as Lave and Wenger[17] leading to the concept of communities of practice.

Lave and Wenger[17] held that all learning occurs in a context and is tightly tied to the context. They used the term 'situated learning' to describe this connection to context. The idea of learning in a social context expands the notion of learning as an individual, internal process, to understand learning as a collective social process that occurs through participation in the authentic, real-life practices of the community. Individuals learn 'to do' and 'in doing'; in that process they come to understand ways of framing, thinking and talking about the profession they are entering. They learn from and contribute to the collective understandings and knowledge building of the community. In this conception, constructivism includes knowledge and skills, attitudes, values and development of a professional identity.

Over the last two or three decades, the concept of 'learning in communities of practice' is commonly used to describe how knowledge, skills, cognition values and so on are learned through active participation in the work of a community.[18] Medical education researchers have drawn on the expertise of social science research colleagues to understand better how learning occurs both at the level of the individual and at the level of the collective or community. The concept of learning and knowledge being socially constructed is also rooted in the constructivist world view.

Studies of learning within the social constructivism paradigm include studies of teamwork, inter-professional learning, identity formation and learning in the clinical setting.[19] Other theories of learning, which are underpinned by constructivism, include Cultural Historical Activity Theory (CHAT), commonly called Activity theory, Actor-Network Theory and the more recent socio-material theories (see Chapters 7, 8 and 9 in this book).

In summary, constructivist outlooks on learning can be seen as encompassing those that focus on the individual learner, as well as those that focus a more collective construction of knowledge. They also include a range of theories from those that are quite applied to those that are more abstract. Figure 6.1 may help to illustrate the range and number of such theories.

From this brief overview of theories of learning that are underpinned by constructivism, we now turn to consider how research is conducted within this worldview.

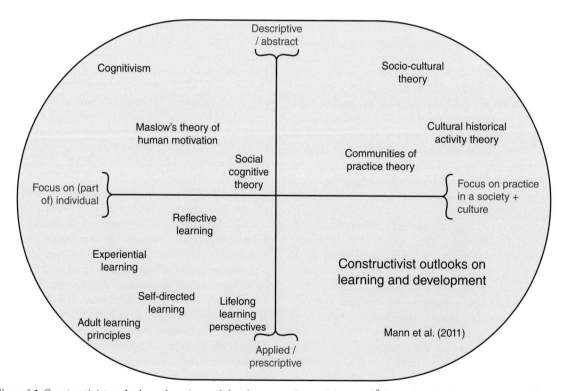

*Figure 6.1* Constructivist outlooks on learning and development. *Source*: Mann *et al.*[3] Reproduced with permission of Elsevier.

## Constructivist approaches to research

When conducting research from a constructivist worldview, it is common to hear discussions of the following three terms: relativist, transactional and subjectivist. These ideas have a significant influence on the way constructivist research is actually conducted. What do they actually mean?

*Relativist*: Relativist ontologies influence constructivist approaches to research. Simply put, there is an underlying philosophical assumption characterising constructivist approaches, that 'there is no objective truth to be known'[20] (p. 278). Relativist assumptions emphasise the wide variety of interpretations that can be applied to a world, which clearly has an important influence on the way constructivists approach the processes of research.

*Transactional*: Transactionalism is at the core of constructivist epistemologies, and deals with issues of truth. From a constructivist approach, truth is a 'transaction' and is the product of these interactions and the individuals' thoughts, leading to what are termed 'constructed realities', or how individuals have constructed their understanding of reality. Transactionalism, therefore, influences the goals of any constructivist research project.

*Subjectivist*: Within constructivist epistemologies, the world is unpredictable. This includes the thoughts, feelings, and psychologies of research participants. As a result, the researcher's work is to construct an impression of the world as they see it, rather than to reveal truth.[21] For these reasons, reflexivity (to be discussed below) is highly important within constructivist approaches.

Let us consider relativist, transactional and subjectivist in the context of a research interview. A constructivist would approach the research interview hoping to gain insight from a research participant rather than to learn the 'true story', because she or he recognises that there is no single truth. This is an example of relativism. Further, the constructivist researcher would accept that the information being shared through the interview process is the result of an exchange between the researcher and the participant, rather than the conveying of 'pure, unfiltered' fact. This is an example of transactionalism. Finally, a research interview constructed with a constructivist worldview would recognise that people – research participants and researchers – are unpredictable. The ways in which people respond to questions, for example, might

be quite different depending upon many different factors. For example, is the participant particularly passionate about the issue at hand and taking the interview in an unexpected direction? Is the researcher feeling a time crunch and trying to get through the interview as quickly as possible? Is the participant regularly consulted about the topic at hand and feeling 'tired' of talking about the same issues? Did the researcher have a particularly good rapport with a particular participant but not with another? These are examples of the subjectivism inherent in the research process that are acknowledged and taken into account in a constructivist worldview.

What do 'relativist, transactional and subjectivist' mean in terms of how to 'do' constructivist research? What does a constructivist research project look like in actual practice? As a rule, constructivist research would display the following five important characteristics:

1 It is (typically) qualitative
2 The literature does not necessarily define the research question(s); rather, it informs the researcher.
3 It involves naturalistic methods (for example, interviewing, observation, document analysis).
4 It includes a dialogue between the researchers and the research participants in order to collaboratively construct meaning.
5 Meaning is emergent through the research process.

Constructivism is based upon the belief that reality is socially constructed and is therefore fluid. Constructivists believe that knowledge is in a constant process of evolution based on the negotiation of important factors such as cultures, social issues and relationships. Therefore, multiple competing, even conflicting, yet valid claims about knowledge exist. We know this all too well within our own disciplines. For example, the Objective Structured Clinical Examination (OSCE) has been hailed as the gold standard in healthcare profession education assessment and a body of research support this claim.[22] A parallel body of literature, however, simultaneously describes OSCEs as a problematic assessment method.[23]

For those who have mainly thought about research from a positivist stance, it may be unsettling and even uncomfortable to be untethered from the safety of traditional approaches in which there are established guidelines and processes in place to determine the rigour and quality of a particular research project. In response to this discomfort and desire for order, Angen[24] proposed a set of criteria to evaluate research conducted from an interpretivist approach, such as constructivism. These include the following:

- A carefully considered and well-articulated research question
- A demonstration that the research was conducted respectfully
- An articulation of the choices and interpretations the researcher makes and evidence that the researcher takes responsibility for those choices
- A persuasive and well-argued account of the research
- A transparent description of the methods and analysis
- A plan and evaluation for the dissemination of results
- An articulation of the validity of the research focusing on:
  - *Ethical validity*: The researcher should be clear that the choices made throughout the process have both political and ethical considerations.
  - *Substantive validity*: The researcher should evaluate the substance of content of an interpretive work.

If a researcher is able to demonstrate that she or he took these dimensions into account in the design, conduct and analysis of the research project, then it is our role, as audience, to make a determination about the quality of the research project based upon the information provided. We will discuss the criteria for ensuring quality of constructivist research in a later section of the chapter; however, for now, let us consider the aforementioned principles using an example.

Jordan *et al.*'s[25] paper 'Thinking through every step: How people with spinal cord injuries relearn to walk' demonstrates the aforementioned seven points. The authors were interested in learning about the experiences of people who have spinal cord injuries; however, this could be quite a broad and unwieldy subject area. The authors fine-tuned their interest posing a well-articulated research question 'If medicine can offer partial recovery from spinal cord injury and therapeutic interventions aim to improve walking ability, how do these efforts impact the everyday lives of people with incomplete spinal cord injuries?' The question focuses the inquiry, making the parameters of the research clear.

The respectfulness of the research is indicated throughout this written account. For example, with respect to participant recruitment, the researchers were one step removed. Physical therapists, with whom participants already had an established relationship, were the first point of contact for recruitment. Likewise, the focus of the article is on the participants themselves, who were encouraged to share their stories and experiences, good and bad, in a sensitive and thoughtful way. Given the difficult subject matter, approaching the research in a respectful manner is particularly important.

The authors provide a careful description of their analytical processes, detailing their decisions with respect to participant recruitment, data collection, data management and interpretation. Actual interview guides are included as appendices and the authors also include a set of notes describing some of their choices. The authors not only describe the 'wheres and whys' of the study, but also make clear the rationale for some of their choices, ranging from practical to theoretical. This provides a detailed picture of their research process and allows readers to draw conclusions about the rigour of the research process. The 'Findings' section of the paper provides a persuasive description of the research findings, presenting the account in a well-argued and concise manner.

While we are seeing the research in its final published stage, as a written account; however, we can make inference about the plan and evaluation of the dissemination. This article is published in Qualitative Health Research, a solid journal with a good impact factor designed to publish the results of qualitative research related broadly to health. In addition, the Discussion section highlights several study findings that could be directly translated into action.

## Five research examples of constructivist research traditions

As medical and healthcare profession educators, we often find ourselves with questions we would like to explore to learn more and understand more fully. In the section that follows, we use an example of a potential medical education issue, which we could explore using the constructivist research approaches. Specifically, we will consider how our issue of interest could be explored using the following methodologies: 1. Narrative; 2. Phenomenology; 3. Grounded theory; 4. Ethnography; and, 5. Case study.[1]

We present two examples of constructivist research with each tradition: a hypothetical example and an actual example from the literature. All of the hypothetical examples are related to one area of interest: how medical students manage their feelings of insecurity and uncertainty throughout their undergraduate education. We provide

*Table 6.2* Dimensions for comparing five research traditions in qualitative research

| Dimension | Narrative | Phenomenology | Grounded theory | Ethnography | Case study |
|---|---|---|---|---|---|
| Focus | Explores an individual's life story | Describes experiences about a phenomenon | Develops theory (theories) based in data from the field | Describes in depth cultural and/or social groups | Provides an in-depth analysis of a single bounded case or multiple cases |
| Data collection | Interviews and documents | Long interviews with approximately 10 people | Interviews with 20–30 individuals to 'saturation' | Observations and interviews over an extended time | Multiple sources – documents, records, interviews, observations, and so on |
| Data analysis | Stories Epiphanies Historical content | Statements Meanings Meaning themes General description of the experience | Open coding Axial coding Selective coding Conditional matrix | Description Analysis Interpretation | Description Themes Assertions |
| Narrative form | Detailed description of an individual's life | Description of the 'essence' of an experience | Theory or theoretical model | Description of cultural behaviour | In-depth description of a bounded case |

*Source*: Based on Creswell.[1]

descriptions of how this issue could be framed from each approach to elucidate the scope of methodological approaches that can be used to explore a single issue within constructivist framework. See Table 6.2 for a summary.

1 *Narrative*: This approach to inquiry retells someone's story over a period of time. It explores what the story means and what some of the potential lessons to be learned might be. A narrative research project would often involve interviews and participants sharing stories in text form. Using our example of wanting to understand uncertainty amongst undergraduate medical students, a narrative approach could involve a series of in-depth interviews with medical students focused on their experiences of not feeling certain of their medical knowledge in given situations.

Bleakley[3] offers a compelling argument for using narrative research in clinical education. He highlights the fact that narrative approaches can illuminate 'hard' data. As an example, Bleakley[3] highlights Rich and Grey's[26] narrative exploration of the effects of trauma surgery amongst young black survivors of penetrating violence. The researchers were interested in learning about how the meaning and circumstances of violent injury might lead to recurrent injury, which they describe as a disturbingly common reoccurrence and note that there is much to learn beyond numbers. This clinician-led program of research included the recruitment of participants while they are still in hospital, offering them the opportunity to tell their story using broad, conversational questions such as 'Tell me what happened to you', and 'How has your getting hurt affected your family?'

2 *Phenomenology*: The goal of phenomenological research is to describe participants' experiences in a specific context in order to understand a phenomenon. For example, given our interest in uncertainty, we could explore the experience of feeling uncertain for medical students with backgrounds from non-scientific disciplines. To explore this, a phenomenologist can use an interview to gather the participants' descriptions of their experience, or the participants' written or oral self-report, or even their aesthetic expressions (i.e. written reflections, poetry).

An example of a phenomenological study from the medical education literature is Dornan and colleagues 'study of clinical teachers' perceptions of problem-based learning. The research team had semi-structured group interviews with clinical teachers to learn about their perceptions of problem-based learning.[19] The researchers asked a broad question of their participants, 'How successful were third-year students at learning from experience?' with some probes. This high-level open-type question allowed for participants to describe their impressions of the phenomenon of problem-based learning in their own words. Interviews were transcribed then opened up to phenomenological reduction, which means that the participant narratives are reduced to a thematic description of key concepts based on the wording of participant responses.

**3** *Grounded theory*: This type of qualitative approach iteratively investigates a process, action or inter-action. The ultimate goal is to develop a theory. As an example, a grounded theory research project might explore feeling uncertain in the clinical clerkship. The researcher might conduct inter-views with students and preliminary analysis of interviews may suggest a theme of 'uncertainty'; this theme could be refined by interviewing par-ticipants who are at various points in their clinical clerkship, who might offer different perspectives on what it means to be uncertain. Analysis of the subsequent phase of data collection will lead to further adaptations of the data collection process to refine and complicate the emerging theory of uncertainty.

Kennedy and colleagues'[27] work on clinical trainees' requests for support is an example of a rigorous grounded theory study in a medical education context. These researchers intended to develop a theoretical explanation of a social phenomenon, in this case learning when and how to ask for help, that was grounded, or based in naturalistic data. The data was obtained through observations and interviews with junior and senior residents, medical students, nurses and attending physicians. The grounded theory approach allowed the researchers to build theory about the many factors, which are more than just clinical, that influence a medical trainees likelihood of asking for support.

**4** *Ethnography*: Arising from early cultural anthro-pology, ethnography is the process of developing an in-depth description of a group done by becoming 'immersed' in their culture through observation and other means of data collection. An ethnographic study may look at the culture of a particular teaching site (i.e. a specific clin-ical ward). The researcher would use multiple data collection approaches, one of which would necessarily be observation, in order to build a rich and nuanced understanding of the formal and informal teaching practices that occur in that ward. The researcher would look for (i.e. observe) examples of practices during which a medical student might feel uncertain, and proceed to explore these in more detail through interviews.

An example of an ethnographic study from the health education literature is Hancock and Easen's[28] study of nurses' decision-making processes when extubating patients following cardiac surgery. The research team spent many hours observing operating room procedures over a course of 16 months. The observations were followed up by interviewing the people they had observed with the goal of understanding how the culture of the operating room influenced nurses' decision making. Their ethnographic approach helped to illuminate the fact that the often taken aspects of a clinical context, things such as relationships, hierarchy, power, leader-ship, education, experience and responsibility, weighed heavily in the complex process of making decisions.

**5** *Case study*: Case study involves exploring episodic events within a definable framework bounded by time and setting. The selection of an appro-priate case to explore is of central concern. Case study research often focuses on questions of 'how'. An example of a case study may be exploring how a student makes use of available resources to find information when she or he is feeling uncertain about a case presentation. The researcher must systematically collect and manage multiple sources of data about practices of information locating and resource appraisal, in formats that can be referenced and sorted so that multiple lines of inquiry and patterns can be explored.

Crowe and colleagues[29] discuss the benefits of case study research in the context of med-ical research, highlighting that the approach allows in-depth explorations of complex issues in real-life settings. They highlight Pearson *et al.*'s[30] work, which uses case study as a mechanism to understand how students from various health-care professions learn about patient safety. This group of researchers reviewed course docu-ments/materials related to patient safety from education programs within a number of different healthcare professions. They then interviewed representatives of each of those professions. Fol-lowing this, case studies were developed and explored with participants from various profes-sions to explore the underlying organisational cultures to which students and new professionals are exposed.

While each tradition offers different methodolog-ical approaches and analytical processes, when approached within a constructivist worldview, each of these approaches shares interpretive epistemo-logical and ontological viewpoints. Specifically, the 'investigator and the object of investigation are … interactively linked so that the findings are literally created as the investigation proceeds'[31] (p. 207). The epistemological and ontological positions adopted in constructivist research thus differ from those in which the researcher's role is to discover the truth that lies within the object of investigation, in which reality is believed to exist autonomously outside of any consciousness[32]. Constructivist approaches challenge the assumption that data are objective 'facts' that exist in the world as well as the position that a researcher has the job of 'discovering' these data and the related theories they might imply. Rather, as Charmaz[32] describes, constructivist approaches place 'priority on the phenomena of study and seeing both data and analysis as created from shared experiences and relationships with participants and other sources' (p. 330). Further, constructivists might actually consider more traditional, objectivist approaches problematic, because these approaches weaken 'the power of the constructivist approach by treating experience as separate, fragmented and atomistic'[32] (p. 331).

Keeping in mind notions of relativism (no objective truth exists), transactionalism (truth is co-constructed) and subjectivism (the world is unpredictable), which we discussed earlier, research conducted from a constructivist worldview and framed as Narrative, Phenomenological, Grounded Theory, Ethnographic, or Case Study, despite their individual approaches to data collection and analysis, would have several common themes.

1 Constructivist research produces 'multiple constructed realities that can be studied holistically; inquiry into these multiple realities will inevitably diverge (each inquiry raises more questions than it answers'[31] (p. 37).

2 People should be the primary data collection instrument[31] since it is difficult to imagine non-human entities (i.e. tools) that could interact with participants in such a way that their multiple constructed realities could be explored.

3 The research should take place in a natural setting related to the issue to be explored as 'the knower and the known are inseparable'[31] (p. 37) and their 'realities are wholes that cannot be understood in isolation from their contexts'[31] (p. 39).

4 'Every act of observation influences what is seen'[31] (p. 39), which reinforces the position that the researcher must be the primary data-gathering instrument in order to understand, respond and describe the interactions taking place within the research setting.

5 Each research participant has her or his own point of view and set of experiences; therefore, the research is focused on identifying the nuanced meaning of these multiple points of view in order to produce a collaborative account from the multiple realities that exist. This means that the research participants are, in effect, co-producers in the research process.

## Methods commonly used within constructivist research approaches

As a form of naturalistic inquiry, constructivist research should be conducted in a natural setting, since context is essential to the process of constructing meaning. We highlight herein three such methods that allow naturalistic inquiry: interviews, observation and document analysis.

### *Interviews*

*There are no facts, only interpretations.*

(Friedrich Nietzsche)

Traditionally, the interview has been considered a vehicle by which the knowledge of the interviewee was passed on to the interviewer.[33] The two distinct parties barely interacted except by means of a structured interrogation. Within a constructivist theoretical frame, however, the interview is considered a conversation with multiple purposes, the format of which is constructed as the interview progresses.

Constructivist notions of subjectivity have focused on important considerations regarding the concepts of the self and individualism, which influence the way researchers think about the process of interviewing. Research participants are not considered uncontaminated and passive holders of knowledge about facts, feelings, experiences, and demographic characteristics. Likewise, research interviewers have a role larger than simply posing questions and facilitating appropriate responses. Within a constructivist approach, interviews are conducted from a perspective that acknowledges the subjectivities of both the participants and the researcher, considering the participant an active contributor and a co-constructor of knowledge--more than a 'fountain of facts.'

From this perspective, a participant cannot 'contaminate' the data that she or he is helping to construct. Rather, the subject is always building knowledge before, during, and after occupying the role of the research participant.[34]

The subjectivity of the research participant and her or his related experience are in a process of continuous assembly and modification, therefore, the 'truth' of interview responses cannot be determined in terms of whether the responses provided by the participant correspond with a supposedly objective 'vessel of answers'. Within a constructivist approach, the value of data from interviews is hence not only in their meaning but also, critically, in identifying the range of meanings and ideas put forth by participants.[34]

### *Observation*

*There is no more difficult art to acquire than the art of observation*

(Sir William Osler)

A constructivist researcher may choose to engage in research observations in order to learn more about a specific scenario in a natural setting. The researcher would observe and collect a set of field notes. While this sounds relatively straightforward, it is in fact an iterative process during which the focus of, methods for, and ideas about our observations might change.

Conceptualising field notes as inert texts designed to accurately describe what was observed falls within the realm of positivism and assumes that there is a single 'accurate' observation. From a constructivist perspective, there is no one correct or true account to be described. Field notes are not truths, but descriptions of social life and social discourse, which reduce the complexities of social phenomena into written accounts that are then analysed.

Related to the concept of subjectivity, it is important for researchers to document their own activities, context, and emotional responses as they are conducting observations, as these factors influence the process of observing and the manner in which they choose to record the lives of others. It is common practice, therefore, for constructivist researchers to maintain a research journal documenting reflections on the observations of the day.

In a constructivist approach, however, drawing a distinction between field note data and personal reaction is misleading as accounts are necessarily transactional (developed as a result of interaction of meanings and events), and relativist (reflecting multiple realities). While the researcher can certainly separate what she or he says and does from what she or he observes, this separation would misrepresent constructivist inquiry in several ways.

First, this separation treats data as 'objective information' that has a fixed meaning independent of *how* that information was elicited or established and by whom. In this way, the [researcher's] own actions, including [her or] his 'personal feelings and reactions' are viewed as independent of and unrelated to the events and happenings involving others that constitute 'findings' or 'observations' when written down in field notes. Second, this separation assumes that 'subjective' reactions and perceptions can and should be controlled by being segregated from 'objective', impersonal records. And finally, such control is thought to be essential because personal and emotional experiences are devalued, comprising 'contaminants' of objective data rather than avenues of insight into significant processes in the setting.[35] (pp. 11–12).

Constructivists hold that including personal reflections enhances interpretive and analytic processes, by encouraging a new, but situated, appreciation and understanding of the events being observed. For that reason, rather than attempting to account for, and limit, strong reactions to particular events, a constructivist researcher would consider these reactions as key points of analysis.

### Document analysis

*[H]ere I sit and govern [Scotland] with my pen: I write and it is done.*

(King James VI (Scotland) and James I (England))

As the quote illustrates, people 'do' things with, through, because of, and in spite of documents. If a researcher is seeking to construct an account of a particular phenomenon, it is her or his role then to understand how relevant documents influence the scenario being studied. Atkinson and Coffey[36] have argued that 'documentary materials should be regarded as data in their own right. They often enshrine a distinctively documentary version of social reality' (p. 59).

Collecting and reviewing important documents that constitute a component of the natural environment is a particularly useful exercise. Within any social organisation, documents do not stand alone. Documents are in a sense 'living things' that can be 'produced and manipulated, used or consumed, and as things that can act back on their creators--very much as Dr. Frankenstein's monster sought to act back on his creator'[37] (p. 77). As Foucault[38] argued, the organisation of artefacts, such as documents, offers insight into basic elements of culture.

Constructivists take documentary sources into account as they are sources of information about the issues being studied. Whether curriculum documents, accreditation standards, program websites, or lists of competencies, documents are important components that offer unique insights.

### The role of the researcher within the constructivist paradigm

Those who espouse a constructivist approach to research appreciate the requirement that the researcher operates from a position of reflexivity. What do we mean by reflexivity?

From a constructivist position, knowledge is socially and culturally constructed and it is therefore necessary for a researcher to acknowledge, and take into account, the many assumptions and views that influence the research process and its related products. Relatedly, reflexivity is not a mechanism to help researchers eliminate their subjectivity(ies), but rather it is intended to support researchers in using, and making sense of their own 'personal interpretive framework consciously as the basis for developing new understandings'[39] (p. 94).The practices of reflexive inquiry address the ways in which meaning is made through research practice and, as Ruby[40] acknowledged 'being reflexive in doing research is part of being honest and ethically mature in research practice' (p. 154). Positions of neutrality and objectivity, within a constructivist worldview, are considered problematic, and have even been described as 'obscene' and 'dishonest'[40].

What does reflexivity look like in practice? Take, as an example, a research interview. Alex and Hammarstrom[41] remind us that within the context of an interview, issues of power are a central consideration. An interview does not occur in isolation; both the interviewer and the interviewee act, speak, respond and interact in particular ways in accordance with their perception of the other and her or his associated power. This might result, for example, in an interviewer choosing to focus on particular aspects of the interview while overlooking, or minimising other aspects. In addition, issues of age, gender, social class, ethnicity, and so on may also influence the dynamic of the interview. Thus, within a constructivist framework, it is important to be conscious of power hierarchies and take into account how those dynamics influence interactions within the context of the interview. 'Despite the best intentions, the interview situation may be experienced as, and may in fact be, a form of abuse. Practicing reflexivity can be one way to minimise such experiences in interview situations' (p. 170).[41] For these, and other reasons, reflexivity should be practised throughout all stages of the research process.

The actual practice of reflexivity requires a conscious effort. A constructivist researcher practising reflexively would think critically about the following four elements according to Alvesson and Skoldberg[42] captured in Table 6.3.

A reflexive researcher would attempt to be explicit in addressing the aforementioned concerns in an effort to identify viewpoints that might influence her or his interpretations and analysis. Being unequivocal in such a manner involves actually stating what has been a focus, what has been minimised, and what may have been left out altogether.

*Table 6.3* Four elements of constructivist reflexive research practice

| Element | Researcher activity |
| --- | --- |
| Interaction with empirical material | Take the empirical into account. This includes concrete matters such as transcripts of interviews, written field notes and other relevant materials |
| Interpretation | Pay particular attention to, and think critically about, the ways in which she/he makes sense of, and interprets data and constructs meeting |
| Critical interpretation | Be tuned into social issues, including important issues such as ideology, power, and social issues |
| Reflection on text production and language use | Think critically about questions of 'ownership'. Who owns the knowledge that is being constructed? Who has the authority? Who determines which voices are heard? |

*Source*: Alvesson and Skoldberg.[42] Reproduced with permission of Sage Publications.

## Approaches to ensure quality and rigour of research

Approaches to ensuring quality of research exist in the constructivist paradigm and have been described by several authors.[43,44] As researchers in the field of medical education, we may be most familiar with the criteria utilised for judging the quality of more quantitative methodologies, arising from the positivist paradigm. Lincoln and Guba[2] and Guba and Lincoln[31] proposed different terms and criteria to assess the quality of constructivist research: *trustworthiness* and *authenticity*. These are explained in the following sections.

## Trustworthiness criteria

Four elements of trustworthiness have been described:

*Credibility*: This criterion asks the questions: Does the account of reality provided by the researcher have credibility? Has the research been conducted using accepted practices and is it accepted by others? Is the interpretation of the researcher endorsed by participants in the research? Credibility is considered as broadly analogous to the criterion of internal validity in the positivist paradigm. Researchers in the constructivist paradigm use two main approaches to ensure the credibility of their findings. The first is member checking, also called respondent validation, in which the researcher returns the findings to the participants, who judge whether they reflect their understanding of and are congruent with the process as they experienced it. The second approach is through triangulation. Triangulation means taking different perspectives on a particular object, event or phenomenon. This helps to ensure that multiple views are presented, and that a major oversight has not occurred. It may also involve more than one method: for example, interviews might be combined with observation.

*Transferability*: The transferability criterion asks the question: Can the findings of this study be useful in other contexts, that are similar, but that differ in some ways? The comparable criterion in positivist research is external validity or generalisability. While constructivist researchers are often reluctant to suggest that their findings may apply across contexts beyond what they have studied, certain forms of constructivist research, for example, constructivist grounded theory, have the goal of developing a theoretical explanation of the processes and relations that may explain their findings in a coherent way. Results of studies such as these may often have utility across contexts, where similar situations exist. Transferability relates to the researcher's ability to provide rich detail, so that a reader can assess the extent to which the conclusions drawn in the study setting can transfer to another setting.

*Dependability*: Dependability in constructivist research is analogous to the reliability criterion in positivist research. While conventional notions of reliability assume that a degree of stability is present in research settings, qualitative researchers assume that real world settings are dynamic and changeable and that replication is not achievable.[44] Judgements of the dependability of research findings consider the extent to which the research process was carried out in a manner that may be reviewed or audited by another. For example, an 'audit trail' is established, which clearly describes how recruitment occurred, what questions were asked of the participants, how the analysis was conducted. The interpretations drawn from the analysis, and their relationship to the data, are also part of establishing dependability. The researcher attempts to distinguish between the instability that is part of the research context, and that which is introduced by the process itself.

*Confirmability*: Confirmability is the extent to which the researcher makes clear his or her personal relationship to the research and the findings, and the contribution that any personal views may have

made to the research. Research conducted in the constructivist paradigm can never be construed as objective. However, researchers should provide enough detail of how they collected and analysed their data that readers can see how their conclusions might reasonably have been reached.[44]

## Authenticity criteria

Authenticity criteria assess the fairness of research within the constructivist domain.[2,31,45] They focus on whether the research increases our awareness (ontological authenticity), educates us (educative authenticity), inspires change (catalytic authenticity) and empowers stakeholders (tactical authenticity). Table 6.4 briefly summarises these criteria.

King and Horrocks[44] describe what they have labelled 'procedures for assessing quality'. They argue that whatever criteria are utilised to assess quality in constructivist research, they must be consistent with the researcher's philosophical and methodological position. They describe four main approaches: independent coders and expert panels, respondent feedback, triangulation and the provision of thick description and audit trails. Although these have been mentioned earlier, a more detailed description may be helpful.

*Independent coding and expert panels*: Some form of independent coding is frequently used as a quality check. The aim of doing so is not to prove reliability (as might be the case in quantitative approaches), but rather to assist researchers to reflect critically on the thematic structure they have developed and the coding decisions they have taken. It helps the researchers to be alerted to alternative understandings of the data. Having

*Table 6.4* A summary of quality and authenticity criteria in constructivist research

| Criteria | Questions asked |
| --- | --- |
| Credibility | Does the researchers' account of reality have credibility? Has the research been appropriately conducted? |
| Transferability | Can the findings of this study be useful in other contexts? |
| Dependability | Was the research conducted in a way that others could replicate? |
| Confirmability | Has the researcher clearly presented his or her relationship to the research? |
| Authenticity | Has the research been conducted fairly? Does it increase our awareness, educate us, inspire change, or empower stakeholders? |

data coded by multiple people can also help to encourage reflection on the interpretations being made. A commonly used approach is what King and Horrocks[44] describe as 'code-defining'. In this approach, members of a research team carry out analysis independently, and then meet to compare and discuss the coding that each has produced. An agreed-upon coding structure may then guide further analysis. In some cases, an expert panel of persons with detailed knowledge of aspects of the research is assembled to scrutinise the results. However, selection of individuals with the appropriate expertise is a challenge for doing this effectively.

*Respondent feedback*: The process of 'respondent feedback', sometimes referred to as member-validation or member-checking, includes taking the analysis back to the participants, to ask how well the interpretation fits with their experience. This is sometimes seen as an ethical obligation, to ensure that participants' voices are well heard. Some concerns have been expressed about this process, as it is possible that either participants may deny an interpretation that engenders discomfort, or alternatively, agree with an interpretation because they do not wish to disagree with the researcher. Use of this process requires that participants are provided an explanation of the analysis, which is clear and accessible and which they can assess.

*Triangulation*: Triangulation refers to using multiple methods of data collection, or multiple sources of data, for example, data from both teachers and learners to study a particular phenomenon. Denzin[46] proposed the following approaches: data and methodological triangulation, using more than one type of qualitative data, or a mixture of qualitative and quantitative methods; investigator triangulation, in which data are collected by different researchers whose different perspectives are purposively selected; and, theoretical triangulation, where different theoretical models are used to make sense of the data. As King and Horrocks[44] note, both qualitatively and quantitatively oriented researchers question whether different methods and worldviews can ever be successfully integrated (cross reference with Cleland and McMillan).

*Thick description and audit trails*: Thick description refers to researchers providing detailed descriptions of what they study and the context in which they study it. This helps readers to judge whether the interpretation presented is consistent with what has been described. Thick description helps readers to understand how researchers reached their conclusions from the data available, and how the analysis was developed. Lastly, it provides the reader a basis to determine the transferability of the findings to another context. Audit trails involve maintaining careful records of all aspects of the research, especially any changes that occur as the project is conducted; this documentation contributes to judgement of the rigour of the research.

## Important points and common pitfalls

No research approach is without its slippery spots and challenges: we present here five common pitfalls and important point to keep in mind, when working in the constructivist or indeed any research approach.

*Language 'slippage' between paradigms*: For those of us working in the healthcare professions, the language of the positivist paradigm – validity, generalisability, subjects, and so on – is familiar. Yet, constructivism and positivism are very different approaches; relatedly, the language of each paradigm is also unique and representative of its associated theoretical underpinnings (see Figure 1.1 in Chapter 1 of this book). For example, constructivists use terms such as research 'participants' rather than 'subjects'. This terminology reflects the fact the people who take part in constructivist research are actually participating in co-constructing meaning. Another example is the word 'hypothesis'. Constructivist research is inductive and aims to understand phenomena within particular contexts. The research findings are bound to particular contexts and are not generalisable. Constructivist research, therefore, does not aim to 'test' and/or 'prove' a researcher's hypothesis.

*The question determines the methods*: Within a positivist theoretical frame, particular methodologies are recognised as 'gold-standards' (i.e. randomised controlled trials) and are, therefore, desirable. Within a constructivist paradigm, there are no gold-standard methodological approaches. The focus, rather, is on developing a well-conceptualised research question/objective and selecting a methodology that will best support the rigorous exploration of that question/objective.

*Role of the literature*: Researchers operating in the positivist paradigm use the literature with a very specific purpose in mind: to develop a hypothesis based on previous published research. Positivist researchers want to be able to develop a knowledge base in order to develop a testable hypothesis and benefit from methodological insights published by colleagues in similar fields. In contrast, the literature serves a different purpose for those operating within a constructivist paradigm. Constructivist researchers require a familiarity with previous relevant research in order to develop their questions and fine-tune research plans so as not to duplicate already existing research. However, constructivists must remain open to emerging ideas and must be careful to not be overly persuaded by existing literature rather than what they are seeing in their own data.

*Time commitment*: Constructivist research is complex and we encourage those considering constructivist approaches to allocate a significant amount of time to complete your research project. It is iterative in nature, which means that the process can become time-consuming. Rigorous constructivist research also requires the authentic involvement of participants, which can be logistically complex. Further, multiple methodological approaches mean that there are often large amounts of data generated, which, in turn, leads to complex analytical processes. Constructivist approaches, therefore, lead to rich insights and understandings, but they can be very time intensive.

*Reflexivity*: Given that constructivist research focuses on the social construction of the world, it is of central importance for a researcher to take into account, and acknowledge, the ways in which her or his understandings of the world, including the research process, the data, and the resulting analysis have been shaped. Reflexivity is a central tenant of constructivism. It is not intended to be a form of 'confessional writing;' rather, it is meant to be a rigorous form of self-assessment designed to illuminate the theory and practice gap. Therefore, reflexivity is considered not an optional strategy, but a moral obligation of the researcher.

## Conclusion

Constructivist approaches to research offer a rich and varied way to build knowledge and understanding of peoples' experience in the world. In using these approaches, researchers are guided by different traditions within constructivist research, and by important considerations of methodology.

In this chapter, we have presented constructivism as a philosophy and situated constructivist theories of learning and constructivist approaches to research within that worldview. As we noted earlier, we believe that alignment between theoretical frameworks and concepts, and research approaches is critically important. If we understand the foundations of the constructivist paradigm, and how it gives rise to theories of learning and approaches to research, our questions can more effectively lead to new understandings that can have beneficial effects for teaching, learning and research.

---

**Practice points**

Constructivist research is naturalistic. This means that it takes place in natural settings and uses naturalistic methods (e.g. interviewing, observation, document analysis).

Constructivist research includes a dialogue between the researcher and the research participants in order to collaboratively construct meaning.

High-quality constructivist research includes the following:
- A carefully considered research question
- A demonstration that the research was conducted respectfully
- A reflexive researcher
- A persuasive and well-argued account of the research
- A plan and evaluation for the dissemination of results

---

## References

1  Creswell, J. (2009) *Research Design: Qualitative, Quantitative and Mixed Methods Approaches*, 3rd edn. Sage, London.
2  Lincoln, Y. & Guba, E. (1985) *Naturalistic Inquiry*. Sage, London.
3  Bleakley, A. (2005) Stories as data, data as stories: making sense of narrative inquiry in clinical education. *Medical Education*, **39**, 534–540.
4  Bleakley, A. (2012) The proof is in the pudding: putting Actor-Network-Theory to work in medical education. *Medical Teacher*, **34**, 462–467.
5  Bleakley, A. (2006) Broadening conceptions of learning in medical education: the message from teamworking. *Medical Education*, **40**, 150–157.
6  Hean, S., Craddock, D. & Hammick, M. (2012) Theoretical insights into interprofessional education: AMEE Guide No. 62. *Medical Teacher*, **34**, e78–e101.
7  Mann, K., Dornan, T. & Teunissen, P.W. (2011) Perspectives on learning. In: Dornan, T., Mann, K., Scherpbier, A. & Spencer, J. (eds), *Medical Education: Theory and Practice*. Churchill Livingstone, Elsevier, Edinburgh.

8 Piaget, J. (1929) *The Child's Conception of the World*. Harcourt, Brace Jovanovich, New York.

9 Schmidt, H.G. & Rikers, R.M. (2007) How expertise develops in medicine: knowledge encapsulation and illness script formation. *Medical Education*, **41**, 1133–1139.

10 Norman, G. (2005) From theory to application and back again: implications of research on medical expertise for psychological theory. *Canadian Journal of Experimental Psychology*, **59**, 35–40.

11 Ericsson, K.A. (2005) Deliberate practice and the acquisition and maintenance of expert performance in medicine and related domains. *Academic Medicine*, **79**, S70–S81.

12 Bordage, G. (1991) Semantic structures and diagnostic thinking of experts and novices. *Academic Medicine*, **66**, S70–S72.

13 Schmidt, H.G. (1993) Foundations of problem-based learning: some explanatory notes. *Medical Education*, **27**, 422–432.

14 Mann, K., Gordon, J. & Macleod, A. (2009) Reflection and reflective practice in health professions education: a systematic review. *Advances in Health Sciences Education Theory and Practice*, **14**, 595–621.

15 Sandars, J. (2009) The use of reflection in medical education: AMEE Guide 44. *Medical Teacher*, **31**, 685–695.

16 Bandura, A. (1986) *Social Foundations of Thought and Action: A Social Cognitive Theory*. Prentice-Hall, Englewood Cliffs, NJ.

17 Lave, J. & Wenger, E. (1991) *Situated Learning. Legitimate Peripheral Participation*. Cambridge University Press, Cambridge, UK.

18 Wenger, E. (1998) *Communities of Practice: Learning Meaning and Identity*. Cambridge University Press, Cambridge, UK.

19 Dornan, T., Scherpbier, A., King, N. & Boshuizen, H. (2005) Clinical teachers and problem-based learning; a phenomenological study. *Medical Education*, **39**, 163–170.

20 Hugly, P. & Sayward, C. (1987) Relativism and ontology. *Philosophy Quarterly*, **37**, 278–290.

21 Ratner, C. (2008) Subjectisim. In: Given, L. (ed), *The Sage Encyclopedia of Qualitative Research Methods*. Sage, London, pp. 840–844.

22 Schuwirth, L.W. & van der Vleuten, C.P. (2003) The use of clinical simulations in assessment. *Medical Education*, **37**, 65–71.

23 Hodges, B. (2003) Validity and the OSCE. *Medical Teacher*, **25**, 250–254.

24 Angen, M. (2000) Evaluating interpretive inquiry: reviewing the validity debate and opening the dialogue. *Qualitative Health Research*, **10**, 378–395.

25 Jordan, M.M., Berkowitz, D., Hannold, E., Velozo, C.A. & Behrman, A.L. (2013) Thinking through every step: how people with spinal cord injuries relearn to walk. *Qualitative Health Research*, **23**, 1027–1041.

26 Rich, J. & Grey, C. (2003) Qualitative research on trauma surgery: getting beyond the numbers. *World Journal of Surgery*, **27**, 957–961.

27 Kennedy, T., Regehr, G., Baker, G. & Lingard, L. (2009) Preserving professional credibility: grounded theory study of medical trainees' requests for clinical support. *British Medical Journal*, **9**, 1–7.

28 Hancock, C. & Easen, P. (2006) The decision making processes of nurses when extubating patients following cardiac surgery: an ethnographic study. *International Journal of Nursing Studies*, **43**, 693–705.

29 Crowe, S., Cresswell, K., Robertson, A. *et al.* (2011) The case study approach. *BMC Medical Research Methodology*, **27**, 1–9.

30 Pearson, P., Steven, A., Howe, A. *et al.* (2010) Learning about patient safety: organizational context and culture in the education of healthcare professionals. *Journal of Health Service Research & Policy*, **15**, 4–10.

31 Guba, E. & Lincoln, Y. (1994) Competing paradigms in qualitative research. In: Denzin, N.K. & Lincoln, Y.S. (eds), *Handbook of Qualitative Research*. Sage, Thousand Oaks CA, pp. 105–117.

32 Charmaz, K. (2006) *Constructing Grounded Theory: A Practical Guide through Qualitative Analysis*. Sage, London.

33 Grbich, C. (2004) *New Approaches in Social Research*. Sage, London.

34 Gubrium, J. & Holstein, J. (2003) From the individual interview to the interview society. In: Gubrium, J. & Holstein, J. (eds), *Postmodern interviewing*. Sage, London, pp. 21–49.

35 Emerson, R., Fretz, R. & Shaw, L. (1995) *Writing Ethnographic Field Notes*. University of Chicago Press, Chicago, IL.

36 Atkinson, P. & Coffey, A. (2004) Analysing documentary realities. In: Silverman, D. (ed), *Qualitative Research: Theory, Method and Practice*. Sage, London, pp. 56–75.

37 Prior, L. (2004) Doing things with document. In: Silverman, D. (ed), *Qualitative Research: Theory, Method and Practice*. Sage, London, pp. 76–94.

38 Foucault, M. (1970) *The Order of Things*. Vintage Books, New York.

39 Levy, P. (2003) A methodological framework for practice-based research in networked learning. *Instructional Science*, **31**, 87–109.

40 Ruby, D. (1980) Exposing yourself: reflexivity, anthropology and film. *Semiotica*, **30**, 153–179.

41 Alex, L. & Hammarstrom, A. (2008) Shift in power during an interview situation: methodological reflections inspired by Foucault and Bourdieu. *Nursing Inquiry*, **15**, 169–176.

42 Alvesson, M. & Skoldberg, K. (2000) *Reflexive Methodology: New Vistas for Qualitative Research*. Sage, London.

43 Bryman, A. (2008) *Social Research Methods*. Oxford University Press, Oxford.

44 King, N. & Horrocks, C. (2010) *Interviews in Qualitative Research*. Sage, London.

45 Lincoln, Y. & Guba, E. (2013) *The Constructivist Credo*. Left Coast Press, Walnut Creek, CA.

46 Denzin, N.K. (1978) *Sociological Methods*. McGraw-Hill, New York.

# 7 Making visible what *matters*: sociomaterial approaches for research and practice in healthcare education

*Tara Fenwick and Graham R. Nimmo*

*It is 8.30 a.m. The doctor on overnight is getting ready to handover to the day team. There are two consultants and three trainee doctors spread around the room. Coffee and tea have been made and fresh handover sheets printed for all. They work through the patients using the printed Handover Report sheets from the electronic patient record and they all face the wallboard, which is populated with demographics of all the patients.*

*The computers and screens give access to the patient's history, clinic letters, drugs as well as blood results and CT images and other imaging ('X-rays'). These materials are not just tools to be passively used in handover. As explained later in this chapter, the materials act on the process in ways that shape and are shaped by the human social dynamics of handover.*

## Introduction

Healthcare as well as educational practice is fundamentally a material as well as a social process. Yet materiality is often taken for granted or overlooked. An example is clinical handover, which is not only ubiquitous across healthcare[1] but also is shaped by the materials involved (see Figure 7.1). Materiality here refers to settings and human bodies as well as objects, technologies and substances of various kinds, from wires to paperwork, that flow through everyday life and practice. These actively work on what humans think and do. Some argue that what matters – what is important in our activity – is what has become materialised: 'matter' is not just things, but the process through which things come into being, which might even be thought of as a 'mattering' process. Materials are enmeshed with social dynamics, such as meaning, interactions and decisions – they do not just 'inter-act' as though they are inherently separate, but they 'intra-act' in a social/material meshwork.[2] The issue of interest for healthcare educators is to understand *how* materiality acts on the social, in healthcare as well as educational practices, and in particular, how it affects learning and knowing. This chapter will introduce the value of sociomaterial approaches for researching education and practice in the medical profession, and describe specific examples of this research in action.

## What is a sociomaterial approach, and why is it useful?

Sociomaterial approaches basically help to make visible the material dynamics in practice situations – the relationships among bodies, tools, technologies and settings as well as human intentions, expertise and communication. It is important to note that there are many sociomaterial approaches, about which more will be said further on.

In education, sociomaterial approaches in education focus not on an individual learner or an individual's skills, but on the collective. In this collective, we need to recognise the ways that materials of all kinds actively influence what people think, what they say and how they behave. 'Stuff' matters, and it is matter. Knowing and capability are not generated and controlled only through humans – they are more-than-human, produced at least partly through the ways things work on humans' perceptions, emotions and judgments.

Yet materials are often missing from accounts of learning. Materials tend to be accepted simply as part of the backdrop for human action, dismissed in a preoccupation with consciousness and cognition, or relegated to brute tools subordinated to human intention and design. Clearly in healthcare practice, a range of materials shape practice and medical knowledge: textbooks and curricula, antibiotics and analgesics, nebulisers and electrocardiograms (ECGs), catheters and laparoscopes, crowded wards and ever present sounds, pagers and policies, databases and protocols. While most

*Researching Medical Education*, First Edition. Edited by Jennifer Cleland and Steven J. Durning.
© 2015 John Wiley & Sons, Ltd. Published 2015 by John Wiley & Sons, Ltd.

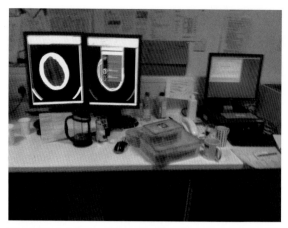

*Figure 7.1* Artefacts and agents of handover: computers, CT images, on call rotas, telephone lists, telephones, coffee and cake, handover print outs, the room.

healthcare practitioners and educators appreciate the importance of their environments of practice, these environments are actually composed of a myriad of technological, natural, manufactured, symbolic and bodily material elements that can easily be taken for granted.

Bleakley[3] contends that lack of attention to materiality frequently puts patient safety at risk. He shows how it is the *relationships* among objects acting together with patients, healthcare personnel, routines, and so on, that transform one another to create risky situations. He uses examples such as a valve nearly left inside an abdominal cavity, or a patient almost falling when a gel mat slid across a frictionless operating table mattress in a steep tilt. These sorts of incidents continue to happen, but we do not seem to learn from them. Bleakley argues that doctors – and we would suggest the members of the whole clinical team – need to learn to attune much more to these micro-details of how materials act in practice.

From a sociomaterial perspective, in research as well as in practice we need to attend holistically to the diverse agents, human and non-human, that interact to produce particular practices including those that are problematic. One example of this may be found in emerging studies of surgical checklists. Amidst the research around these checklists, it has been found that 53–70% of errors relating to surgery occur *outside* the operating room.[4] These researchers have called attention to the multidisciplinary inputs into the checklist (ward doctor, nurse, surgeon, anaesthetist and operating assistant) and the different stages of operative care (preoperative, operative, recovery room, intensive care and other postoperative). Across these stages, the researchers draw attention to diverse material networks that

should be included in the checklist. For example, they suggest, including a review of imaging studies, an accounting of all necessary equipment and materials, the marking of the patient's operative side, the handover of postoperative instructions and the provision of medication prescriptions to the patient at hospital discharge.

Recent studies of professional learning in work[5] are using sociomaterial approaches to show the relationships among non-human as well as human elements that produce everyday activity. They establish that professional knowledge, such as practice and even identity, is not only a human capacity. It is performed in activity, through an array of objects and architectures and technologies as well as through human reflection and decisions, human discussions and emotions. That is, researchers increasingly are turning now to understand practitioners' changing micro-practices and meanings as *constitutively enmeshed* with everyday details of materiality and ecologies of environment.

## Common elements across sociomaterial perspectives

A range of perspectives can be described as sociomaterial, and they are briefly introduced in the next section. Although they are all distinct and have important differences, we could argue that they share at least four broad common elements as explained below:

1 *There is a deliberate focus on materials.* This focus does not erase human activity, but just helps highlight the ways materials shape and extend human activity. In professional education and learning, for example, we often focus on cognition and meaning-making, or dialogue or reflection. We tend to lose sight of how physical settings shape the possible meanings and solutions, how tools embed knowledges and elicit particular ways of using them and how particular bodies evoke particular forms of dialogue. We also tend to focus on individual human beings as though they act separately from the material objects, technologies and settings that penetrate us and one another, 'intra-acting'[2] to bring forth what appear to be solid separate things. This is what Orlikowski[6] describes as 'the constitutive entanglement of the social and material in everyday life'. Orlikowski shows, for example, how simulation education is a dynamic sociomaterial configuration performed in practice among various actors, materials and technologies (designers, engineers, students, tutors, mannequins, computers,

algorithms, networks, etc.). Capacities for action are relational, distributed and enacted.

2 *All phenomena are viewed as sociomaterial collectives.* They are gatherings of heterogeneous natural, technical, human and non-human elements. What appears to be an independent 'object', such as a surgical checklist or calibrating instrument, is not a static thing with inherent properties that sprang into being. Rather, it has been brought about through a history of negotiations among these gatherings, which generated its design and accumulated uses. If we examine this checklist now, in a particular situation, we realise again that is not separate from the particular ways in which it is being used. It is performed into being in this gathering of human and non-human dynamics – it is an *effect* of these sociomaterial relations. Researchers examine these gathering, asking how and why some elements became combined, some become included and others excluded, and most important, how elements change as they come together, as they *intra*-act. Bleakley's[3] examples mentioned earlier show how it is these *relationships* among elements that transform one another in healthcare practice to create risky situations. He argues that sociomaterial analyses (such as actor–network theory (ANT)) are so useful to medical education. He is surprised they are not commonly used to highlight these relationships and how they produce new problems or possibilities.

3 *Things are viewed as effects of connections and activity.* Everything – such as standard protocols, professional identities and surgical skills as well as objects and environments – is performed into existence in webs of relations. Materials are enacted, not inert; they are matter and they matter. They *act*, together with other types of things and forces, to exclude, invite and regulate activity. This is not arguing that objects have agency (the capacity to act): a needle does not pop into a vein by itself. But in cannulation, for example, many things act with the clinician's hands and coordination to: vein diameter and depth, patient movement, cannula diameter, the number of previous cannulations thus increasing difficulty, bacteria on the skin, the urgency in treating the patient's condition, competing clinical demands requiring prioritisation and invoking untimely interruptions[7] and so on. Any medical practice, even one as commonplace as venous cannulation, is a collective sociomaterial enactment, not a question solely of an individual's skills, cognitive and practical.

4 *Practice and learning are fundamentally uncertain.* Most sociomaterial perspectives – in different ways – accept uncertainty as an operating principle in everyday life, as well as in the knowledge, tools, environments and identities that are continually produced in it. Uncertainty is not just ambiguity: it means that chance is always operating in the unfolding configurations, which are always opening a multiplicity of possibilities.

Unpredictable novel patterns are always emerging. Mol[8] confesses her astonishment that in clinical practice, anything worthwhile actually happens: 'Once we start to unravel ontology-in-practice there are no longer any stable variables. All variables vary from one site to another. The miracle to explain is, how, even so practices somehow hang together' (p. 143; by ontology we mean the nature of being, or understanding 'what is' ). This may be a familiar notion, but sociomaterial theories offer specific analytic tools that can examine much more precisely just how these new assemblages, or combinations of things, are emerging – why they come together to produce and mobilise particular effects, and when they do not.

## Differences among sociomaterial perspectives

Within these broad common elements, there are very different approaches and views among sociomaterial perspectives. One is ANT (including the broad field of STS or science and technology studies, as well as what is often called 'after-ANT' studies): Fenwick and Edwards[9] offer a comprehensive overview of ANT in educational research, and Latour's *Reassembling the social*[10] is a seminal text. Another sociomaterial perspective is complexity theory, which is examined very accessibly in educational research by Davis and Sumara in their book *Complexity and education*[11]; see also Osberg and Biesta's *Complexity theory and the politics of education*.[12] 'New materialisms' are outlined in Coole and Frost's *New materialisms: ontology, agency, and politics*.[13] Activity theory can also be considered a sociomaterial approach, and a key author here for healthcare practice and education is Engeström.[14] Spatiality studies come from human geography, and an author that we particularly recommend here is Massey[15] (particularly, her book *For space*). Another key spatiality theorist who has influenced educational research is LeFebvre.[16] These perspectives each have very different and often conflicting theoretical and ontological roots, and hence it is very problematic to simply refer to 'sociomaterial theory'. This brief chapter cannot provide extended explanations or examples for this wide range of theories, but there are books available that do. Interested readers are encouraged to consult these sources for comprehensive descriptions and examples of educational research using these approaches.[4,12] The intent here, in the following paragraphs, is to provide a quick overview to illustrate some key theoretical distinctions among these perspectives.

ANT emerges from post-structural orientations and STS, and is more a methodology than a theory: it offers questions to ask and tools for tracing things, rather than frameworks for explaining them. ANT works within a networked view of reality, and treats human and non-human elements as equal contributors to the heterogeneous 'networks' that continually assemble and reassemble to generate particular activities, objects and knowledge.[16] When anyone speaks of a system or structure, ANT asks, how has it been compiled? Where is it? What is holding it together? All things are assemblies, connected in precarious networks that require much ongoing work to sustain their linkages. ANT traces how these assemblages are made and sustained, how they order behaviours as well as space and objects, but also how they can be unmade and how counter-networks or alternative forms and spaces can take shape and develop strength. ANT, therefore, is very good at examining taken-for-granted practices, such as surgical checklists or ward rounds to look at problems that are held in place through materials and that may be overlooked.

Complexity theory is much different in orientation and offers a range of approaches emerging chiefly from evolutionary biology and physics, cybernetics and general systems theories. Complexity theorists in education, such as Davis and Sumara[11] and Osberg and Biesta,[12] have suggested that we examine dynamics of emergence, nested systems and self-organisation in practices of knowing. Phenomena, events and actors are viewed as mutually dependent, mutually constitutive and actually *emerge together* in dynamic structures. Emergence requires there to be many, many interactions among diverse elements that have some overlap, some constraining rules or boundaries and multiple feedback loops. The researcher's focus in examining emergence is not upon isolated actors and objects foregrounded against some contextual backdrop, but on the dynamic, non-linear actions and connections flowing *between* all these parts. Yet all is not simply flow: living systems are distinct, and move within and alongside one another as *nested systems*. A human body, for example, relies

on highly specialised subsystems that not only each respond to different circumstances and different needs, but also have learnt to co-habitate and communicate with one another. Emergence not only enables continuous adaptive change, but also enables *self-organisation*. Through the multiple interactions among diverse elements, usually according to local rules and not to some global pattern, a clear structure emerges without being imposed through any authority or planning. Complexity theory is increasingly evident in medical education and practice studies,[17–19] and see Bleakley and Cleland (this volume).

New spatiality studies examine the material spaces and places of professional practice. They show how spaces help produce the social, but are also produced by human activity and meaning.[20] Issues for education include how spaces become learning spaces, and how they are constituted in ways that enable or inhibit learning, create inequities or exclusions, or open and limit possibilities for new practices and knowledge. Particularly in new educational arrangements incorporating rapidly developing media and communications technologies, the ordering of space-time has become a critical influence on and way of analysing curriculum and pedagogy. Spatial theories raise questions about what knowledge counts, where and how it emerges in different time-spaces, how identities are negotiated through movements and locations and how learning is enmeshed as and in the making of spaces. Studies might examine, for instance, how different built environments and particular practices influence each other, and give rise to particular educational practices for professionals: think of bedside teaching and ward rounds for medical students compared to business students learning to publicly argue a case analysis in a large lecture theatre.

Yet another branch of studies that is gaining a lot of traction in education is calling itself the 'new materialisms'.[21] These are particularly interested in bodily meshings with materials of all kinds, and often work from the ideas of philosopher Gilles Deleuze of continuous 'becoming' to examine how particular social and material forces bring forth very different ways of being. Finally, it is important to mention the growing educational interest in 'practice theory'. This works from conceptions of 'knowing-in-practice', where knowing is a continuous enactment performed through assemblages that are more-than-human,[21,22] A wide range of research using these theories is tracing professional practice in different organisations. Studies might ask, how do different professional groups negotiate ways to work together when each is shaped by very different logics, instruments, material procedures and so on? Or, how does the introduction of a new technology, such as laparoscopic robotic surgery reshape not only how professionals work, but also their relations to their patients, their identities and their knowledge?

(Cultural-historical) activity theory (CHAT) is also becoming very common in healthcare research, particularly to understand learning across intersecting units or organisations. Here the focus is on examining the systems that come together in practices, the internal contradictions and cultural histories of these systems and the artefacts that mediate the knowledge that circulates. CHAT foregrounds a sociopolitical analysis of human activity, including constructs such as division of labour and the rules of a community, which have developed over time in a particular activity system. Research using CHAT might begin with what people identify to be a particular problem in their system, such as chronic work overloads. Then researchers will lead people through a series of exercises to analyse their everyday work to figure out what are the underlying objectives (not just the stated purposes) and contradictions driving the system – and how materials and settings sometimes reinforce these contradictions and disconnections in purpose. When these are explicit, people together can re-envision – expand – the system's purposes, in a process of expansive learning, both for themselves and the system. Many healthcare and educational researchers have used these Developmental Work Research protocols that have been developed from CHAT.[23]

In general, sociomaterial theories help us to examine old, established practices that have become entrenched as black boxes: ward rounds, theatre operating lists, handovers, clinics and so forth. The focus is on the relations between things: how things influence and alter one another in ways that are continuously opening as well as foreclosing new possibilities. The starting point is the assumption that learning and practice is more-than-human. To understand these educational processes, we need to move beyond preoccupations with human meanings and human agency.

## What does a sociomaterial approach look like in action? Materialities of clinical handover in intensive care

To illustrate a sociomaterial approach, this section presents brief excerpts from a doctoral research project examining front line clinical practice. This research was situated in a busy intensive care unit (ICU) in a tertiary referral centre university hospital in Scotland focussing on handover, across the professions involved, and examining how handover is enacted. Handover is the act, the praxis, where a patient or patients are passed on from one clinician or group of clinicians to another. Handover has been identified as a perilous time with implications for patient safety, but it is also a place of concatenation, of bringing together strands in the patient's journey. It is ubiquitous in all of clinical practice and is happening all the time across all sectors of the healthcare system.

In order to study handover, Nimmo[24] adopted a mixed methods approach, and fieldwork was done in the ethnographic mode. That is, systematic observation of clinicians in everyday practice over a number of weeks was conducted and recorded through field notes. Conversations with actors *in situ* were conducted to probe their meanings and experiences of the situations that were observed. Data were audio recorded and transcribed and analysed to explore the clinical handovers of patients by doctors and nurses in this ICU. Texts of both handovers were reviewed and the artefacts and geography of handover photographed and examined. This study explores the role of material artefacts and texts, such as the intensive care-based electronic patient record, the whiteboards in the doctor's office, and in the ward, in the narratives of handover. Through analysis of the data, some of the material entanglements of handover are explored, with a view to understanding the difficulties and improving the process (Figs. 7.2–7.5).

## Multiple ontologies of handover of critically ill patients

It is between 8 and 9 a.m. in the ICU. Three formal handovers are occurring. The overnight staff are passing on the patients and the things of intensive care. In their office the Charge Nurses start:

| | |
|---|---|
| Jane | 'Em, have you looked at the off duty?' |
| Heather | 'No not yet' |
| Jane | 'You've got thirteen plus one' |
| Heather | 'OK' |
| Jane | 'Em, and you've got six Level threes and five Level twos, em, moved a couple of folk about last night but they should have been updated on Wardwatcher' |
| Heather | 'OK, yeah' |
| Jane | 'I'll do all the housekeepery stuff later on' |

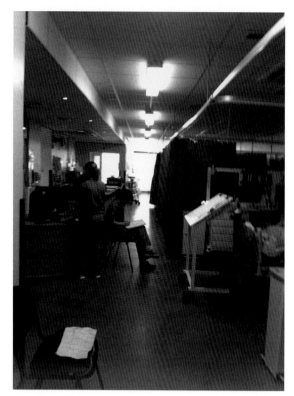

*Figure 7.2* Material artefacts and text in an intensive care unit.

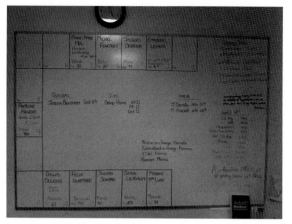

*Figure 7.3* Whiteboard in doctors' room. Charge nurse handover is 'through the wall'.

Heather    'Yep'

In the room next door, directly through the wall, the doctors are finishing their handover:

Ian        'OK, em, there is also a guy up in 21 (surgical ward) that we went to see earlier, Jim Carter who has been in (ICU) previously, Hartmann's (bowel operation) back in March, rehab in hospital Y. Came in with a fistula between bowel and bladder'

David      'Is this the chicken bone guy?'

Angus      'The chicken bone guy'

Ian        'Oh Right'

Angus      'He has been back on the ward for a couple of weeks and has developed pulmonary oedema'.

And at a patient's bed space in the ICU, the staff nurses talk through the patient's physiology, support and treatment while the handover is being enacted by the attendant artefacts:

Mike       'I'll just start from the top. Respiratory wise I put him on external CPAP at quarter past 2 PEEP of eh 7.5 (means adjusting ventilatory support) and he's lasted on that quite well. He's just on 30% FiO$_2$ (oxygen) and his saturations have been fine em and his respiratory rate has been OK. They haven't said about putting him back onto the ventilator overnight, I haven't switched him back as he seemed, seemed reasonably settled ... '

Callum     'Yes, settled'

The charge nurses immediately focus on the staffing levels within the unit and the severity of critical illness, which is reduced to numbers: level 1, level 2 and level 3. The doctors, on the other hand, having discussed all of the patients in the ward, turn to those around the hospital, the so-called *outliers*. The language used in the medical handover is also different with the clinical and the vernacular mixed up. Critical illness emerges as diagnosis and labelling. The bedspace nurses do critical illness through handover of physiology and organ support. In all of these spaces, handover is enacted through the assemblage of the sociomaterial things that matter: printed Handover Report sheets, patients, whiteboards, staff, charts, computers, pens and paper towels (Fig. 7.5). The multiple ontologies of handover are enacted by the disparate practices of the clinical entity, that is, critical illness.

Multiple handovers can be seen to be taking place across the different physical spaces of intensive care. But this is not only a geographical separation. There are clinical-, managerial-, philosophical- and professional-related differences amongst and between the practices of handovers and the practitioners engaged in it. In these different spaces, different realities are happening, 'the architectural divide is duplicated by a divide between human

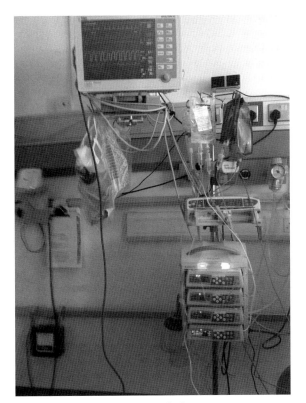

*Figure 7.4* Some of the *matter* at a bed space.

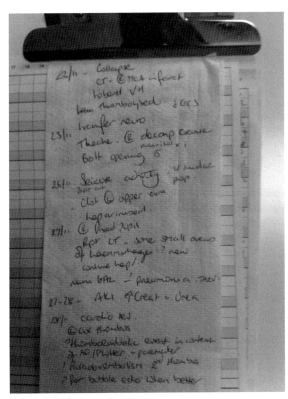

*Figure 7.5* Paper towels: floating texts in handover.

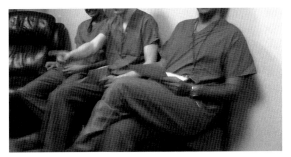

*Figure 7.6* Even clothing intra-acts in handover.

populations'.[8] The multiple ontologies, the distributed realities, of handover are revealed in the multiplicity of the clinical entity, that is, critical illness.

Evening handover between trainee doctors involves another materiality, that is, floating texts (Fig. 7.6).

Jackie    'Em I don't know em you know, he sort, you know he's been a wee bit better. Well there's not been any issues. The microbiologist phones, I took some cultures from him, it must have been before I went home yesterday 'cause he had a wee pyrexia, they phoned to say he had Gram-negative bacilli in his blood cultures'

Susan    'Oooh'

Jackie    'And he is started on whatever I've got written on my leg here, Meropenem, and em, I think it's probably significant in that it's not a contaminant but I mean it's probably contributing to his confusion but I'm not sure if it explains about his seizure. He's a bit old for a febrile convulsion' (laughs).

Jackie has been called by the microbiologist in the laboratory to let her know the result of a blood culture, which has grown Gram-negative bacteria. Like all of the other trainees (and the bedspace nurses and some of the consultants), she wears surgical scrubs (often called 'blues' or 'greens'). Information and messages are commonly written onto the trousers of these. The crucial information, which is to start a powerful, broad spectrum antibiotic, is transferred through handover from this floating text on Jackie's trousers. While questions might be raised about these and other 'floating text' practices, they are not uncommon in the heat of action – part of the utility of this research was in making visible how much clinicians 'make do' with what is to hand, in addition to and sometimes instead of following approved protocol strictly. At the end of the shift, Jackie will change back into her normal clothes and consign her scrubs to the linen basket from which they will be transported to the laundry for washing, potentially erasing that text for all time. This is the kind of thing that happens in 'messy' clinical practice all of the time.

## Implications for clinical education

In light of the analysis of the empirical data from this study, it is proposed that attention is given to handover as a reflective space in the professional development of nurses and doctors and probably others. Handover is thus signposted as a potential educational space for all staff. Supported debriefing of handovers could facilitate this. (This point is widely discussed in the literature. See Nimmo[24] for a full summary and list of references.) The different professionals attending each other's handovers might improve interactions, as could raising the patient to the surface as person through diaries, photos and other sources of knowledge of their life. The critical role of things, objects, official and marginal texts in handover has been highlighted and deserves inclusion in any educational initiatives. Sharing understanding of the working and enactment of handover, between professions and across the different spaces where it happens, could be achieved by postgraduate clinical staff and undergraduate students attending handovers involving other professional groups.

## Research in practice

There are many challenges, as we can see in these examples of sociomaterial approaches to research. The first challenge is simply how to look more closely at materials and their entanglements with learning, which is not something that education researchers tend to focus upon. This challenge is not only how to attend to the key materials that are at work in any moment of 'sociomaterial' practice, but also to understand how in fact these materials are acting on the unfolding action. The second challenge is to discern the relationships among materials, technologies, bodies and environments with human dynamics, such as analysing, decision making, including making a diagnosis, and emotion management. These are complex, and working them out is difficult. There are, of course, limitations in these approaches, which are described at the end of this chapter as 'Notes of Caution'.

The most common approach, as we saw in the previous section, is through methods borrowed from ethnographic research: systematic observation of practice and conversations with people participating in practice. (Quantitative methods, such as non-linear regression and stochastics, have also been used, in a recursive iterative way, working with complexity theory to examine interaction effects and collinearity of variables.)[25] Both methods have been described in great detail in texts about ethnographic research such as Hammersley and Atkinson, along with critical issues such as the observer's partial perceptions and frames of reference, the observer's position as an inside/outsider and the effects on the activity being observed, the ethics of observing others and the importance of tracking these issues as well as the action. Even when the observer is working with video records of practice in action, which is common in medical education research, what one sees is highly mediated by expectations, priorities, prior experience and the language one is using to describe the action. The researcher's task is to continually interrupt the illusion that what we commonly assume is the 'real' in our observations is in fact highly constructed through our own interventions.

In sociomaterial research, these methods of ethnographic observation and informal plus formal interviews are often amplified through other approaches to gathering data about materials. Three are briefly explained below: photo elicitation, participant mapping and interview to the double, all drawn from the studies presented by Fenwick and colleagues.[26]

## Photo elicitation

How can we show the human and non-human 'things', and the relations among them, in clinicians' practice? One way of communicating an understanding of these relationships is for the researcher to photograph the materials that appear to be significant in practice, however mundane, in the way that Nimmo[24] did in his study of handover in intensive care. He photographed the built environments, including specific elements in these such as the whiteboards in the separate rooms, as well as a range of materials such as printed handover sheets and paper towels that seemed to be connected somehow with handover. The participants can be invited to discuss these materials. Harper[27] tells researchers to 'break the frame' when taking photos to elicit participant experience, avoiding or altering images representing what participants see or use every day. The goal is to promote participants to adopt 'a reflective stance vis-à-vis the taken-for-granted aspects of work and community'. Many researchers also ask participants to take photos themselves of materials in their practice, which may be unnoticed but that influence action somehow. Here is one participant from Scoles' study of professional learning in practice (in Fenwick *et al.*[26])

> They're things that I wouldn't think of but … when you become part of the system you don't really see it from the outside and you just see your little bit and I think that's definitely it. You go, this is just my day to day, just do this and this … but when you actually look at it a bit more you go, well that's my whole target, what I'm going for, there's a bit more behind that.

Researchers often report that discussion of these photos, whether participant- or researcher-produced, opens the interview to unexpected ground and often makes visible surprising new details of materiality in practice.

## Participant mapping

In conversational interviews with the actors of a particular practice setting, researchers can sometimes get beneath the words by having these participants draw maps right in the interview situation. These maps are to show the relationships between themselves and the various objects, technologies, events and other humans that affect their everyday practice. The researcher might ask participants to simply draw a mind map, noting all the people and objects with whom they come into contact on an average day or in a particular practice in that day to get their work done. As noted in Fenwick *et al.*,[26] if this is done in the interview situation itself, participants often talk about the links between themselves and the objects they use to get their work done. Many observe that they find themselves sketching out materials that they had not thought about before.

## Interview to the double (ITTD)

This is a technique developed extensively by Nicolini.[22] The interviewer asks a participant to narrate what they do in everyday practice, as if giving detailed instructions to someone who is going to impersonate them without being suspected by colleagues. Scoles describes how she used this method in her research.[26] The instructions she gave to participants were something like this:

> Imagine that tomorrow, an alien that looks exactly like you – your double – has offered to come to work to take your place (you get a free day off). In order not to betray the switch and alert your colleagues, the alien must conduct himself exactly as you behave, down to the smallest detail of personal habits. Therefore, please give detailed instructions to me as if I were your double, on precisely what I must do from the moment I enter your workplace. Start with 'First you must ….'

Scoles found that some participants struggled to remain at the micro-level. Therefore, she directed them to describe a particular practice. This seemed to work much better, with greater detail and rich instruction, perhaps because there was concrete focus and boundaries provided by the delimited time frame. Overall, she found ITTD very useful for illuminating the small tasks and connecting materials that make up practitioners' everyday work, as well as their unique and often proudly defended approaches to these tasks.

In each case, these researchers have found that sociomaterial understandings of the everyday worlds they are studying offer an important counterpoint to the human-centric traditions of studying professional learning, which tend to emphasise cognitive, emotional and social dimensions. Although these dimensions are important, they are inherently wrapped up with materialities in particular ways and with particular effects that ethnographic work can help to make visible.

## Implications for practice in research

Of course, these and other sociomaterial methodologies and conceptions are only valuable in terms of the work that they do to help us examine the educational issues that call for research. In the end, the important thing is not the techniques we use but the questions that we ask. In educational research, sociomaterial perspectives suggest questions such as the following:

- How is the range of actors – material and virtual, human and non-human – influencing what is enacted in education?
- What kinds of learning are promoted through particular sociomaterial assemblages? What kinds of pedagogies?
- How do some educational practices become stabilised and durable (and not others)?
- When do sociomaterial 'black boxes' create problems, and how? (e.g. inclusions and exclusions)

- What material elements *limit possibilities* for education and learning? When/why do these resist efforts to change them, and why? When do they escape notice?
- How do sociomaterial assemblages produce particular identities, boundaries and centres of power?

Medical education research informed by sociomaterial perspectives might adopt approaches such as the following:

1 Interrupt the notion of 'human actors' as self-evident. Focus instead on the *relationships* among things, spaces, bodies, protocols and human action that together produce this action.

2 Unsettle other preconceptions, such as particular categories that already define the field of vision and the problem: diagnosis, disease, control, standard, treatment, professional and patient. Big categories may be helpful to delineate general patterns, but they also shine powerful lights on certain elements and obscure the rest.

3 Attempt to focus on what seems to be banished from view: what is ignored as if it is unimportant, and what is made 'other' through a particular focus of the research or the practice itself. Sometimes what is 'invisible' is not actively ignored but simply unnoticed, such as domestic staff or hospital porters (who, according to researchers Fuller et al.,[28] hold a range of vital knowledge about patients that is rarely accessed).

4 Unpick assemblages, highlighting the role played by different participants whether human or non-human.

## Implications for practice in education

In sociomaterial perspectives, learning and knowing are also enactments, not mental activity or received knowledge. Mind, after all, is a matter of continuous neurological connections with the myriad matter of environments. Sociomaterial perspectives shift the attention from an individual learning subject to the larger collective – not just the social and cultural collective of people or a community of practice, but the sociomaterial collective including spaces, bodies, technologies and tools. Capability is understood to be distributed, not a case of individual expertise.

For example, Mol[29] spent 1 year observing clinical practices in diabetes care taking shape and shifting. She concluded that despite neat and systematic treatment plans and protocols, unruly materialities continually disrupted daily care: technologies malfunctioning, patients forgetting and all sorts of

smelly, messy, frightening and tedious activities. She concludes that 'Control is an illusion *even if you master the tasks*' (p. 1757). The main task, Mol learns, is 'of attuning everything to everything else, one way or another'. What to fiddle with and what to keep fixed, is rarely obvious. What you try to do, may not work out. Try something else. Keep on tinkering. Doctoring. Caring' (p. 1757). Nimmo describes his own practice in the ICU in similar terms. He recalls that during his MD research as he was manipulating a patient's physiology with drugs, fluids and ventilators the nurses would handover by saying, 'Oh, he's just fiddling'.

When we accept this view of the world full of agency, *doing* things, learning shifts away from a sole emphasis on acquiring packages of knowledge or practicing isolated clinical skills. Instead, education becomes about preparing for this world: preparing to participate wisely and resiliently in certain and uncertain situations. Learning issues become more focused on how to attune to minor fluctuations and surprises, how to interrupt matters that seem settled and hold open controversies for matters of concern, how to track one's own and other's effects on the emerging sociomaterial situation or how to improvise solutions.

## Notes of caution

There is a danger in becoming overly fascinated with sociomaterial conceptions without asking why such analysis is any more productive than other perspectives in understanding and responding to educational concerns. Like all theories, different sociomaterial approaches have been debated and critiqued by educators. Complexity theory, for example, has been questioned in terms of its critical capability. Important issues need to be examined about how power flows through education or any other practice. We need to ask not just how materiality affects the action, but what are the power relations of these effects. Educators also need to ask: What knowledge and activities are given the greatest visibility and influence over the movements and directions of the system? Whose interests are most advantaged or disadvantaged by the practices that emerge? How can better practices – more generative, open, fair and life-sustaining – be induced, or at least be available as possibilities? ANT, too, has enjoyed its fair share of critique, as explained by Fenwick and Edwards.[20] Much of this has opened new questions and directions for ANT – around which 'actors' are being studied and which are being excluded, about the problems of humans representing human–non-human heterogeneity, and about the limits of a 'network metaphor'.

Educators working in sociomaterial areas also continue to raise the question of human subjectivity, and human meaning. When we move away from the individual human, are we then in a world of techno-determinism? Or, from a different set of concerns, do sociomaterial approaches simply remain at a systemic level that omits the person and the personal that are crucial in education? For some, sociomateriality represents a post-human orientation. However, this is not an anti-human nightmare of technological enhancements and digitised bodies. Rather, this is a post-humanism that refuses to accept the predetermined centrality of human beings and human knowledge in defining the world. It accepts the value of transgressing boundaries and disrupting conventional ideas about what it means to be human. It also suggests expanding the current limitations of human being-ness to 'becoming more-than-human' in Braidotti's[30] terms, a relational conception of humans in tune with the continually emerging possibilities of their sociomaterial worlds.

## Towards future sociomaterial research

Sociomaterial research in medical and other healthcare professions education is relatively recent, but is already expanding. One of the most prolific developers is Bleakley[2,31] who has been exploring ways to improve diverse forms of practice from surgical teams and interprofessional practice to developing practitioners' awareness of healthcare systems' various dynamics on the emerging complexity of their everyday work. Interprofessional education in the healthcare professions is an obvious area to introduce students to the sociomaterial dynamics – not just the social dynamics – that create boundaries between very different worlds within which each practitioner group works. One PhD project[14] shows how teaching students and educators some principles of complexity theory can produce significant positive change in Institute for the Psychology of Eating (IPE) design and coaching. Simulation education is another area where sociomaterial researchers are experimenting with new ways to brief, coach and assess students, as well as to understand the many competing material layers and locations that students must negotiate in simulated scenarios. In medical education research, more broadly there is increasing evidence of sociomaterial approaches. For example, Ajjawi and Bearman[32]

use a sociomaterial reading to draw attention to the ways power is enacted and resisted through all kinds of human–material interactions in primary care. Finally, in developing countries, a sociomaterial approach could be very helpful in adapting particular healthcare protocols and instruments to sites where available materials and settings are very different. Even cultural differences are more helpfully addressed through a sociomaterial analysis, because it digs into the specific, nuanced ways that particular people's knowing and interactions are enmeshed with the particular objects, languages, substances and technologies of their settings. In focusing on how materials combine with and work on human activity, sociomaterial help to highlight where materials are holding in place important beliefs, and where are the opportunities for introducing new materials and technologies to bring about change in practices.

## Main messages

We have written this chapter in the belief that sociomaterial perspectives could be very useful to research and practice in healthcare education. As yet, there is only a little work available to demonstrate what these perspectives can do for healthcare. However as the reference list shows, there is lots of material available in professional education more widely demonstrating sociomaterial research approaches. These perspectives are each unique and their distinctions are important to note. However in this short discussion, the emphasis was on some common elements shared across these perspectives, as follows:

- A focus on *materials* as dynamic and enmeshed with human activity in ways that act on everyday practice.
- Emphasis is not on individual things and their characteristics (such as individual clinicians' skills or particular technologies), but on their *relationships* and what these produce.
- Practices themselves are continuously changing *gatherings* of human and non-human forces, technical and cognitive/affective, organic and inorganic elements and so on, that constitute one another while bringing forth particular situations and knowledge. Human cognition, meanings and agency are not privileged – practices and learning are understood to be *more-than-human*.
- The *whole system* is important to understand any particular activity, analysing how human/non-human action and knowledge are entangled in systemic webs.

## Conclusion

In conclusion, sociomaterial approaches provide resources to systematically examine the power of materials in everyday practice – bodies, tools, technologies, settings – and how they relate with social dynamics to produce certain forms of knowing and action. These approaches offer different research methods that are useful to recognise and trace the everyday struggles, negotiations and accommodations among social and material dynamics in practice. In tracing these dynamics and relations, sociomaterial analyses make visible those forces that produce what practitioners often take for granted as inevitable and immutable categories, events, objects, rules, hierarchies and so forth. Finally, sociomaterial perspectives offer important approaches for understanding the power relations and politics that constitute learning. Their analytic tools can interrupt and trace the ways powerful webs become assembled as knowledge, but also point to affirmative ways to intervene in, disturb or amplify these webs.

For teaching practice, sociomaterial perspectives have implications for designing medical education environments, and scenarios, for coaching students before, during and after educational exercises, such as simulation and for assessing student activity. At the very least, medical educators have found that simply introducing key concepts of sociomaterial complexity to students can affect their learning. They, too, are concerned about becoming capable of practicing competently in messy situations of material unpredictability, fast-changing technologies, increasing multidisciplinarity and conflicting sociomaterial demands.

> ### Practice points
>
> Sociomaterial approaches suggest that in medical education, we might consider incorporating activities that promote processes of situation awareness such as the following, as summarised by Fenwick[33]:
>
> - Attending to minor, even mundane, fluctuations and uncanny slips.
> - Attuning to emerging ideas and action possibilities in everyday 'mattering' processes.
> - Noticing one's own and others' effects on what is emerging.
> - Tinkering amidst uncertainty.
> - Interrupting black boxes of practice to hold open their controversies and disturbances.

> The point here is not to displace current practice in medical education, but to reorient and enrich it by developing students' awareness of the sociomateriality of their practice.

## References

1 Singer, J.I. & Dean, J. (2006) Emergency physician intershift handovers. An analysis of our transitional care. *Pediatric Emergency Care*, **22**, 751–754.

2 Barad, K. (2007) *Meeting the Universe Half-way*. Duke University Press, Durham, NC.

3 Bleakley, A. (2012) The proof is in the pudding: putting actor–network theory to work in medical education. *Medical Teacher*, **34**, 462–467.

4 de Vries, E.N., Prins, H.A., Crolla, R.M.P.H. *et al.* (2010) Effect of a comprehensive surgical safety system on patient outcomes. *New England Journal of Medicine*, **363**, 1928–1937.

5 Fenwick, T. & Nerland, M. (eds) (2014) *Reconceptualising Professional Learning: Sociomaterial Knowledges, Practices, Responsibilities*. Routledge, London.

6 Orlikowski, W.J. (2007) Sociomaterial practices: exploring technology at work. *Organization Studies*, **28**, 1435–1448.

7 Nimmo, G.R. & Mitchell, C. (2008) A preliminary audit of interruptions in intensive care: implications for patient safety. *Journal of Intensive Care*, **9**, 240–242.

8 Mol, A.-M. (2002) *The Body Multiple: Ontology in Medical Practice*. Duke University Press, Durham, NC.

9 Fenwick, T. & Edwards, R. (2010) *Actor-Network Theory in Educational Research*. Routledge, London.

10 Latour, B. (2005) *Re-assembling the Social: An Introduction to Actor-Network Theory*. Oxford University Press, Oxford.

11 Davis, B. & Sumara, D.J. (2006) *Complexity and Education: Inquiries into Learning, Teaching and Research*. Erlbaum, Mahwah, NJ.

12 Osberg, D. & Biesta, G.J.J. (eds) (2010) *Complexity Theory and the Politics of Education*. Sense Publishers, Rotterdam.

13 Coole, D. & Frost, S. (2010) *New Materialisms: Ontology, Agency, and Politics*. Duke University Press, Durham.

14 Engeström, Y. (1987) *Learning by Expanding: An Activity-Theoretical Approach to Developmental Research*. Orienta-Konsultit, Helsinki.

15 Massey, D. (2005) *For Space*. Sage, London, Thousand Oaks.

16 Lefebvre, H. (1991) *The Production of Space*. Blackwell, Oxford.

17 Mennin, S. (2010) Self-organisation, integration and curriculum in the complex world of medical education. *Medical Education*, **44**, 20–30.

18 McMurtry A. (2007) *Complexity science and the education of interdisciplinary health teams*. unpublished doctoral thesis, University of Alberta, Edmonton, Canada.

19  Sturmberg, J.P. & Martin, C.M. (eds) (2013) *Handbook of Systems and Complexity in Health.* Springer, New York.

20  Fenwick, T., Edwards, R. & Sawchuk, P. (2011) *Emerging Approaches in Educational Research: Tracing the Sociomaterial.* Routledge, London.

21  Hager, P., Lee, A. & Reich, A. (2012) *Practice, Learning and Change: Practice-Theory Perspectives on Professional Learning.* Springer, Netherlands.

22  Nicolini, D. (2013) *Practice Theory, Work and Organisation.* Oxford University Press, Oxford.

23  Edwards, A., Daniels, H., Gallagher, P., Leadbetter, J. & Warmington, P. (2009) *Improving Inter-Professional Collaborations: Multi-agency Working for Children's Wellbeing.* Routledge, London.

24  Nimmo G.R. (2014) *Materialities of clinical handover intensive care: challenges of enactment and education.* Unpublished doctoral thesis, University of Stirling, Stirling, UK.

25  Gilstrap, D.L. (2013) Quantitative research methods in chaos and complexity: from probability to post hoc regression analysis. *Complicity,* **10**, 1–14.

26  Fenwick, T., Doyle, S., Michaels, M. & Scoles, J. (forthcoming) Matters of learning and education: sociomaterial approaches to ethnographic research.

In: Bolle, S., Seele, C., Honig, H. & Neumann, S. (eds), *Multi-Pluri-Trans, Emerging Fields in Educational Ethnography.* Columbia University Press, Berlin.

27  Harper, D. (2002) Talking about pictures: a case for photo elicitation. *Visual Studies,* **17**, 3–26.

28  Fuller A, Laurie I, Unwin L (2013) *Learning at work as a low-grade workers: the case of hospital porters.* Lakes research paper no. 25, Institute of Education, University of London. http://www.llakes.org/wp-content/uploads/2011/07/25.-Fuller-Laurie-Unwin-reduced.pdf

29  Mol, A. (2009) Living with diabetes: care beyond choice and control. *The Lancet,* **373**, 1756–1757.

30  Braidotti, R. (2013) *The Posthuman.* Polity Press, Cambridge.

31  Bleakley, A. (2010) Blunting Occam's razor: aligning medical education with studies of complexity. *JECP,* **16**, 849–855.

32  Ajjawi, R. & Bearman, M. (2012) Sociomateriality matters to family practitioners as supervisors. *Medical Education,* **46**, 1141–1151.

33  Fenwick, T. (2014) Sociomateriality in medical practice and learning: attuning to what matters. *Medical Education,* **48**, 44–52.

# 8 Sticking with messy realities: how 'thinking with complexity' can inform healthcare education research

*Alan Bleakley and Jennifer Cleland*

*The male changing room has an odour of urine and sweat. As I change into newly laundered, slightly stiff and itchy blue scrubs I wonder quite where I will put my reading glasses. I search in vain for a pair of scrub trousers that will fit. I slip on a pair of white clogs and a hat. My buddy notes that I have taken a favourite pair of clogs belonging to one of his colleagues – I look at them and they are clearly marked with a name. Once in the operating theatre (room), I feel even more like a fish out of water. I am introduced to the surgical team and make my first mistake – I offer my hand for a handshake; but of course in operating theatres that is unnatural, breaking the rules of sterility. I learnt something on my first day – to suspend habits and study the context more carefully.*

## Introduction

The highly stylised world of surgery and its companion world of surgical education are complex. Multiple teams – surgical, anaesthetic, recovery, ward, instrument sterilisation, porters, laboratory, pathology, radiology and physiotherapy – network around patients and with each other. The numbers of exchanges, both connections and misconnections, between such teams is vast. In turn, those teams' clinical practices are embedded in, and shaped by, highly dynamic cultures whose impact is keenly felt. The first of these cultures is hospital management with its raft of directives shaped by national policy. The second is the culture of healthcare *education*, with its various models of what constitutes 'learning'. Academics, clinicians and patients who engage in *researching* this healthcare educational culture constitute a third complex culture. These three contexts interweave, often in unpredictable ways.

How can healthcare education researchers meaningfully engage with such highly complex contexts? Complexity theory informs and shapes a group of research methods – how they are conceived, utilised and developed, and how several methods can be productively combined without losing focus.[1,2] However, the application of complexity thinking to clinical education and its research wing is in its infancy. This chapter shows how 'thinking with complexity theory' can be a conceptual lens or framework[3] to give greater power to research in the general field of healthcare education.

In the first half of the chapter, complexity theory is defined and some core concepts introduced. Drawing on a number of illustrative examples, the second half shows how complex clinical and educational contexts have been researched through applications of complexity theory. Limits to thinking with complexity and future trends in complexity theory are both noted. By the end of this chapter, readers will have a greater appreciation and understanding of the use of complexity theory in healthcare education research.

## Background

### What is complexity?

What is 'complexity'? If you piece together a jigsaw, even a complicated one, as long as all the pieces are there you will predictably complete the puzzle. What is more interesting is what happens to you – will you show patience and endure until all the pieces are in place; call for help and complete the jigsaw in collaboration; give up entirely in boredom or lose your cool and go in to a tantrum as a child might, frustrated and scattering the pieces on the floor in a mess? The difference between you and the jigsaw is stark – the jigsaw is a static, linear puzzle where the whole is equal to the sum of its parts; you, on the other hand, are dynamic, complex and adaptive. Compare a jigsaw to a game of scrabble, where both the players and the game are unpredictable, where outcome depends on innovation in terms of responding to both the letters on the board and the letters which come out of the bag.

*Researching Medical Education*, First Edition. Edited by Jennifer Cleland and Steven J. Durning.
© 2015 John Wiley & Sons, Ltd. Published 2015 by John Wiley & Sons, Ltd.

As another example, I(AB) look out of my office window at the trees and the road beyond, with increasing levels of traffic moving in a heavy and sudden downpour of rain, people are waiting to cross the road, getting soaked by the rain. A man, presumably frustrated by the fact that there is no gap in the traffic stream, makes a hair-raising bolt for the other side of the road between speeding cars. ... Simultaneously, without knocking, three colleagues enter the room and interrupt me, ready to convene a meeting. ... Unexpectedly, the fire alarm for the building goes off – we have no idea if this is a planned rehearsal or a real emergency. All of this is happening dynamically through time.

This episode can be read as a sequence of discrete events. However, if you focus in a different way, you will see complex systems at work with non-linear elements just as is the case in a game of scrabble. The multiple relationships and connections between people and systems, and the consequences of these, need to be understood. Understanding such complex problems and systems requires awareness of the alternatives, simple or complicated problems, and of the core concepts of linearity and non-linearity.

## Simple, complicated and complex problems/systems

Table 8.1, reproduced from Glouberman and Zimmerman,[4] illustrates the distinctions and identifies some of the characteristics of simple, complicated and complex systems.

Even though these are presented as different categories of activities, it is more accurate and useful to think of them as degrees of constraint and conditions that have particular consequences.

Simple problems may require some skills or techniques, but once these are mastered, success is likely. Complicated problems multiply up the number of components and potential interactions but maintain the element of rules. For example, space travel is complicated, but achievable because the

components and their potential interactions and the consequences of those interactions can be mapped. On the other hand, complex systems are made up of multiple interconnected elements, with the adaptive capacity to change such that the system as a whole learns from experience. The components in the system co-evolve through their relationships with other components. Complex systems cannot be fully understood by an analysis of their parts, as the interactions between these parts and the consequences of these interactions are equally significant. A complex problem, such as raising a child, has a large number of components and potential interactions between components, which are dynamic and malleable. The outcomes of these interactions are often unpredictable or unknown. While complex problems can include both complicated and simple subsidiary problems, they cannot be reduced to either because of their inherent nonlinearity (see later).[5]

Complex systems are also likely to generate the most potential creativity – in terms of high levels of reformulation in adapting to rapidly changing environmental contexts – at maximum complexity at the edge of chaos (EOC).[6] In this context, chaos, with reference to chaos theory,[7] refers to an apparent lack of order in a system that nevertheless obeys particular laws or rules. Systems exist on a spectrum ranging from equilibrium to chaos. A system in equilibrium does not have the internal dynamics to enable it to respond to its environment and will slowly (or quickly) die. The most productive state to be in is at the EOC where there is maximum variety and creativity, leading to new possibilities.[8] Imagine a junior doctor on her first placement in a busy hospital Accident and Emergency Department at 2 a.m. She faces traumatised and irascible patients, impatient colleagues, endless paperwork and fatigue. She is prescribing, inserting central lines, suturing wounds, breaking bad news, calming an injured child and working to clinical guidelines while also improvising, meeting targets and attempting to contact an orthopaedic surgeon.

*Table 8.1* Simple, complicated and complex problems

| Following a Recipe | Sending a Rocket to the Moon | Raising a Child |
| --- | --- | --- |
| The recipe is essential | Formulae are critical and necessary | Formulae have a limited application |
| Recipes are tested to assure easy replication | Sending one rocket increases assurance that the next will be OK | Raising one child provides experience but no assurance of success with the next |
| No particular expertise is required. But cooking expertise increases success rate | High levels of expertise in a variety of fields are necessary for success | Expertise can contribute but is neither necessary nor sufficient to assure success |
| Recipes produce standardized products | Rockets are similar in critical ways | Every child is unique and must be understood as an individual |
| The best recipes give good results every time | There is a high degree of certainty of outcome | Uncertainty of outcome remains |
| Optimistic approach to problem possible | Optimistic approach to problem possible | Optimistic approach to problem possible |

This is work at a high level of complexity at the edge of, but not falling into, chaos.

Complex, adaptive systems can reorganise through self-organisation, when close to chaos, via adaptability and innovation: indeed, self-organisation is at the heart of complex adaptive systems and learning. For example, if a complex medical school timetabling system breaks down, the classes could stop if the system was not self-organising. However, all those involved in teaching and timetabling, working within the complex wider university and healthcare systems, with their many constraints and conditions, will muddle through and find a solution (e.g. the creation of an alternative, possibly better timetabling system). On the other hand, healthcare staff are bound by protocols and professionalism that promise patient safety, but, in ordering the work too strictly through regulation, the potential for self-organisation (innovation and adaptation) may be squashed and the system may crystallise. Complex adaptive systems need to incorporate manageable elements of risk and invention for innovation to occur (e.g. going 'off protocol' to potentially save a life). The 'system' here is not an autonomous force but a product of intentions and reflections, serendipities and the unexpected, in continuous and recursive flow.

Put individuals together to make a team, and the numbers and potential quality of interactions between elements increase as a higher level of complexity emerges. Put many teams together as an organisation and complexity again increases as the number of interactions between elements multiplies.

## Linearity and non-linearity

What about linearity and non-linearity? These too are core concepts when understanding and using complexity theory. An example of a linear system is a heating system. This works through feedback from a thermostat or regulating device where there is a linear relationship between input and output $(a + b = c)$.[9]

All systems that are not linear, which have fewer constraints, are called non-linear systems. In these systems, the change in a variable at an initial time can lead to a change in the same or a different variable at a later time that is not proportional to the change at the initial time (called the butterfly effect, see later). A non-linear system is one where the whole cannot be expressed as the sum of its parts, whereas a linear system is additive. Going back to our analogy of scrabble, the score is not directly proportional to the values of each letter, but to how these are used, which is in turn unpredictable as

this depends on what is already on the board and the order in which the letters come out the bag. An 'x' can be worth 8, 16 or 24 depending on where it is put down, and the overall value of the word in which it is used can also change depending on the other letters in the word and its position on the board.

Linear problems or systems can be broken up into little pieces, each piece solved separately and then put back together to make the complete solution.

Non-linear problems or systems, on the other hand, cannot be broken up into little pieces and solved separately. They have to be dealt with in their full complexity. This has implications for how they are researched (see later).

Linear systems are not 'bad' and non-linear systems 'good'. We need predictable outcomes and certainty just as we need innovation through unpredictability. The critical factor is that the system and processes are congruent. For example, drawing on the Canadian Medicare system as a case study, Glouberman and Zimmerman[4] point out that linear problem solving approaches to organisational change are flawed because, where the system is complex, the solution has to be as complex as the problem itself. Under certain circumstances – whether space flight, military operations or firefighting – command-and-control, logics-based, protocols-based, linear, hierarchical and authority-led management processes are used. Most healthcare situations, however, require greater flexibility than this, especially where there is a high level of potentially open-ended decision making, necessary ambiguity over potential practice – including a need for innovation – and a high level of emotional investment. Under these conditions, command-and-control tactics involving hierarchical structures are inappropriate as they do not allow new ways of working to emerge (see later for discussion about the emergent properties of complex systems).

Another example from healthcare education is the differentiation between competence and capability. Fraser and Greenhalgh[10] suggest that the focus on 'competence' in healthcare education and its research wing is an example of regression to linearity in the face of a non-linear reality. Where competence[11] literally means to be 'good enough', Fraser and Greenhalgh[10] (p. 801) suggest that 'capability' (what may unfold as potential) is a more accurate descriptor for what we need to achieve in healthcare education. Capability aligns with complexity thinking, where it introduces unknown and unpredictable future elements (potential). Competence aligns with 'training' that is largely focused on acquisition of content, where capability aligns with education that is largely focused on interactions between elements, process or learning to learn.

Going back to looking out of my window on a rainy day, what are the significant *connections between* events rather than the events themselves? The sudden downpour makes driving conditions more hazardous. People waiting to cross the road are getting soaked and the traffic is getting heavier. Interactions are intensified as driving conditions and the behaviour of pedestrians caught in a rainstorm become more unpredictable. Somebody impulsively making a dash across the road may cause others to follow leading to an accident. Meanwhile, will the group of us obey fire instructions and proceed to the assembly point, which is outside the building, in the middle of a heavy rainstorm?

Focusing on the number and quality of interactions, rather than on discrete linked events, brings alive Mennin's[12] (p. 20) definition of complexity as 'the study of the dynamics, conditions and consequences of interactions'. 'Thinking with complexity' reveals a fabric of the habitual and the serendipitous, the expected and the unexpected, with a focus on the dynamics of interactions and both planned and unplanned consequences. This is the world of the non-linear rather than the linear, the complex rather than the merely complicated, where things simply do not follow each other in an orderly fashion – nevertheless patterns and networks are revealed.

### Origins of complexity theory

For many years, scientists saw the universe as a linear place. One where the rules of cause and effect applied and everything in it could be predicted and controlled. However, some things did not behave as expected, or rather seemed to be behaving according to a very different set of rules to cause and effect. Gradually as scientists of all disciplines explored these phenomena, a new theory emerged – complexity theory. Complexity theory is therefore a confluence of several historical developments across science disciplines leading to 'complexity science' and a further set of developments across the arts and humanities better described as 'complexity theory'. (See[6,13-15] for the history of the emergence of complexity science and theory from disparate disciplines).

Some authors see complexity theory as having wide application, including the social and cultural spheres of human life[16], while others see this widening of application as a dilution of complexity science's origins in mathematical or computational modelling of natural phenomena[13]. This chapter adopts the liberal line that complexity models can have wide application.

Healthcare has drawn on complexity science to inform clinical practice and to model decision-making.[17-20] However, the application of complexity thinking to clinical education and its research wing is in its infancy.[1,2,12,21-28] This may be connected with the fact that researching complex contexts does not invite reductive breaking down into linear elements that can be put back together as a complicated jigsaw. Rather, holistic complex research designs capture complexity as patterned forms of relationships between elements rather than discrete elements themselves. The latter part of this chapter gives illustrative examples of how the challenge to match researching complex contexts with complex research designs has been met.

## Key features of dynamic, complex adaptive systems

The key features of linearity and non-linearity, simple, complicated and complex systems are introduced earlier in this chapter. Here we briefly introduce adaption through change, emergent properties, the butterfly effect, nested and interacting systems and fuzzy boundaries.

### 1. Adaptation through change

Dynamic, complex, non-linear systems – such as biological systems – have an added component that takes them beyond linear systems: they adapt to the environment or context through learning.[29] Local interactions and self-organisation lead to system-wide adaptive change (see earlier). Systems change because the tension that accumulates in them cannot be sustained due to the differences among the agents, the way they are contained or bounded together and the nature of their exchanges. In other words, systems change because they learn and learn because they change – otherwise known as transformational learning. Innovation and creativeness are inherent in the unpredictable future-orientation of dynamic systems (i.e. systems which evolve with time) but this means coping with change, tolerating the uncertainty of being at the EOC and learning how feedback and reflection are key to managing the conditions for change and innovation at high levels of uncertainty and ambiguity.

A good model for reconfiguration of a complex system at a higher level of complexity is human learning. As we develop and learn, particularly as children acquiring language, the complex system of the human child develops and evolves, and hence reconfigures at a new level of complexity. Although we can map the broad stages of child development physically and cognitively, we cannot predict how this trajectory will emerge for each individual child, where the complex adaptive system of the child will have emergent properties (see below).

## 2. Emergent properties

Complex living systems exhibit behaviours and characteristics that are different from the behaviours and characteristics of the parts or members. This phenomenon, where the whole is greater than the parts, and where there is a continuous feedback loop (e.g. people shape the organisation and the organisation shapes the people), is called emergence. Rather than being planned or controlled, components in the system interact in semi-autonomous ways, apparently unpredictable ways. Under particular circumstances and conditions, new patterns emerge, which inform the components within the system and the behaviour of the system itself. Adaptation of dynamic, complex systems to changing contexts is thus not simply functional but creative and 'fit for function'. In a clinical example, in our timetabling example earlier, the emergent outcome would be the new, better timetabling system. As a clinical team faces a challenge, if communication is open then the effect of a network of feedback is to shift the system into a higher level of functioning beyond the sum total of the elements in that system. This is an emergence of a new property of the system. This phenomenon is covered well in several papers about team working.[30–32] Note that emergence of new properties can happen even in a dyadic (rather than team) system, such as a general practice consultation.[33]

## 3. Butterfly effect: small changes can produce big results

Drawing from chaos theory, the butterfly effect is the sensitive dependency on initial conditions in which a small change at one place in a non-linear system can result in large differences in a later state. The name of the effect, coined by Edward Lorenz, is derived from the theoretical example of the details of a hurricane (exact time of formation, exact path taken) being influenced by minor perturbations equating to the flapping of the wings of a distant butterfly several weeks earlier. An example of this in healthcare education would be the impact of duty-hours regulations in Europe and North America on training and practice, and patient care, for example, increasing the frequency of handover ('hand-off') leading to fears about increased error rates, miscommunication and poor continuity of care.

## 4. Attractors

Despite the lack of detailed predictability in complex systems, there are often general patterns, or 'attractors', that allow one to make useful statements about the behaviour of the system under the given conditions. An example of an attractor that is variably stable would be an effective team that knows how to work together and can be adaptive to varying conditions (e.g. absence of a member, a change of operating theatre) and still remain effective. Attractor is an important term as it orients us to the work of the environment in shaping activity rather than to the individual cognition of practitioners dictating events.[34]

Attractors are sets of physical properties, such as nodes of activity that typify effective practice or patterns of physical spaces that house practices such as wards or a nursing station. In patient-centred clinical education, the patient is, by definition, the main attractor. (Note that attractors can be in conflict. For example, in healthcare, economic efficiency and patient care are attractors that may clash, causing perturbations in the overall system.) A system tends to evolve towards an attractor, or multiple attractors, regardless of the starting conditions of the system. In this way, attractors shape the system. Forecasting through knowledge of historical patterns of a system is thus important as knowing the patterns of the past can help in terms of illuminating and understanding what is happening in a system.

Attractors act both to maintain stability of a system and to lead the system into EOC, as dynamic systems move through various 'state spaces' or transformations through time. State spaces can be short term and local, such as the 'list' in an operating theatre, or a specific ward round, or longer term such as the life of an organisation.

## 5. Nested and interacting systems and fuzzy boundaries

Delineating a dynamic, complex adaptive system is arbitrary because systems are both nested (i.e. located within other systems, as a ward is nested within a hospital, which is in turn nested within a healthcare provider, within a political and social system) and interacting. Thus, while we can readily delineate a cell in a larger biological system, such as an organ in a body, boundaries between systems become fuzzy (i.e. have meaning(s), which can become clearer only through further elaboration and specification, including a closer definition of the context in which they are used[35]) when we think about social relationships such as those between a person as patient, as a citizen, as a family member, as a caregiver and so forth. When we study a team in clinical education research and take this as the unit of analysis, the boundaries to the team and the nature of interactions with other elements in the total process of patient care are necessarily fuzzy. At the same time, it is the fuzzy boundary which forms the container that holds the elements together so that they can interact and exchange energy to form new emergent structures.

This suggests that such relationships are best researched through qualitative, descriptive methods, to retain and articulate this quality of 'fuzziness'. One approach suitable for articulating 'fuzziness' would be third-generation activity theory ([36]; see Chapter Nine).

## Applications of complexity theory

### Where the unit of analysis for learning is the social

Where traditional learning theories focus upon what is learnt or accumulated by an individual and how that is retained and reproduced, sociocultural learning theories focus upon processes of participation, collaboration, means of access to distributed knowledge, how knowledge and practices acquire legitimacy and meaning, knowledge production rather than reproduction, socialisation as a process of learning and identity construction as a learning outcome.[37,38] For example, two decades ago, the focus of much research in medical education was on the characteristics of effective clinical teachers, as individuals.[39] Now, such research is more likely to focus upon the social contexts for effective teaching and learning.[40,41] This shift from the individual to the social as the unit of analysis for research increases complexity as it increases the potential number and quality of interactions between components. It requires that we shift our focus in researching learning from studying individual traits to studying patterns of collectives such as teams, implying a shift in gears in terms of studying complexity.

Three main traditions have developed under the broad umbrella of complex sociocultural and sociomaterial learning theories[42]: communities of practice,[43,44] cultural–historical activity theory[36,45,46] and actor–network theory.[47–49] Research informed by sociocultural learning theory tends to stress ontologies over epistemologies, experiences and meanings over theoretical insights,[50] and the importance of the individual's context, previous experience and knowledge, attitudes and beliefs (see Chapter 10). (For example, Mol's[51] ethnographic study of atherosclerosis reveals that what is described to patients in information leaflets as 'the gradual obstruction of the arteries' is conceived differently by doctors, vascular surgeons and nurses, and is further modulated by differing professional and lay languages, and through varieties of imaging artefacts such as microscopes, X-rays and ultrasound.[52,53]

## Researching with complexity in mind

Complexity of context should not present an obstacle to research, but rather a challenge to meet complex situations through thinking complexity in research designs. Lorelei Lingard and colleagues[54] (p. 869) describe a model piece of clinical education research in which they aim to 'represent complexity well' in researching complex settings in healthcare. The rationale for the project was that complex clinical settings are often researched in a piecemeal fashion that misses the richness of relationship between elements. Using collaborative practice on a distributed, solid organ transplant team as a model, the research employed a binding perspective of complexity theory, a methodology or 'theoretical lens' of activity theory, and embedded methods of ethnographic observation and interviews with key practitioners. The aim of the research was to reconfigure current approaches to inter-professional clinical practice and education.

The research focused upon patterns and interactions. A major finding was that the core transplant team's collaboration with other services, such as pathology, radiology and cardiology was not linear and predictable and often problematic. Research results were offered as a paradigmatic and illustrative 'single story' of such problematic interactions in deciding whether or not a patient is suitable for transplant. Assumptions about stable roles and identities across professionals underpin conventional inter-professional collaboration models, but such stability is assumed. The ontologies of practice show shifts in stability within a dynamic system. Further, teams do not necessarily share a 'unifying objective' of patient care, but work is formed and patterned dynamically through multiple and contested objectives. 'Everyday' collaborative work then remains intricate and not readily explained through linear input–output models. In this section, two further pieces of enquiry are briefly described, each setting out to research complex contexts through complex designs, reinforcing the value of Lingard's aim to represent complexity well.

## Thinking with complexity in researching surgical teamwork

Returning to where this chapter started, investigating how to improve teamwork in surgical environments, Bleakley and colleagues[32,55–61] designed the research using a combination of ethnography (to map out the territory), participatory action research (to empower team members to flatten hierarchies and establish democratic work habits), sociocultural learning theories (to explain learning in terms of participation) and complexity theory (to gain an overall grasp of the dynamic system being researched).

This aforementioned design is depicted in Figure 8.1 as nested forms of research. This figure should not be read hierarchically. Complexity as a 'meta-methodology' is not placed 'over' the other methodologies of sociocultural learning theories and participatory action research; nor is it placed over the methods of ethnography and auto-ethnography. Rather, again as Davis and Sumara[1] (p. 8) suggest and Haggis[2] reinforces, complexity is 'meta' in the sense that it describes a nested association amongst methods and methodologies. In the research described, these methods and methodologies come in and out of focus according to context, all the while dynamically producing complexity through multiplying interactions.

Ethnography and auto-ethnography[62] and ethnomethodology,[63,64] as research *methods*, are nested inside participatory action research, an approach to research in communities that emphasises participation and action (PAR).[65–67] PAR is nested in sociocultural or sociomaterial learning theories that are, in turn, nested in complexity theory. This has clear resonance with Lingard and colleagues' research design described earlier.

The overarching challenge in the research process described in Figure 8.1 was to introduce democratic processes into surgical teamwork. In this context, 'democratic' describes teamwork in which there is equity between members of the team and equality of opportunity, for example, to engage in appropriate decision-making.

The research programme hypothesised that the introduction of face-to-face, democratic briefing and debriefing in operating theatres would initiate longer term changes in working patterns. While working across all surgical groups, the researchers specifically observed and videotaped activity in orthopaedic theatres, and used edited videotaped examples of key incidents as a stimulus to debriefing at the end of lists. In brief, the introduction of briefing and debriefing significantly changed team members' perceptions that a safer surgical environment was being provided through improving teamwork, as shown by a longitudinally administered Safety Attitudes Questionnaire (SAQ).[68] Interviews and observational data demonstrated that such values were translated into practices. However, this progress or change was thwarted by an international revolution in surgical practice: the introduction of surgical checklists.[69,70] The checklist's introduction was never meant to replace face-to-face briefing and debriefing, but to supplement these forms of democracy. Our study indicated that this was not what happened in our local hospital. Rather the adoption of the instrumental use of the checklist had an unintentional outcome: it displaced a more complex and richer potential for face-to-face encounters, briefing and debriefing. Surgeons were relieved of the need to encounter and wrestle with social learning theory educational interventions associated with the introduction of face-to-face briefs and debriefs. Complexity, in turn, was reduced with a slide back to more linear, instrumental accounts of practice.

This example illustrates how thinking with complexity provided a meta-methodology that shaped, informed and creatively enriched the other levels of complexity that it encircled. Our research illustrated how democratising work was resisted through tactics that can be equated with the shift from complex, non-linear thinking to complicated, linear thinking, in the context of the operating theatre.

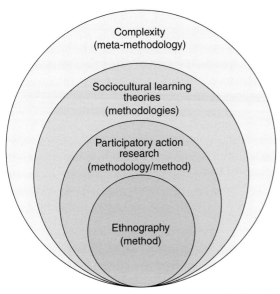

*Figure 8.1* Embedded and interacting elements of a dynamic, complex system of healthcare education research.

## Thinking with complexity in researching cross-cultural applicability of problem-based learning in undergraduate medicine curricula

Problem-based learning (PBL) was developed in a Western/Northern European cultural context that values self-direction or autonomy and facilitated (non-directive) learning rather than closely directed pedagogies. Commentators point out that such methods may not translate readily across cultures.[71]

Frambach and colleagues,[72] from Maastricht University in the Netherlands, recently tackled this complex issue through a research design involving several differing cultural sites. Instead of asking 'does PBL work in different cultural contexts?' (a linear question with prior assumptions that PBL is a universal method to be applied uncritically), the research team asked 'how might PBL be adapted to work in differing cultural contexts?' (a complex, open-ended question with multiple possibilities; see Ref. [4]). Further, they also aligned complexity thinking with sociocultural learning theory as a framework for designing the research. The authors studied how PBL had been applied in undergraduate medical education in three medical schools located in the Middle East, East Asia and Western Europe. The first level of research and the most deeply nested (as per Fig. 8.1) was the data collection *methods*. The researchers triangulated ethnography and interviews within a comparative case study framework. The informing *methodology* is activity theory, part of the portfolio of sociocultural learning theories; and the encompassing *meta-perspective* is thinking with complexity, or complexity theory. Again, these are interdependent and arise among one another, rather than being arranged hierarchically or in a linear sequence. Complexity is not the sum of the other research processes but an emergent property of their multiple interactions.

Frambach and colleagues' research investigated how students across the three cultures 'internalise' PBL or made sense of the method through their cultural frames, and how they 'externalise' their cultures in learning through PBL – or how cultural views come to shape PBL practices and give local flavour. Networks of interactions were compared and contrasted within the activity systems delineated across the three cases.

The research found that PBL was elastic and could be internalised and adapted through forms of learning suitable for the cultural contexts. Again, the complexity question was not closed ('does PBL work?'), but open ('how might PBL be adapted?'). Externalisation factors that challenged 'pure' PBL

included cultural issues, such as how a 'group' is conceived, not losing face with peers, respecting hierarchy and tradition, coping with uncertainty, and integrating achievement and competition. Internalisation factors included variations in forms of self-directed learning, and types of discussion and communication skills. The authors reported contradictions in terms of adopting 'purer' forms of PBL, transformations of rules according to local context, and differences in division of labour across the three medical schools. Data were reported innovatively, as narratives and visualisations that reflected the dynamics of the activity systems across the three contexts.

### Notes of caution in using complexity theory

This section offers some brief notes of caution concerning the application of complexity theory to clinical education research.

First, complexity is not a research method but a lens and a synthesising structure in which complexity itself is an emergent effect and not a dominant discourse or totalising perspective. Researchers must still decide on methods and methodologies within the overall structure of a complexity approach.

Second, complexity introduces a new language that it is important not to dilute. Neologisms, such as 'attractors' and 'phase spaces', do important metaphorical work by shaping the imagination. Third, researchers must be prepared to suspend the desire to focus on discrete phenomena in a shift to interactions between phenomena. This is not simply a cognitive shift of understanding, but also an affective shift of appreciation that is major because it asks for a shift in worldview (see MacMillan in this book). Fourth, do not be lulled into thinking that the dynamic movement of systems with emergent properties is an autonomous force leaving you, the researcher, as a mere spectator. Fifth, persons with their intentions and reflections are integral to systems and to researching these systems. Sixth, match the research design and methods to the theory – do not resort to reductive, linear approaches in the face of non-linearity. Complexity approaches ask for rich 'overview' descriptions that place value upon the aesthetics of research, such as describing patterns.

### Future directions in clinical education research drawing on complexity theory

There are a number of challenges in applying complexity approaches to healthcare education and its research wing. First, there is still a danger that systems are dismantled through reduction to linear parts, continuing the tradition of learning to objectify patients through clinical education and designing medicine curricula on discrete organs rather than interconnected processes (such as the life cycle). Interest in elements themselves may remain dominant, frustrating the study of relations between elements. One way to avoid this is to frame research questions in non-linear ways. This shifts focus from either/or to both/and questions.[4]

Second, medical and other clinical education curricula must respond to the call from those who have been involved in reconceptualising the curriculum itself as a dynamic complex system[12,26,73,74] so that the focus shifts from discrete syllabi content to integrated curriculum process.[10] Such curriculum innovations, should they occur, will need to be evaluated appropriately. Patton's developmental evaluation (DE) is one approach to doing so.[75]

Third, clinical education researchers must collaborate on larger, more intensive projects if they are to meet complex contexts with research designed with complexity theory in mind. Researchers will need to form multi-skilled networks and programmes of research (See the chapter by Taylor and Gibbs later in this book). Such programmatic research will not only require an educational initiative for establishing skilled, knowledgeable and innovative researchers, but will require some unlearning of habitual practices that could frustrate the development of complexity approaches, such as the tendency to revert to linear and reductive approaches.

Fourth is the ontological issue that clinical education researchers tend to form exclusive identities through their familiar bounded research fields (e.g. so-and-so studies professionalism, so-and-so is a qualitative researcher). This is exercised in boundary setting, competition for resources and academic spats. Collaborative, transdisciplinary research[28] emphasising thinking with complexity requires a plural appreciation and fluidity in identities. Just as complexity theory focuses on multiplicity and quality of interactions, so research collaborations must follow suit. Complexity-based research is best conducted holistically and democratically, without research approaches (and then researchers) being placed in hierarchies.

Fifth, and finally, appreciation of form and patterns, especially connections and networks, is central to complexity approaches. This can translate into experimentation with media for both research and presentation of data to include story, film, performance, television scripts and auto-ethnographies.

## Conclusion

From the examples given earlier, it should be clear that the key issue in complexity approaches is how transformational learning is achieved. This is a fresh way of describing the generation of creativity and innovation as emergent, based on appreciating connections between elements rather than thinking discrete elements. Drawing creatively on complexity theory and the associated methods described in this chapter, researchers and practitioners can move the fields of healthcare professions education and education research forward significantly through work based on iterative cycles of enquiry (so what, now what[76]).

---

### Practice points

- When dealing with complex situations, researchers must shift focus from discrete phenomena and activities to interactions/connections between phenomena and activities.

- Complexity theory, and an understanding of its key features and core concepts, can provide a conceptual framework through which to view and understand such contexts.

- Complexity theory also informs and shapes research questions and research designs – how studies are conceived, utilised and developed, and how several methods can be productively combined.

- Complexity of context should not present an obstacle to research, but rather a challenge to meet complex situations through thinking complexity in research designs.

- Working with complexity may require a shift in thinking for the researcher.

---

## Recommended reading

Davis, B. & Sumara, D. (2006) *Complexity and Education.* Lawrence Erlbaum Associates, Mahwah, NJ.

Doll, W.C., Fleener, M.J., Trueit, D. & St Julien, J. (2008) *Chaos, Complexity, Curriculum, and Culture: A Conversation.* Peter Lang, New York, NY.

Haggis, T. (2009) Beyond 'mutual constitution': looking at learning and context from the perspective of complexity theory. In: Edwards, R., Biesta, G. & Thorpe, M. (eds), *Rethinking Contexts for Learning and Teaching: Communities, Activities and Networks.* Routledge, London, pp. 44–60.

Mennin, S. (2010a) Self-organisation, integration and curriculum in the complex world of medical education. *Medical Education*, **44**, 20–30.

# References

1 Davis, B. & Sumara, D. (2006) *Complexity and Education*. Lawrence Erlbaum Associates, Mahwah, NJ.
2 Haggis, T. (2009) Beyond 'mutual constitution': looking at learning and context from the perspective of complexity theory. In: Edwards, R., Biesta, G. & Thorpe, M. (eds), *Rethinking Contexts for Learning and Teaching: Communities, Activities and Networks*. Routledge, London, pp. 44–60.
3 Bordage, G. (2009) Conceptual frameworks to illuminate and magnify. *Medical Education*, **43**, 312–319.
4 Glouberman, S. & Zimmerman, B. (2002) *Complicated and Complex Systems: What Would Successful Reform of Medicare Look Like?* Commission on the Future of Healthcare in Canada: Discussion Paper No. 8. http://c.ymcdn.com/sites/www.plexusinstitute.org/resource/collection/6528ED29-9907-4BC7-8D00-8DC907679FED/ComplicatedAndComplexSystems-ZimmermanReport_Medicare_reform.pdf [accessed on 15 June 2014].
5 Goodwin, B. (1994) *How the Leopard Changed its Spots: The Evolution of Complexity*. Touchstone, New York.
6 Kauffman, S. (1995) *At Home in the Universe: The Search for the Laws of Self-Organisation and Complexity*. Viking, London.
7 Lorenz, E. (1963) Deterministic non-periodic flow. *Journal of the Atmospheric Sciences*, **20**, 130–141.
8 Grassberger, P. (1986) Towards a quantitative theory of self-generated complexity. *International Journal of Theoretical Physics*, **25**, 907–938.
9 Lorenz, E. (1995) *The Essence of Chaos*. University of Washington Press; Reprint edition (March 30, 1995).
10 Fraser, S.W. & Greenhalgh, T. (2001) Coping with complexity: educating for capability. *British Medical Journal*, **323**, 799–803.
11 Hodges, B.D. & Lingard, L. (2012) *The Question of Competence: Reconsidering Medical Education in the Twenty-First Century*. Cornell University Press, New York, NY.
12 Mennin, S. (2010a) Self-organisation, integration and curriculum in the complex world of medical education. *Medical Education*, **44**, 20–30.
13 Coveney, P. & Highfield, R. (1995) *Frontiers of Complexity: The Search for Order in a Chaotic World*. Faber & Faber, London.
14 Luhmann, N. (2013) *Introduction to Systems Theory*. Polity Press, Cambridge.
15 Wheatley, M. (1992) *Leadership and the New Science: Learning about Organization from an Orderly Universe*. Berrett-Koehler, San Francisco, CA.
16 Estrada, E., Fox, M., Higham, D.J. & Oppo, G.-L. (eds) (2010) *Network Science: Complexity in Nature and Technology*. Springer, Dordrecht.

17 Paley, J. (2010) The appropriation of complexity theory in health care. *Journal of Health Services Research & Policy*, **15**, 59–61.
18 Plsek, P., Sweeney, K. & Griffiths, F. (2002) *Complexity and Healthcare: An Introduction*. Radcliffe, Oxford.
19 Sweeney, K. (2006) *Complexity in Primary Care: Understanding Its Value*. Radcliffe, Oxford.
20 Holt, T. (ed) (2010) *Complexity for Clinicians*. Radcliffe, Oxford.
21 Plsek, P. & Greenhalgh, T. (2001) Complexity science: the challenges of complexity in healthcare. *British Medical Journal*, **323**, 625–628.
22 Dickey, J., Girard, D.E., Geheb, M.A. & Christine, K. (2004) Using systems-based practice to integrate education and clinical services. *Medical Teacher*, **26**, 428–434.
23 Dornan, T. (2010) On complexity and craftsmanship. *Medical Education*, **44**, 2–3.
24 Greenhalgh, T., Plsek, P., Wilson, T., Fraser, S. & Holt, T. (2010) Response to 'The appropriation of complexity theory in health care.'. *Journal of Health Services Research & Policy*, **15**, 115–117.
25 Mennin, S. (2007) Small-group problem-based learning as a complex adaptive system. *Teaching and Teacher Education*, **23**, 303–313.
26 Mennin, S. (2010b) Complexity and health professions education. *Journal of Evaluation in Clinical Practice*, **16**, 835–837.
27 Bleakley, A. (2010) Blunting Occam's razor: aligning medical education with studies of complexity. *Journal of Evaluation in Clinical Practice*, **16**, 849–855.
28 Bleakley, A. (2014) *Patient-centred Medicine in Transition: The Heart of the Matter*. Springer, Dordrecht.
29 Davis, B., Sumara, D. & Luce-Kapler, R. (2008) *Engaging Minds: Changing Teaching in Complex Times*. Routledge, New York.
30 Arrow, H. & Henry, K.B. (2010) Using complexity to promote group learning in health care. *Journal of Evaluation in Clinical Practice*, **16**, 861–866.
31 Guastello, S.J. (2010) Self-organization and leadership emergence in emergency response teams. *Nonlinear Dynamics, Psychology, and Life Sciences Psychology, and Life Sciences*, **14**, 179–204.
32 Bleakley, A., Allard, J. & Hobbs, A. (2013) 'Achieving ensemble': communication in orthopaedic surgical teams and the development of situational awareness. *Advances in Health Sciences Education: Theory and Practice*, **18**, 33–56.
33 Innes, A. (2010) Complexity and the consultation. In: Holt, T. (ed), *Complexity for Clinicians*. Radcliffe, Oxford, pp. 37–48.
34 Clark, A. (2008) *Supersizing the Mind: Embodiment, Action, and Cognitive Extension*. Oxford University Press, Oxford.
35 Markusen, A. (2003) Fuzzy concepts, scanty evidence, policy distance: the case for rigour and policy relevance in critical regional studies. *Regional Studies*, **37**, 701–717.
36 Engeström, Y. (2009) The future of activity theory: a rough draft. In: Sannino, A., Daniels, H. & Gutiérrez,

K.D. (eds), *Learning and Expanding with Activity Theory*. Cambridge University Press, Cambridge, pp. 303–328.

37  Crook, C. (2002) Learning as cultural practice. In: Lea, M.R. & Nicoll, K. (eds), *Distributed Learning: Social and Cultural Approaches to Practice*. Routledge/Falmer, London, pp. 152–169.

38  Edwards, R., Biesta, G. & Thorpe, M. (eds) (2009) *Rethinking Contexts for Learning and Teaching: Communities, Activities and Networks*. Routledge, London.

39  Irby, D.M., Ramsey, P.G., Gilmore, G.M. & Schaad, D. (1991) Characteristics of effective clinical teachers of ambulatory care medicine. *Academic Medicine*, **66**, 54–55.

40  Cook, V., Daly, C. & Newman, M. (eds) (2012) *Work-Based Learning in Clinical Settings*. Radcliffe, London.

41  Cooke, M., Irby, D.M. & O'Brien, M. (2010) *Educating Physicians: A Call for Reform of Medical School and Residency*. Jossey-Bass, San Francisco, CA.

42  Jonassen, D.H. & Land, S.M. (2000) *Theoretical Foundations of Learning Environments*. Lawrence Erlbaum, Mahwah, NJ.

43  Lave, J. & Wenger, E. (1991) *Situated Learning: Legitimate Peripheral Participation*. Cambridge University Press, Cambridge.

44  Wenger, E. (1998) *Communities of Practice: Learning, Meaning, and Identity*. Cambridge University Press, Cambridge.

45  Engeström, Y. & Middleton, D. (eds) (1998) *Cognition and Communication at Work*. Cambridge University Press, Cambridge.

46  Blunden, A. (2012) *An Interdisciplinary Theory of Activity*. Haymarket Books, Chicago, Ill.

47  Law, J. & Hassard, J. (1999) *Actor Network Theory and After*. Wiley Blackwell, Oxford.

48  Latour, B. (2007) *Reassembling the Social: An Introduction to Actor- Network-Theory*. Oxford University Press, Oxford.

49  Fox, S. (2005) An actor-network critique of community in higher education: implications for networked learning. *Studies in Higher Education*, **30**, 95–110.

50  Mol, A. (1999) Ontological politics. A word and some questions. In: Law, J. & Hassard, J. (eds), *Actor Network Theory and After*. Blackwell, Oxford, pp. 74–89.

51  Mol, A. (2002) *The Body Multiple: Ontology in Medical Practice*. Duke University Press, Durham, NC.

52  Mol, A. (2008) *The Logic of Care: Health and the Problem of Patient Choice*. Routledge, London.

53  Mol, A. *et al.* (2010) *Care in Practice: On Tinkering in Clinics, Homes and Farms*. transcript Verlag, Bielefeld.

54  Lingard, L., McDougall, A., Levstik, M., Chandok, N., Spafford, M.M. & Schryer, C. (2012) Representing complexity well: a story about teamwork, with implications for how we teach collaboration. *Medical Education*, **46**, 869–877.

55  Bleakley, A. (2012) Establishing patient safety nets: how actor-network-theory can inform clinical education research. In: Cook, V., Daly, C. & Newman, M. (eds), *Work-Based Learning in Clinical Settings*. Radcliffe, London, pp. 143–166.

56  Bleakley, A. (2012b) The proof is in the pudding: putting actor-network-theory to work in medical education. *Medical Teacher*, **34**, 462–467.

57  Bleakley, A. (2013) Working in "teams" in an era of "liquid" healthcare: what is the use of theory? *Journal of Interprofessional Care*, **27**, 18–26.

58  Bleakley, A., Hobbs, A., Boyden, J. & Walsh, L. (2004) Safety in operating theatres: improving teamwork through team resource management. *Journal of Workplace Learning*, **16**, 83–91.

59  Bleakley, A., Hobbs, A., Boyden, J., Allard, J. & Walsh, L. (2006) Improving teamwork climate in operating theatres: the shift from multiprofessionalism to interprofessionalism. *Journal of Interprofessional Care*, **20**, 461–470.

60  Allard, J., Bleakley, A., Hobbs, A. & Vinnell, T. (2007) Who's on the team today? Collaborative teamwork in operating theatres should include briefing. *Journal of Interprofessional Care*, **21**, 189–206.

61  Henderson, S., Mills, M., Hobbs, A., Bleakley, A., Boyden, J. & Walsh, L. (2007) Surgical team self-review: enhancing organisational learning. In: Cook, M., *et al.* (eds), *Decision Making in Complex Environments*. Ashgate, Aldershot.

62  Roth, W.-M. (2005) *Auto/Biography and Auto/Ethnography: Praxis of Research Method*. Sense Publishers, Rotterdam.

63  Garfinkel, H. (1967) *Studies in Ethnomethodology*. Prentice-Hall, Englewood Cliffs, NJ.

64  Gibson, W., Webb, H. & vom Lehn, D. (2012) Ethnomethodological workplace studies and learning in clinical practice. In: Cook, V., Daly, C. & Newman, M. (eds), *Work-Based Learning in Clinical Settings*. Radcliffe, London, pp. 167–188.

65  Reason, P. & Bradbury-Huang, H. (eds) (2014) *The SAGE Handbook of Action Research: Participative Inquiry and Practice*, 2nd edn. Sage, London.

66  Chevalier, J.M. & Buckles, D.J. (2013) *Participatory Action Research: Theory and Methods for Engaged Inquiry*. Routledge, London.

67  Koshy, E., Koshy, V. & Waterman, H. (2014) *Action Research in Healthcare*, 2nd edn. Sage, London.

68  Sexton, J.B., Helmreich, R.L., Neilands, T.B. *et al.* (2006) The Safety Attitudes Questionnaire: psychometric properties, benchmarking data, and emergency research. *BMC Health Services Research*, **6**, 44.

69  Gawande, A. (2009) *The Checklist Manifesto: How to Get Things Right*. Profile, London.

70  Pronovost, P. & Vohr, E. (2010) *Safe Patients, Smart Hospitals: How One Doctor's Checklist Can Help Us Change Health Care from the Inside Out*. Hudson Street Press, New York, NY.

71  Bleakley, A., Bligh, J. & Browne, J. (2011) *Medical Education for the Future: Identity, Power and Location*. Springer, New York.

72  Frambach, J.M., Driessen, E.W. & van der Vleuten, C.P.M. (2014) Using activity theory to study cultural complexity in medical education. *Perspectives in Medical Education*, **3**, 190–203.

73  Doll, W.C., Fleener, M.J., Trueit, D. & St Julien, J. (2008) *Chaos, Complexity, Curriculum, and Culture: A Conversation.* Peter Lang, New York, NY.

74  Treuit, D. (ed) (2013) *Pragmatism, Post-modernism, and Complexity Theory: The "Fascinating Imaginative Realm" of William E. Doll, Jr.* Routledge, London.

75  Patton, M.Q. (2010) *Developmental evaluation. Applying complexity concepts to enhance innovation and use.* Guildford Press, New York.

76  Eoyang, G.H. & Holladay, R.J. (2013) *Adaptive Action. Leveraging Uncertainty in Your Organization.* Stanford University Press, Stanford, CA.

# 9 Activity theory: mediating research in medical education

*Jenny Johnston and Tim Dornan*

*In your mind's eye, picture a day's hospital rounds. Even if you are a not a healthcare professional, you will likely be familiar with how a ward round is conducted because you have been a patient in hospital or, at the very least, watched a medical drama on the television. There is always a patient, probably in bed and connected to drips, monitors and other machinery, surrounded by a bevy of staff who move as a pack. There is a consultant, who is patently the leader of the pack; junior doctors striving to keep up; nursing staff bustling about and maybe other healthcare professionals, such as pharmacists or physiotherapists. Everyone plays a well-rehearsed part in this* activity, *whose stated object is to care for the patient and assure their recovery. Keep this picture in your head; we will come back to the ward round analogy later to illustrate how activity theory (AT) (or, to give it its full title,* cultural-historical AT)[1] *can be used to explore what goes on in an* activity system.[2]

## Introduction

When people talk about AT, they are referring to a school of thought which first emerged in Russia in the early twentieth century, and which has had a major impact on Western thinking since it became available to English language readers in the 1970s.[3] Broadly speaking, AT offers a way of understanding human action and human learning, which takes into account not just an individual but also his/her social and cultural context. AT has travelled a long way from its beginning and will probably continue to develop beyond our current understanding. We briefly outline its story as it arches across the 20th century and into the 21st. We introduce some basic principles, clarify some potentially confusing terminology and outline the three generations of AT.[4] We discuss its strengths and weaknesses and how it relates to some other social theories commonly used in education. We finish with a look at how it may be used to tackle empirical research problems in health sciences education, and discuss how education

researchers can use AT to move beyond simple observation towards engineering social change.

## The sociocultural construction of meaning

Any exploration of the concept of activity begins with Lev Semyonovich Vygotsky, including (in true sociocultural style) his life and context. Vygotsky lived and worked in Soviet Russia from the 1920s until his untimely death in 1934.[5] While our Western conception of Vygotsky's Russia is heavily coloured by dictatorship and the Cold War, post-revolutionary, pre-Stalinist Russia seems to have been a time of great intellectual creativity. Despite his short working life and suppression of his works to Western readers until the 1970s, it would be hard to overestimate Vygotsky's impact on modern educational theory.[6] Together with his colleagues Leontiev and Luria, his work revolved around extending Marxist principles to the field of science, in the hope of creating a better future.[7] Their project was to theorise a model of human development, which extended Marx and Engel's concept of dialectical materialism: the idea that all progress occurs as a result of the clash between two opposites, and that it happens in response to our material needs.[8,9] With this in mind, Vygotsky developed a distinctive new wave of thought known variously as 'the cultural-historical school', 'sociocultural theory' and even (somewhat unbelievably) as 'socioculturohistorical theory'.[10] Despite the confusing nomenclature, all of these refer to the same core ideas. Vygotsky's concept of sociocultural learning was revolutionary and spawned a huge amount of scholarship; AT developed as one such strand of thinking.

The sociocultural perspective makes a paradigm shift in thinking about how people learn, moving from a focus on the internal workings of the individual towards one encompassing their social and cultural surroundings. Vygotsky understood meaning, the development of consciousness, to be mediated through people's interactions with others and the wider world.[11] While humans, like animals, are born with innate 'lower' functions, the higher mental functions needed for conscious thought are acquired through cultural means.[12] As we grow and develop, we learn rote actions from our teachers without understanding their purpose, and later we come to internalise what the action really means. This happens in a shared space between learner and teacher (or community), which Vygotsky called the *zone of proximal development* or *zoped*.[12] On the ward round, a junior student learning respiratory examination for the first time goes through the motions, copying the physical actions of the consultant. Later, with time and experience, they will understand what they are hearing and how to interpret the information they have gained.

Such a concept of learning challenges many taken-for-granted ideas about how we learn and even, fundamentally, who we are. Much modern medicine, science and educational theory has a positivist, individualist focus, founded on a philosophical concept known as *Cartesian dualism* – the idea that our minds are separate from our bodies.[13] Vygotsky's work rejects Cartesian dualism in favour of the idea that our conscious experience of the world is inextricably bound with our physical presence in it. The process of becoming the person we are happens in response to our relationships with other humans and our environment – 'Through others, we become ourselves'.[14]

## The principle of mediated action

For Vygotsky, the development of meaning is mediated by our relationship with the world. In turn, this relationship is always an indirect one. Our actions in the world require mediation by cultural *tools* or *artefacts*,[3,12] which may be either technical or psychological.[15] Technical tools are physical props which help us accomplish tasks: think of how we use a spade to dig the ground, or a stethoscope to examine someone's chest. Psychological tools are ways of mediating thought, the most important of which is language (*semiotic mediation* or mediation by *signs*).[12] Just like physical tools, we use language as a mediator to help us to accomplish a task. Vygotsky's basic concept of action, mediated by technical or psychological tools and orientated towards a specific objective, is the basis for the development of cultural-historical AT. Indeed, in AT terms it has been reframed over time as *first-generation AT*. This model is shown in Figure 9.1.

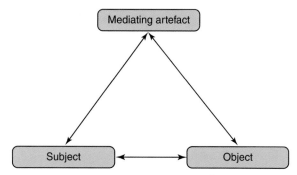

*Figure 9.1* 'First-generation' activity theory.[3]

## Semiotics and meaning

In Vygotsky's work, semiotic mediation assumes particular importance. He was preoccupied with the dialectic relationship between language and consciousness, in the sense that our language use does not simply reflect our consciousness, but helps to construct it: 'Thought is restructured as it is transformed into speech. It is not expressed but completed in the word'.[11]

Consider language use and meaning in the activities of clinical medicine. We use language not just to convey information, but also to perform a myriad of other important social actions, such as identity building and maintaining or challenging structures of power. Medical jargon, for example, is a social language of its own. Medical students' early professional learning about the core activities of the consultation, such as taking a history, interpreting signs and symptoms and formulating a differential diagnosis, investigations and treatment plan, is all the while conducted in the appropriate clinical jargon. Students' learning about how to think and work as doctors is mediated by the language of clinical medicine. Furthermore, understanding medical jargon is an important symbol of belonging, and as potent as a stethoscope slung round the neck to signify membership of the tribe.

If we think about the clinical encounter between doctor and patient, we can illustrate another important aspect of semiotic mediation. Language mediates both the doctor's actions (taking a history) and the patient's actions (telling their story) as they engage in a joint activity aimed at diagnosis and treatment. However, the meaning of the language used is specific to the context in which it is used and the intentions of the person who uses it. This introduces an element of risk into everyday communication, and into the performance of the shared activity. Therefore, the medical jargon, which provides a useful shorthand when speaking with colleagues, becomes a barrier when communicating with patients. Junior doctors soon learn that clinicians and patients often take different meanings from commonly used words[16]: a patient discussing a 'numb' feeling might mean a pins and needles sensation, while the listening doctor interprets it as indicating a complete loss of sensation. Good communicators learn that communication happens in the space *between* two people.[17] Once a speaker has tried to make his/her meaning clear, it is up to the listener to interpret what was said. The meaning of the encounter is negotiated between the two and will affect the outcome of the activity.

## Historicity and cultural change

Closely tied to the sociocultural construction of meaning, the concept of *historicity* is a final relevant aspect of Vygotsky's work. Both as individuals and as societies, the history of how an activity has developed determines its current shape and scope. In examining any cultural aspect of social life, we need to consider where it has come from, where it is going and where we stand ourselves in relation. Human experience and human learning are not absolute. Our understanding of any social concept is tied to its place in time and how we interpret it through the lens of our own culture and experience. Meaning is defined experientially and dialectically by how we (individually and collectively) construct our past and future in relation to present events.[18]

Individually, as a clinician with 10 years' experience (JJ), I reinterpret the experiences I had as a medical student through the things I have learnt about medicine since then. At a more societal level, as a community of clinicians we define ourselves against our profession's place in society; hence scandals in the healthcare profession shake our sense of professional identity and change how we relate to others outside the profession. Vygotsky's zoped provides a vehicle for the transmission of cultural norms from one generation to the next, but it also provides a means for society to engage in collective change and development. Life does not stand still, and we are constantly adapting to meet the needs of our surroundings. In this sense, cultural-historical theory is dynamic, able to encompass the flux of everyday life and its development over time and fundamentally optimistic, because it assumes that humans can continue to grow and change in positive ways. It is also quintessentially Marxist in the sense that growth happens through a dialectical process. We will return to the significance of the clash of opposites as a catalyst for change later in the chapter.

Appropriately enough, AT itself cannot be thoroughly understood without some appreciation of its historical development. Perhaps more explicitly than any other theory of learning, its meaning is inextricably bound up with its historical antecedents and context. Each generation of AT is tied to its sociocultural context, and our understanding of it tied to our own context. Some reflexivity, therefore, regarding our own vantage point is helpful in translating AT principles into real-world research.

## Moving towards the collective and the material

In the worsening political climate of the 1930s, some of Vygotsky's main collaborators, including Leontiev, left Moscow for the provincial city of Kharkov.[19] This divergence resulted in a new emphasis in Leontiev's work, as he refocused his empirical work away from semiotics and consciousness and towards material activity (activity directed towards a physical object). He also broadened the basic AT model to encompass the collective effort of a community of people working towards a shared objective.[10] Leontiev's ideas were later consolidated by Engeström, working in modern-day Finland.[20] Leontiev's extension towards collective activity and its subsequent reformulation by Engeström have become known as *second-generation AT*.[21] The diagram that Engeström formulated to connect the different aspects of Leontiev's theory of activity is shown in Figure 9.2.

This *activity system* is a more sophisticated interpretation of Vygotsky's original idea, in which an individual subject engages in mediated action towards a particular object. While this concept is still central, here sociocultural context assumes much greater importance with the addition of Rules, Community and Division of labour, all acting as mediators in their own right and being mediated in turn by other aspects of the activity system. Figure 9.2 shows how the various elements depend on one another.[22] The bidirectional arrows represent the dialogic nature of interaction and emphasise that many social voices are in dialogue with one another (*multi-voicedness*).

In extending the theory, Leontiev's thinking reflects Marxist notions of labour as a collective, practical human activity in which we engage with and try to change the natural world.[23] In this sense, labour is essentially creative. Engaging in it is a way of transforming ourselves, the dialectic materialist

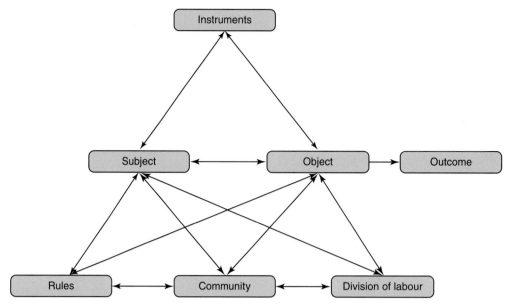

*Figure 9.2* 'Second-generation' activity theory.[20]

view of human progress we referred to earlier. When looked at from that perspective, the tools we use to mediate between ourselves and nature take on a special significance, because they come to define our very humanness. In addition, because labour is a collective activity, it is not only mediated by physical tools, but also by our social relationships with other humans. The way a community of individuals divides up labour will, in Marxist terms, affect the ultimate value of the commodities produced.[8]

Famously, Leontiev used the metaphor of a 'primeval hunt' to exemplify his model of collective activity. He also used this example to divide activity into a three-level hierarchical model.[24] At the highest level, the overall *activity* is directed towards meeting a collective need, and is determined by an overarching motive. In the metaphor of the primeval hunt, the overall collective activity of a hunt is motivated by a collective need for food and clothing. In pursuit of the overall object (motive), a number of smaller, coordinated *actions* have to be undertaken; for example, during the hunt, someone must frighten the game out of the bushes. Actions constitute a middle level and are *goal-oriented*, whereas activity is *object-oriented*. The goal of an action is more immediate, and is not necessarily the same as the ultimate motive for the overall activity. The bottom level consists of *operations*, smaller steps which are undertaken in response to prevailing conditions. In the context of the hunt, beating a stick to make a frightening noise constitutes an operation.[25] We can see a focus here on using physical tools to

mediate, which contrasts with Vygotsky's emphasis on psychological tools.

Let us now go back to the ward round example with which we opened the chapter, and conceptualise it in these AT terms. Everyone on the ward round is motivated by the shared activity of patient care, accomplished via a series of coordinated actions and operations, such as undertaking a respiratory examination and attaching an oxygen saturation monitor. They use psychological tools, such as history taking, and material ones such as stethoscopes and laboratory tests. The rules of the activity are fairly stringent: the hospital is an institution with a rigorous social structure defining the terms of activities taking place within. On the ward round, the consultant is in overall charge, and other staff have clearly defined roles within hierarchical relationships. Labour is divided among the various team members according to the requirements of patient care: the junior doctors organise further tests, while nurses check observations and administer medication and the physiotherapist assesses the patient's mobility. All are cogs in an apparently well-oiled machine.

Consider how medical students entering this environment learn from more senior doctors how to dress, how to talk and how to act. They are learning more than just how to use their stethoscope; amongst other things, they are learning how to occupy their place in the medical hierarchy and how to negotiate the complex web of social rules and relationships within the healthcare setting. Consider, too, how the simultaneous experience of

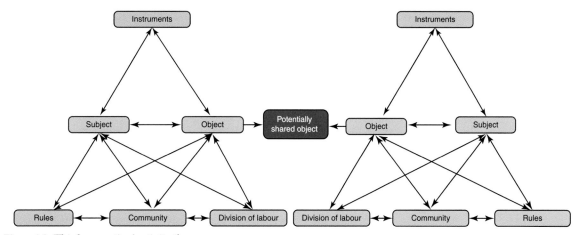

**Figure 9.3** 'Third generation' activity theory.

nursing students in the same space differs from the medical students. They have different role models and are learning different ways of dressing, talking and acting. For example, in nursing, uniform and the need to conform to proscribed standards of appearance assume a greater (or at least more tightly defined) importance.[26] Interactions with patients and colleagues proceed from a different viewpoint, although the same relations of power must be negotiated.

The dialectic between different professional groups, working closely together and all with their own cultural norms, is a potential source of conflict within the activity system. When we next return to this example, however, we will consider how such conflicts offer the potential to bring about cultural change and improved interprofessional working practices.

## Contradictions and expansive learning

While the early generations of AT became very influential in the Soviet sphere, one consequence of the political turmoil of the Cold War was that the works of Vygotsky and Leontiev were not introduced to the West until the 1970s. Around the same time, the 'paradigm wars' were emerging, as qualitative researchers began to challenge the dominance of an individualist, rationalist/scientific paradigm for studying social interaction. The new sociocultural context to which AT was exposed in the West lit a revolutionary spark in human sciences, allowing the theory to gain momentum and resulting in an entirely new wave of work in the field. A central proponent of this modern take on AT is Finnish educationalist Yrjö Engeström. As we discussed earlier, Engeström and his collaborators

were responsible for consolidating and moving forward the second generation of AT. Since then, Engeström has sought to push the theoretical limits with a *third-generation* expression of AT, called *activity systems analysis*.[3] This approach looks at how different activity systems interact with each other (Fig. 9.3).

Engeström's approach to AT is largely concerned with harnessing its creative potential to facilitate social change and forward movement. We mentioned earlier how Marxist theory views labour as a creative force in our lives. Things do not have to always be the same – we can change and develop as we work our way through life. Indeed, we *need* to be constantly moving forward. The struggle for improvement is part of what defines us as human, and it is never finished.

In AT, this process is conceptualised as arising from the resolution of dialectically opposing positions, which are in tension with each other. Tensions can arise either within or between systems. The tensions are termed *contradictions*[27] (see the first of our empirical research exemplars for a practical example of this term) and the process of creating something entirely new from their resolution is called *expansive learning*.[2] Activity systems are inherently *multi-voiced*, and contradictions come from the differences between people, their interactions and their cultural development over the course of history.[28] Contradictions do not always lead to expansive transformation but, when they do, the original activity shifts its entire axis to encompass a completely new purpose, with all the new possibilities that can open up.[3]

In the meantime, returning to our earlier ward round analogy will help us illustrate some of Engeström's major concepts. Thinking of the ward round as an activity system, we can first look at the potential for internal contradictions. Remember that the most obvious object of the healthcare team's activity is patient care; so far, so good. In reality, though, we are confronted with a complex activity that involves a number of different and potentially conflicting motives and goals. For example, at the macro level, the publicly funded UK National Health Service is under constant pressure to ration resources and reduce expenditure. North American healthcare systems, in contrast, often encompass commercial concerns. Thus, in different contexts, financial considerations may compete with the apparently more altruistic (and socially acceptable) motive of patient care. At the more fundamental level of staffing, different subjects are likely to maintain somewhat different objects. Consider how medicine and nursing have had traditionally different viewpoints, cultures and practices, even though the stated aim of both is care and well-being of patients. This is a source of contradiction in which we can see the influence of an accumulation of the weight of history in the cultural differences between the two groups.

We could then start to think about how the ward round team interacts with other activity systems. Assume that the patient who is the focus for their activity is diagnosed with tuberculosis. This will bring the team in contact with other professional groups, such as the public health department, or the patient's family doctor, each working within their own activity system. Each new system, even with the overall shared objective of patient care, will have different focus, different rules and different priorities, all potential sources of contradiction. Now we begin to get just a glimpse of the complexity of modern healthcare! Nevertheless, all parties must find a way to overcome their differences and work together successfully for the patient's benefit. If the clash between them is resolved by developing new, more effective working patterns, then expansive learning will take place. In this case, the original object of the activity has shifted slightly as a result of the engagement of its subjects.

Expansive learning is a very different way of thinking about learning, compared to other pedagogical theories, which have been popular in the last 100 years – contrast AT with a behaviourist or cognitive approach to learning. In fact, so profoundly different is expansive learning that we have to think twice about what we actually mean by the word learning. In this case, we are not defining learning narrowly as something which is undertaken by students and guided by a teacher in a classroom. Instead, we define learning broadly as a constant comparative process of adaptation in

which we are all involved through the entire course of our lives. For this reason, the Finnish strand of AT has become a popular way of investigating and interpreting the ways in which people adapt and learn within the daily rigours of the workplace.[29] AT, in its most modern incarnation, has more ability than most theoretical positions to take in this richness and complexity and to appreciate it in its entirety as well as its constituent parts. This makes it of particular interest to those of us researching healthcare professions education, because so much of this learning is not classroom based, but takes place in the workplace.

In applying AT to workplace learning, the Centre for Activity Theory Research in Helsinki sought a way to stimulate positive (expansive) change and came up with a specific format for AT-grounded action research, called the Change Laboratory (CL).[30] Typically, participants meet several times in workshop fashion and utilise a range of tools to look critically at problems within the work environment. Progress is cyclical, based on identifying and describing issues in their contexts, then reformulating them within potential creative solutions.[31] A successful CL requires participants to be open and creative outside their normal work parameters. Because it is led by participants, it emphasises their own ability to be agents of change within their environments. In the section on empirical research, we discuss an example of this approach within healthcare and its ability to bring about meaningful social change.

## Linking activity theory to other theories of learning

Having outlined the evolution of AT over three generations and almost a century of scholarship, it is worth considering how this particular theoretical perspective fits with others, which may commonly be encountered in medical education research. Social theories are built on other social theories; understanding the many and various linkages between all the influential thinkers of the last century would require a whole book (or a whole library). Having said that, there are some antecedents and subsequent lines of thought that link so strongly to AT that it is worth bringing them out a little. There is significant cross-pollination, and understanding one aspect can help us to understand another aspect better.

In tracing its origins, we showed earlier that AT is a sociocultural theory of learning which emerged from Marxist theory. It is deeply constructionist in its epistemological orientation, by which we mean that it is committed to a view of truth and knowledge as being constructed by people, and not imposed by a fixed, external reality. Immediately, this aligns it with one particular line of educational theory, and places it far away from others. Popular 20th century behaviourist and cognitive theories of learning, such as operant conditioning (learning as reflex, where learning is reinforced by positive and negative stimuli),[32] learning styles (learning as defined by individual attributes and preferences)[33] or even social cognitive theory (individual learning by modelling the actions of others)[34] are not natural bedfellows with AT. On the other hand, AT is closely related to other sociocultural theories emerging from Vygotsky's work. One theory in this tradition that has risen to particular prominence in medical education research is Communities of Practice theory.[35] Lave and Wenger's work has attained particular prominence in the medical education literature in recent years and has intuitive appeal for health sciences education.[36] A different line of research stretching back to Vygotsky focuses on the construction of worlds through discourse (semiotic mediation); Holland's figured worlds theory is a sociocultural discourse theory of identity, which has also come to recent prominence in medical education research.[37,38]

All sociocultural theories draw ultimately on similar theoretical backgrounds, though with different emphases. Vygotsky is a key scholar whose work we have discussed at length. Another work which we have touched on several times in passing but not elaborated is that of Bakhtin. Throughout this chapter, we have referred to the Marxist concept of 'dialectic', referring to the clash of two different positions resulting in some sort of forward movement, because this is a fundamental principle in AT. Bakhtin, also working in Soviet Russia in the 1920s and 1930s, has been equally influential with a similar but not an identical idea. For Bakhtin, the focus was less on the clash and more on the interaction – the idea of *dialogism*.[17] When we spoke earlier about the uncertain nature of communication, we were referring to a quintessentially Bakhtinian idea – meaning lies somewhere between what the speaker intends and the listener hears. Speech is inherently dialogic, and monologue is more or less a contradiction in terms (as you might imagine, this emphasis on multi-voicedness did not go down well with the Soviet authorities, resulting in exile to Siberia). Bakhtin was and continues to be exceptionally influential in modern AT and elsewhere. The multi-voicedness of activity systems in second-

and third-generation AT is a concept lifted directly from Bakhtin.[3]

In a different aspect of AT – its systems-level focus on the web of connections between people – we can discern a pathway to even other areas of research. Third-generation AT shares some concerns with the field of cybernetics, as conceptualised by Gregory Bateson, in that both share a commitment to constructivist explanations of human behaviour and a focus on the dynamic organisation of systems.[39] Meanwhile, Latour's actor–network theory (a way of connecting human action with non-human actors, such as computers) provides another systematic way of thinking about our relationship with the material world, by assigning agency to things as well as people.[40] Along with AT, these approaches are increasingly being used to explore our relationships with modern technologies, and are hence equally applicable in a healthcare setting.[41,42]

This brief 'family tree' provides just a taster of the potential of these diverse and enriching areas of scholarship. We urge anyone interested to start with the antecedents of activity (beginning with Marx and Engels)[8,9] and work their way forward from there!

## Using activity theory in empirical research

In the following, we discuss different ways in which researchers have used AT empirically using a number of case studies from health sciences education research.

### 1. Using activity theory to explore conflicting activities in undergraduate medical education

De Feijter *et al.* used AT to explore students' understanding and experiences of patient safety issues at the time when they were beginning to transition between university and work.[43] In the Dutch university, where the research was done, students undertook clinical clerkships in their final years before graduating and taking up positions as residents in specialty training. Although still technically students, participants had reached a stage of training where they were enmeshed with the world of work and where the distinction between the student and junior doctor was somewhat blurred.

An initial inductive thematic analysis was followed by a top-down analysis using the principles of third-generation AT. Two competing activities were identified: 'learning to be a doctor' and 'taking care of patients without doing harm'. Contradictions arose whenever the two clashed. Important aspects of each activity (rules and division of labour) could conflict with aspects of the other activity, such as when a student rather than an experienced doctor performed a procedure. In this case, while students were provided with a good training opportunity, patient care was potentially less safe. Students (as subjects) were forced to negotiate a solution when faced simultaneously with the two activities – the responsibility for balancing their training with maintaining patient care lay primarily with them. It is worth reflecting that students' expansive learning may have been more about how to compromise than how to be either a good doctor or a good learner.

Here, De Feijter *et al.* used AT as a post hoc way of elaborating the findings of a thematic analysis. using social theory in this manner is one way of adding depth to results, pulling together seemingly disparate themes into a more cohesive and explanatory framework, and sparking ideas for future research projects. This type of research, which has also been used in mathematics education, opens up a rich vein of enquiry into transitions between university and work.[44] Given the amount of time spent learning in the workplace as a student doctor, and the even greater time for student nurses before graduation, this is not a straightforward proposition and offers some interesting research questions for which AT may be a useful conceptual framework.

## 2. Using activity theory to explore teamwork in a healthcare setting

In their 2012 paper, Lingard *et al.* used AT to explore the complexity of teamwork amongst staff in an organ transplant unit in a major Canadian teaching hospital.[45] The analysis involved two different procedures: one a classic inductive, data-driven thematic analysis and the other conducted by patient case. The latter method enabled the researchers to follow the threads of a particular case chronologically through all the different instances of teamworking and complexity involved in providing care. In AT terms, this allowed the various strands of knotworking (the dynamic way in which people come together and apart to solve problems in daily work activities)[46] to be unpicked. Team members had to strategise and improvise in order to solve everyday problems, which because of the nature of their work became high-stakes issues and put patient well-being at risk. The authors conclude by undermining two commonly held notions in teamwork research: that professionals take on stable roles/positions within teams and that patient

care is the only object (in reality, other objects such as protection of resources and the need to provide training for juniors compete with patient care).

AT allowed the authors to undertake a piece of work that is methodologically sophisticated, grounded in real-world activities and addresses issues of complexity, which are commonly put to one side. Even in qualitative research, with its potential for elucidating the richness and detail of social life, it is more usual to focus on certain aspects of phenomena. AT allows researchers access to the complexity and dynamism of real-life scenarios, such as those involved in healthcare. Because we are rediscovering the fact that learning for the healthcare professions happens most significantly 'on the job', it is hard to overstate how important it is to research what actually happens on the job. Furthermore, this example offers a good illustration of how our conception of learning itself is expanded by AT: learning is not just something that happens in classrooms with students, but a necessary process of adaptation and evolution which we are all doing day in, day out in order to achieve our work and life goals.

## 3. Using the Change Laboratory approach to improve working conditions in a secondary care setting

Kerosuo *et al.* from the Centre for Activity Theory research in Helsinki published a case study in 2010, which illustrated how the CL method can be used within healthcare.[47] The setting for the research was a hospital surgical unit in Finland. Participants were drawn from a range of professional backgrounds, including medicine, nursing and management. The aim was to identify tensions and difficulties in everyday working practices (contradictions) and develop potential solutions, which could be reified into a new model of working.

In the preliminary phase, researchers conducted 5 days of ethnographic observation (including following a number of patients through the unit), together with 17 interviews with key staff. These data were used in the first stages of the CL approach (in which researchers facilitated five CL sessions and two follow-up sessions) to present a 'mirror' of the current activity, thereby revealing areas of tension. Some of the areas of difficulty highlighted in this manner included theatres being closed even though patients were waiting for surgery, anaesthetists not being immediately available because of work demands elsewhere in the hospital and operating lists mixing elective and emergency cases. The work of anaesthetists and surgeons was eventually conceptualised as consisting of two different but interacting activity systems, each with a different object. The interaction of these differing objects was a source of contradictions.

By uncovering and discussing challenging aspects of daily work, potential openings for positive change were uncovered. Over the course of the sessions, participants worked to develop a new leadership and management strategy for the unit that addressed the issues which had arisen. Part of the project involved formalising these in the form of a document, which was then implemented at the end of the CL intervention. The new model was 'owned' by the unit staff and remained grounded in their everyday working practice. Subsequent external evaluation of the unit demonstrated high performance.

CL takes AT research beyond explaining activity to bring about change in large-scale social systems. While change is often the implicit aim of human sciences research, CL makes the move towards change explicit and, unlike much other AT research, offers tools for getting started. Researchers act as facilitators, not as observers or controllers of output. Genuine change or innovation comes from the participants themselves, whose agency and ability to tackle difficult situations is foregrounded and even reinforced by the research process.

## In summary: AT and empirical research

The aforementioned examples illustrate a few potential applications of AT research in both education and healthcare. It is applicable to the undergraduate, postgraduate and professional development contexts. Getting started with AT only requires knowledge of basic qualitative methods, an open mind and a commitment to understanding learning as a social process and an agent of social change. Some examples have been given. Other suitable projects might include examining the interaction of different activity systems and the borders between them, such as the relationship between residents' work and their education, or differences between skills taught outside workplaces and the same skills in real-work contexts. Our earlier ward round example gives just a flavour of the multiple and conflicting activities in any healthcare setting, and should hopefully stimulate you to consider how you might get started with this sort of research in your own context.

## Strengths and limitations of activity theory

For AT research projects, qualitative methods are a good epistemological fit and offer the potential for exploring and unravelling the complex social interactions of mediated activity, rather than measuring or testing using quantitative methods. Part of the rigour of qualitative work comes from fully understanding the implications of choosing a particular theoretical framework. Every theoretical position has its strengths and weaknesses. Understanding where these lie is an important practical aspect of the research process, so we will finish our exposition of the theoretical aspects with a look at this area.

For most of the past century, social science has come down heavily on one side or the other of the 'structure-agency debate' – either individuals are responsible for their own fate (agency) or they have very little say in the matter, which instead is largely determined by macro social structures. In sociocultural approaches such as AT, the gap between the individual and society is bridged and we have a potential way of resolving the structure-agency debate, at least on a case-specific basis. All the generations of AT overcome the traditional Cartesian division; AT does not view people as 'minds in bodies'.[48] It is phenomenological in the sense that people's experiences within the world directly influence their cognitive development; people's consciousness arises from their relationships with themselves, other people and the world around them.

While not disregarding the influence of social structure, AT provides a lot of space for human agency. The potential for expansive learning in particular allows for the possibility that out of difficult situations we can generate creative responses with the power to improve the world around us. The CL approach, which reifies these principles into a fairly concrete methodology with the explicit aim of social improvement, is a particular instance of this strength.[30] In the sense that AT sees human life as essentially capable of progressing forward in a positive manner, we could say it is an optimistic theory (compared, for example, to the relative nihilism of much postmodernist thought, such as that of Foucault or Lyotard).[49]

Another major strength of AT is its dynamism – its capacity to accommodate change, and to stretch and grow in unexpected directions. Consider how its evolution over time encompasses revolutionary roots in Vygotsky and Leontiev, a completely new context in Engeström and most recently an influential position in researching Western work-places. In working with AT, we acknowledge the importance of history, which is so often ignored in analyses, as crucial to our contemporary cultural life. Appropriately enough, the history of AT itself acts as a heuristic here. If we did not know how AT had evolved in a post-revolutionary, pre-Stalinist Russia, where Marx's ideas seemed to offer hope and inspiration for the future, or understand how the transfer of ideas from this context is influenced by their transfer to Western contexts and modern times, then we would not understand AT at all. The latest generation of AT is also dynamic in a more immediate sense, which is that it has space to accommodate the ebb and flow of real-life activities. Life is complex, and activity is by definition in constant movement.

In terms of limitations, a common criticism is that AT lacks explanatory power. It is relatively straightforward to use it as a tool to describe a social situation, but more challenging to undertake empirical research, which leads to theory development. Perhaps one reason for this may be that AT appears quite conceptual, with no hard and fast rules about how to translate theoretical principles into research – a second major criticism. AT lacks a concrete research methodology, which, for some who are new to this type of research, may present a significant barrier. CL offers a partial solution, but the fact remains that choosing AT as a theoretical framework does not come handily packaged, as in phenomenology or grounded theory, which both offer clear epistemological and methodological positions rolled into one. However, we can frame this more positively as offering researchers some flexibility within their interpretative process.

## Conclusion

In this chapter, we have traced AT over almost a hundred years and thousands of miles. We followed the story of Vygotsky and mediation, through Leontiev and the collective, and ended up with Engeström and the dynamic interaction of activity systems. We discussed how AT puts the voices of participants at the vanguard of change. By definition, it is multi-voiced and draws much of its strength from its democratic and multidisciplinary orientation. It continues to evolve and, as medical education researchers, we can help shape the next generation of AT by using it in our own work. We hope the chapter has given you a taste of what AT can do and the enthusiasm to get started on your own AT journey.

---

**Practice points**

- Existence is a constant struggle for improvement. We learn and change by engaging in *activity*.

- Activity is mediated by *physical tools* (such as a stethoscope) or *psychological tools* (such as history taking).

- An *activity system* connects individuals and communities with their social and cultural context as they act in pursuit of an *object*.

- The clash of perspectives (*contradictions*) between different voices in or between activity systems can stimulate change, resulting in a new object – *expansive learning*.

- Expansive learning can be used in workplaces to implement action research projects, facilitating participants themselves to promote change.

## References

1  Cole, M. (1996) *Cultural Psychology*. Belknap Press of Harvard University Press, Cambridge.

2  Engeström, Y. (1987) *Learning by Expanding: An Activity-Theoretical Approach to Developmental Research*. Helsinki, Orienta-Konsultit.

3  Engeström, Y., Miettinen, R. & Punamäki, R.L. (eds) (1999) *Perspectives on Activity Theory*. Cambridge University Press, Cambridge.

4  Engeström, Y. (1996) Developmental work research as educational research. *Nordisk Pedagogik: Journal of Nordic Educational Research*, **16**, 131–143.

5  Wertsch, J.V. (1985) *Vygotsky and the Social Formation of Mind*. Harvard University Press, Cambridge.

6  Davydov, V.V. & Kerr, S.T. (1995) The influence of L. S. Vygotsky on education theory, research, and practice. *Educational Researcher*, **24**, 12–21.

7  Bickley, R. (1977) Vygotsky's contributions to a dialectical materialist psychology. *Science & Society*, **41**, 191–2.

8  Marx, K. (1990) *Capital, Volume I*. Penguin Books, London.

9  Engels, F. (2012) *Dialectics of Nature*. Wellread, London.

10  Wertsch, J.V., del Rio, P. & Alvarez, A. (eds) (1995) *Sociocultural Studies of Mind*. Cambridge University Press, Cambridge.

11  Vygotsky, L.S. (1987) *Thinking and Speech*. Plenum, New York.

12  Vygotsky, L.S. (1978) *Mind in Society: The Development of Higher Psychological Processes*. Harvard University Press, Cambridge.

13  Kenny, A. (1968) *Descartes: A Study of his Philosophy*. Random House, New York.

14  Vygotsky, L.S. (1997) History of the development of the higher mental functions. In: Rieber, R.W. (ed), *The Collected Works of LS Vygotsky*. Plenum, New York.

15 Lock, A. & Strong, T. (2010) *Social Constructionism: Sources and Stirrings in Theory and Practice*. Cambridge University Press, Cambridge.

16 Mishler, E.G. (1984) *The Discourse of Medicine, Dialectics of Medical Interviews*. Ablex Publishing Corporation, Norwood, New Jersey.

17 Bakhtin, M.M. (1981) *The Dialogic Imagination: Four Essays*. University of Texas Press, Austin.

18 Mead, G.H. (1938) *The Philosophy of the Act*. University of Chicago Press, Chicago.

19 Yasnitsky, A. & Ferrari, M. (2008) Rethinking the early history of post-Vygotskian psychology: the case of the Kharkov School. *History of Psychology*, **11**, 101–121.

20 Engeström, Y. (2001) Expansive learning at work: toward an activity theoretical reconceptualization. *Journal of Education and Work*, **14**, 134–156.

21 Yamagata-Lynch, L. (2010) *Activity Systems Analysis Methods: Understanding Complex Learning Environments*. Springer, New York.

22 Marx, K. (1959) *Economic and Philosophical Manuscripts of 1844*. Progress Publishers, Moscow.

23 Leontiev, A.N. (1978) *Activity, Consciousness and Personality*. Prentice-Hall, Englewood Cliffs.

24 Leontiev, A.N. (1981) *Problems of the Development of the Mind*. Progress Publishers, Moscow.

25 Shaw, K. & Timmons, S. (2010) Exploring how nursing uniforms influence self image and professional identity. *Nursing times*, **106**, 21–23.

26 Il'enkov, E.V. (1977) *Dialectical logic: essays in its history and theory*. Moscow, Progress.

27 Bakhtin, M.M. (1993) *Problems of Dostoevsky's Poetics*. University of Minnesota Press, Minneapolis.

28 Engeström, Y. & Kerusao, H. (2007) From workplace learning to inter-organizational learning and back: the contribution of activity theory. *Journal of Workplace Learning*, **19**, 336–342.

29 Engeström, Y., Virkkunen, J., Helle, M., Pihlaja, J. & Poikela, R. (1996) The Change Laboratory as a tool for transforming work. *Lifelong Learning in Europe*, **1**, 10–17.

30 Virkkunen, J. & Newnham, D.S. (2013) *The Change Laboratory: A Tool for Collaborative Development of Work and Education*. Rotterdam, Sense.

31 Skinner, B.F. (1963) Operant behavior. *American Psychologist*, **18**, 503–515.

32 Honey, P. & Mumford, A. (1982) *Manual of Learning Styles*. P Honey, London.

33 Bandura, A. (1991) Social cognitive theory of self-regulation. *Organisational Behaviour and Human Decision Processes*, **50**, 248–287.

34 Lave, J. & Wenger, E. (1991) *Situated Learning. Legitimate Peripheral Participation*. Cambridge University Press, Cambridge.

35 Mann, K.V. (2011) Theoretical perspectives in medical education: past experience and future possibilities. *Medical Education*, **45**, 60–68.

36 Holland, D., Lachicotte, W., Skinner, D. & Cain, C. (1998) *Identity and Agency in Cultural Worlds*. Harvard University Press, Cambridge, MA.

37 Vågan, A. (2011) Towards a sociocultural perspective on identity formation in education. *Mind, Culture, and Activity*, **18**, 43–57.

38 Bateson, G. (1972) *Steps to an Ecology of Mind: Collected Essays in Anthropology, Psychiatry, Evolution, and Epistemology*. University of Chicago Press, Chicago.

39 Latour, B. (2005) *Reassembling the Social: An Introduction to Actor-Network-Theory*. Oxford University Press, Oxford.

40 Prout, A. (1996) Actor-network theory, technology and medical sociology: an illustrative analysis of the metered dose inhaler. *Sociology of Health & Illness*, **18**, 198–219.

41 Fenwick, T. (2014) Sociomateriality in medical practice and learning: attuning to what matters. *Medical Education*, **48**, 44–52.

42 de Feijter, J.M., de Grave, W.S., Dornan, T., Koopmans, R.P. & Scherpbier, A.J.J.A. (2011) Students' perceptions of patient safety during the transition from undergraduate to postgraduate training: an activity theory analysis. *Advances in Health Sciences Education*, **16**, 347–358.

43 Williams, J.S. (2012) Use and exchange value in mathematics education: contemporary cultural historical activity theory meets Bourdieu's sociology. *Educational Studies in Mathematics*, **80**, 57–72.

44 Lingard, L., McDougall, A., Levstik, M., Chandok, N., Spafford, M. & Schryer, C. (2012) Representing complexity well: a story about teamwork, with implications for how we teach collaboration. *Medical Education*, **46**, 869–877.

45 Engeström, Y. (2007) From communities of practice to mycorrhizae. In: Hughes, J., Jewson, N. & Unwin, L. (eds), *Communities of Practice: Critical Perspectives*. Routledge, London.

46 Kerosuo, H., Kajamaa, A. & Engeström, Y. (2010) Promoting innovation and learning through Change Laboratory: an example from Finnish health care. *Central European Journal of Public Policy*, **4**, 110–131.

47 Merleau-Ponty, M. (2002) *Phenomenology of Perception*. Routledge, London.

48 Foucault, M. (2003) *The Birth of the Clinic*. Routledge, Abingdon.

49 Lyotard, J.F. (1984) *The Postmodern Condition: A Report on Knowledge*. University of Minnesota Press, Minneapolis.

# 10 Social cognitive theory: thinking and learning in social settings

*Dario Torre and Steven J. Durning*

*JS is a new staff physician (attending physician) in internal medicine. This is his first day working with his team, which consists of two interns (doctors in the first year post-qualification), a resident (registrar) and two third year medical students. He would like to provide bedside instruction to the team and is very interested in cardiac disorders, in particular congestive heart failure (CHF). The service is busy with a high number of patients on the team, and JS wonders how much sleep his team members have had recently. There are two patients on the team with a diagnosis of CHF and both may be discharged home later today. He is used to giving lectures to students, but has not had the opportunity to provide bedside instruction. Given the aforementioned factors, what should JS consider when planning a bedside teaching opportunity in CHF?*

## Introduction

Social cognitive theory refers to a group, or family, of theories that consider learning and performance as inherently social. This means that individuals, the environment and interactions between individuals and the environment matter in learning and performance situations. Furthermore, social cognitive theories argue that the uniqueness that each situation brings (in terms of the environment, participants and their interactions) can often lead to different learning and performance experiences and outcomes.

These ideas are distinguished from individual cognitive theories (such as information processing theory or IPT) that pervade healthcare profession education nowadays. IPTs, such as cognitive load theory (see the chapter by Leppink and colleagues), have historically assumed that learning and performance are primarily, if not solely, determined by knowledge acquisition and organisation. While leading to critically important advances in our understanding of cognition (e.g. decision making),[1] IPTs often downplay (or ignore) the possible contribution of other participants, the environment

(setting) and the interaction between individuals and the environment in learning and performance. Thus, from the IPT perspective, the main focus of JS in the opening scenario would be on conveying knowledge regarding CHF to the team, probably best done via a mini-lecture. Indeed, from the information processing standpoint, JS might even question the need for the bedside teaching: IPT could/would argue that it is equally effective to provide the team with information and examples in a seminar room. The value of the bedside and watching the learners interact with the patient and the patient's perspective would often be questioned from this perspective. From social cognitive theories (SCTs) perspective, on the other hand, there are a number of other factors that are likely to contribute to learning in addition to knowledge – the environment, the participants and their interactions – and all these factors would be considered in planning the bedside teaching. We will return to this in more detail later in the chapter.

In this chapter, we describe selected SCTs that we believe apply to healthcare profession education today. We will begin with the historical development and theoretical foundations of this family of theories. Next, we discuss three different theoretical lenses that fall within the family of SCTs: situated cognition, distributed cognition and situated learning. In the last section, we provide some of the applications of these theories, and indicate future research and practice directions. At the end of this chapter, the reader should be able to list underpinnings and key historical developments of SCTs, describe examples of SCTs and their application in healthcare profession education and be aware of some of the future directions for SCT research and teaching.

## Theoretical foundations of SCT

When Bandura[2] championed SCT, behaviouralism was arguably the prevailing theory of learning. The goal of behaviourism was to 'condition' desirable responses in educational programs, much like Pavlov's dog in the classic example of this theory. SCTs made a notable separation from this theory in placing an important role on processes such as goal setting, judging outcomes, emotions and reflection. Thus, one way SCTs differ from behaviourism by recognising that we exert choice as opposed to just responding to educational or other 'stimuli'.

A second difference between behaviouralism and SCT is that the latter argues that we also learn from observation, or 'watching', and, because of this, learning and performance can differ. Although much learning occurs by doing, we also learn by observing others perform the relevant activities that we wish to learn. From the SCT perspective, a medical student could learn from observing JS perform a history and physical examination in a patient with heart failure. This notion of learning through observation is also in line with emerging work from neuroscience on learning.[3]

Finally, from an SCT perspective, whether we ever perform what we have learnt depends upon a variety of factors present in the situation at hand (individuals, the environment and their interactions). This situational notion to performance is in line with the finding of context specificity in medicine, meaning that a physician can see two patients with the same (or nearly identical) history, physical examination, laboratories and diagnosis and yet the physician comes to two different diagnostic decisions.[4,5] Something beyond the 'facts' needed to establish the diagnosis is therefore impacting the physician's decision (in our aforementioned example, this could be the location of the evaluation or the interaction between the patient and the ward team members). SCT's situation-based nature to cognition, learning and performance raises challenges for assessment of learning and transfer, which we will discuss later.

A key development in SCT arose when Bandura[2] introduced the concept of human behaviour as occurring within the framework of *triadic reciprocality* (Figure 10.1). This core concept underpins SCT and its assumptions.

In triadic reciprocality, human behaviour is viewed as being caused by the interaction of three main sets of determinants: personal factors (which include cognition, affective and biological events), behaviour (e.g. choice of tasks, persistence and self-efficacy) and the environment (which can be imposed, selected and/or constructed).

In this work of Bandura,[2,6–8] we begin to see the interaction of cognition and the context in which it

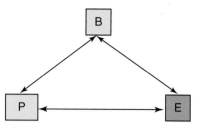

**Figure 10.1** The schematisation of the reciprocal interactions among the three determinants: B=behaviour; P, C=personal and cognitive factors and E = environment.

occurs, with an emphasis on the social process of learning. From a social cognitive view, all human ability is mediated by the interaction of people with the environment, which includes their motivational and cognitive abilities. To return to our example at the beginning of this chapter, merely providing the 'stimulus' of content is not sufficient for optimising learning. Personal factors (such as how well rested the team is), behaviour (is there a patient on the team with CHF who would serve as a prompt, or interest in learning) and the environment (is the room conducive to bedside rounds, etc.) would all be considered important for teaching bedside rounds.

An important element of behaviour in triadic reciprocality is the concept of self-efficacy. (Note that self-efficacy plays a key role in several other theories described in this book, such as self-regulation and motivation and emotion theories [see chapters by Artino and colleagues as well as McConnell and Eva]). Self-efficacy is the belief in one's capabilities to exercise control over one's level of functioning and execute courses of action to obtain a given goal.[9] Self-efficacy is believed to be a major determinant in how people think, feel and act. From an SCT perspective, self-efficacy mediates cognitive development and functioning in three ways: cognitive, motivational and affective.[10] In the cognitive area, a higher level of self-efficacy allows for more thoughtful decision making. This is believed to occur through enhanced integration of self-appraisal, planning, time management and performance feedback. Furthermore, self-efficacy plays a powerful role in metacognition (thinking about thinking), allowing for better use, control and understanding of cognitive strategies needed to achieve academic goals. Self-efficacy has important motivational effects: Bandura states that 'self-efficacy has its most powerful effects thought the process of cognized goals'[10] (p. 56). The setting of high goals derived from high self-efficacy can provide direction, self-management and positive expectations through evaluating and judging the adequacy and effectiveness of one's effort to achieve his/her goals. For example, a stronger perceived self-efficacy should lead to higher goal challenges and greater commitment to goal achievement.[6] Learners who have a high sense of self-efficacy can also provide positive supports for performance and less self-doubt in achieving their goals.[11] Furthermore, two people with the same knowledge and skills (e.g. teaching bedside rounds) may perform differently based on differences in their self-efficacy beliefs.

Self-efficacy can also have larger social effects, such as influencing the management of a learning organisation (SCT of organisational theory[12]). Larger social effects also include collective efficacy. Collective efficacy is a property of the group that generates a collective power, which allows the achievement of the goals of that group. Similar to individual self-efficacy, high perceived collective efficacy results in greater group resilience to setbacks, higher motivation and performance attainments, in educational systems, business organisations or athletic teams.[13,14] This is believed to be one of the several reasons that can underpin why a team that should be beaten by another based on individual player match-ups (looking better on paper than on individual-by-individual bases) but yet the victory goes to the 'underdog'.

## Bruner: culture is an important element in SCT

While Bandura emphasises the role of the environment as a crucial determinant of the reciprocality of learning, Bruner[15] takes this concept further, recognising that the construction of meaning is deeply entrenched in culture, which is a key element of the people and their environment. Bruner's work emphasises the cultural processes in learning and education, introducing the concept of cultural situatedness and the link between human mind, meaning and culture.

In Bruner's view, learning and thinking are always situated in a cultural setting, and their meaning has its origins in the culture in which they are generated. In the culturalist approach, education is part of the large world of culture and is shaped by the role it plays in the environment, group or community. For example, in the bedside encounter previously described, the resident may tell the students before entering the patient's room that is important to correctly perform cardiac auscultation in front of the attending physician. One should not perform auscultation through the gown. It is possible that, if any of the students comes from a culture where such action may be seen as inappropriate (and

hence is not comfortable doing so), the impact of performing auscultation through the gown could undermine the educational value of the encounter. The focus may shift to proper auscultation technique as opposed to 'pearls' for diagnosing and treating CHF. This situation could contribute to creating tensions and misunderstandings within the team, cause the patient to be uncomfortable and hinder the attending physician's teaching performance. In other words, it is important to be aware of how culture may affect the meaning of the cognitive processes of different individuals in a specific context.

In culturalism, meanings are created and shaped by the culture in which they are created. Culturalism gathers insights from a number of areas, such as human sciences, linguistics and psychology to ultimately create new meaning-making activities in cultural communities.[16] Culturalism has two dimensions: one dimension looks at the culture as system of values and opportunities (or affordances, see the chapter by Billett and Sweet in this book) and the other dimension entails the educational demands that the cultural setting has on the individuals within that setting. These two dimensions are interdependent. For example, the meaning of being knowledgeable in a surgical team might be different than that in a general medical team, because the meaning of the event (e.g. working in an operating room or team bedside rounds) and how the individuals should interact within the event are situated in different cultural settings. Having knowledge in the culture of a surgical environment may entail being proficient at ligating an artery in the operating room, whereas in a medical setting it might be related to the ability to develop a differential diagnosis.

Bruner emphasises the role that culture plays in making meaning within communities. The work of Lave and Wenger takes this further by relating learning through participation in *communities of practice* (CoPs).

## Lave and Wenger: learning is social and collaborative

Lave and Wenger[17] underscore the role of learning as a social, collaborative and interactive process through posing the theory of situated learning and its core component parts CoPs[18] and legitimate peripheral participation (LPP).

Learning takes place (e.g. is situated) in a CoP. In addition, members share resources (such as experiences, books) and develop relationships that lead to binding members together into a social entity. The CoP develops around mutual goals and interests over time, such as caring for the patients on a ward team as in our original example. A CoP develops methods, ideas, knowledge and practices to solve common problems in the community. Thus, COPs can become self-organised and self-sustained entities that share practices and models of approaching a problem among members.

In such CoPs, there are core members, who have more experience, are more familiar with the practices, history and culture of that community and there are more peripheral members who are newcomers to the community and who are trying to advance their learning and practice through a greater involvement in the community through LPP. In our example at the outset of this chapter, the ward resident (registrar) could be considered to be a more core member, whereas a medical student would be a more peripheral member.

LPP is an important aspect to the development of a COP. In LPP, learning involves a process of participation, and is built upon previous learning in a social context. This participation creates relationships and mutual experiences and leads to new and meaningful learning. From our initial example, LPP is manifest by the different responsibilities of the different educational 'levels' of the ward team (students, resident or registrar and the attending physician). Members within this educational hierarchy are given different patient care responsibilities. Similarly, members within a level of the hierarchy (e.g. students) are typically given increasing responsibility as they get to know the team, and are successful in their role in the care of patients on the service.

LPP explains the concept of peripherality of participation as a positive term. For example, a less-engaged individual in the group is in an empowering and active position as he/she is not disconnected from the learning process. Peripherality, therefore, is a dynamic concept, that when enabled, 'suggests an opening, a way of gaining access to sources for understanding through growing involvement'[17] (p. 37). From this perspective, effective bedside instruction on CHF requires seeing a patient with CHF, interacting with him/her and engaging in a discussion of the various manifestations of the disease. These experiences cannot be readily obtained through a lecture.

LPP is the way to become an integral part of a CoP, where learning occurs not within individual masters or experts but is rather situated in the organisation, structure and culture of a community. It is the intricate structure of the community, its resources and the interactions between these elements that provides the learning. The connection

of LPP and CoPs may be shown in this example. The team of physicians and students, described in the beginning, may constitute a community of practice (which may be part of larger CoPs, which might include the residency program or medical school). Within this community of practice, the attending physician and the resident may have a more central role while given their experience and time within the community, new group members (interns/house officers/foundation year doctors or medical students) begin to understand the practice and become part of it. In other words, it is participation in daily rounds, working and communicating with the patients, nursing staff and other parts of the healthcare team, that allows community participants to share an understanding about their practice, give meaning to their experience and become more 'central' members of the community. Participation shapes the experience, the practice and the identity of the learner. Learning about CHF requires seeing patients and participating in a community (the ward team's) care of such patients.

## Situated cognition, distributed cognition and situated learning: theory and principles

Each of these three SCTs encompasses a situation-specific social approach to understanding thinking, learning and performance. The first two theories focus on thinking (cognition), but they differ in that the theory of situated cognition, while viewing the entirety of the situation, places emphasis on individual thinking and action. On the other hand, the theory of distributed cognition places greater emphasis on group thinking and performance. Situated learning, which is sometimes confused with situated cognition, places special emphasis on learning. The readers are also encouraged to refer to chapter by Mann and colleagues on social constructivism and chapter by Artino and colleagues on self-regulation for more details about other SCT.

## Situated cognition

Situated cognition theory is based on the idea that thinking (as well as learning and performance) is situated or located in the specifics of an event. Often the specifics of the situation are divided into components or factors that are believed to interact. Thus, from this theoretical viewpoint, cognition emerges from relationships among participants (e.g. teachers, learners and patients) and relationships with specific properties of the environment.[19–23] Situated cognition theory allows for 'unification of the world, the individual and the relations among these reciprocal components'[24] (p. 360). In our introductory example, one could consider the following components for beside teaching rounds: teacher (e.g. his knowledge, experience and well-being), the learners (their sleepiness, knowledge, interest in subject and self-efficacy), the patient (e.g. her/his health literacy, education and acuity of illness) and the environment (e.g. lighting, ambient noise and space). These factors (and their component parts, some listed as 'examples' above) are believed to interact, and, from this, the outcome (e.g. learning) emerges. We will discuss this in more detail in the following sections.

Historically, situated cognition draws upon the work of leaders such as Dewey,[25] Vygotsky[26] and Greeno.[27] It shares many features with, but is arguably distinct from, situated learning, critical theory and critical discourse analysis. For the purposes of this chapter, we will discuss both situated cognition (or thinking) and situated learning, to help in terms of distinguishing between the two approaches.

In situated cognition, the primary goal of cognition (thinking) is to describe the thinking of a professional in a given context.[28] From a situated cognition perspective, thinking and learning are situated (or located) within the larger physical and social context. This theory shifts the focus from the individual participant to the social and cultural activity in which the participant interacts, and places important emphasis on these interactions. Situated cognition not only acknowledges the interplay between participants and the environment, it puts *equal emphasis* on these two components.[29] This assumption, in fact, builds upon the cognitivist approach of a participant *in* environment to participant *and* environment.[19] In addition, all individuals (and the environment) are potentially changed by this interplay. The numerous participants, social settings, cultures and interactions (and emergence of these interactions) can necessitate non-linear and/or multi-level approaches to analysing what occurs (which we will return to later in the implications section below). The focus of learning from a situated cognition perspective is on having the learner move towards expertise in authentic and potentially complex experiences. Such a learning goal is potentially useful for healthcare profession educational research, especially in situations where there are multiple participants and the activity is authentic (e.g. clinical education).

Key assumptions of situated cognition include those listed in Box 10.1. Going back to our earlier discussion of IPT, knowledge is something transferred from the teacher to the learner (e.g. a "pouring" from one mind to the other) and becomes stored in the learner's memory for use later. From a situated cognition perspective, on the other hand, knowledge is not an inert, self-sufficient, abstract, self-contained, symbolic 'substance' independent of the *situations* in which it is learnt and used. Instead, from a situated cognition perspective, knowledge is akin to a tool.[30,31] The readers may indeed have several tools in their garage that they do not know how to use (one might say that such tools are 'inert'). Using the tool helps build an increasingly rich understanding of how and when the tool use is appropriate, and further, both the tool and the world change as a result of its use. Think of how an internist and a surgeon might approach the use of a scalpel – the internist would typically tend to avoid its use and when needing to use a scalpel in the care of a patient (e.g. dermatologic procedure), tend to approach its use more slowly and perhaps timidly while the surgeon's use of the scalpel is second nature. As another example, consider a stethoscope's use in a clinic as opposed to a busy and noisy emergency room situation. In other words, the tool, the participant(s) using the tool, the environment, the specific context and the culture are all *interdependent* – situated cognition would argue that one cannot meaningfully understand one of these components without understanding the others; they are situated. Thus, knowledge is a tool applied in certain circumstances or situations as opposed to an abstract object existing in the mind of the individual.

An example of the use of situated cognition in healthcare profession education entails exploring context specificity. Context specificity refers to how a physician can see two patients with the same chief complaint, essentially the same (or identical) history and physical and have the same diagnosis and yet the physician comes to two different diagnostic conclusions. Clearly something other than content (the facts) is driving the decision. By using the theoretical framework of situated cognition, one is able design experiments that look at more than the facts and also how the participants interact (physician and patient) with the environment. Indeed, the work of Durning and colleagues has demonstrated that the environment (or context) matters – performance is based on more than acquisition of facts and has provided some rationale for why variation in physician performance occurs from a situated cognition perspective.[32–34] This theoretical framework has helped with proposing mechanisms (such as cognitive load) through which these dynamic interactions and subsequent performance emerge.[32–34]

---

### BOX 10.1  Situated cognition key assumptions

- Human thinking is situated in and shaped by the environment
- The actions of individuals and the context in which they operate are not separable
- Knowledge is a tool (vs. a static object) that is accrued through lived practices and engagement
- Performance emerges through interactions between participants and the environment
- Situated cognition puts equal emphasis on the importance of participants and the environment in a situation

---

## Distributed cognition

The second social cognitive theory is distributed cognition. Distributed cognition seeks to understand 'the organisation of cognitive systems'[35] (p. 175) as opposed to individuals. Distributed cognition extends beyond the cognition of the individual 'to encompass interactions between people and resources and material in the environment'[35] (p. 175).

Distributed cognition rests on two basic theoretical principles. First, as opposed to the traditional views of cognition where the unit of analysis is the individual's thinking, here the unit of analysis is the entire system. This system is comprised of (numerous) individuals and the environment in which they operate and perform. For example, in an airline cockpit, the pilots and the artefacts (information) in the environment represented by the cockpit instrumentation constitute the unit of analysis as opposed to an individual pilot. Similarly, in our bedside rounds example, the unit of analysis would be each individual team member, the patient and the environment or artefacts provided by the specific social setting. Besides the individual cognitive properties of each individual pilot (or ward team member), there is therefore a new, larger cognitive unit of analysis, consisting of the pilots (ward team) and the instrumentation together, whose cognitive properties are crucial to fly the plane (or care for a patient with CHF).

The cognitive process that occurs in a distributed cognition system is created by a number of functional relationships among its elements. For example, the dynamic process that occurs in an airline cockpit involves interaction and coordination of a number of subsystems that allow accomplishing a number of functions. There is a pattern of cooperation and coordination of actions among a cockpit fly crew that is considered at one level as a structure for propagating and processing information and at another level as an activity system in which shared cognition emerges.[36] In a similar way, consider the interactions and coordination among the team members, the patient and the ward room that allow the accomplishment of learning and patient care.

Second, in distributed cognition, there is a broader range of mechanisms that occur, compared to individual cognitive events. For example, in our bedside teaching example of the attending residents and students, there is a rich interaction among the internal cognitive processes of each member. Not all the cognitive processes occur in the brain of any one individual; there are cognitive processes that take place and are unique to the cognitive processes of a system or a group of individuals. As another example, the administration of a medication to a patient entails the physician ordering the medication, clarified by a pharmacist and then administered by a nurse. Each of these individuals will utilise areas of knowledge, and 'an implicit understanding to transform, interpret and act on the order, ultimately resulting in administration of medication to the patient'[37] (p. 540). Thus, distributed cognition deals with the cognitive activities of a system rather than with those of an individual. In this model, cognition is better understood as a social phenomenon as opposed to one localised at the individual level.[38]

The concept of distributed cognition may involve three kinds of distribution of cognitive processes:
- Cognitive processes that may be distributed among members of a group (for example, the diverse cognitive properties of each member of the medical team described in the vignette).
- Cognitive processes distributed in such a way that involves the coordination between members of the medical team and the surrounding environment (for example, the medical team making a decision and entering an order in the electronic medical record, or the medical team working in the emergency room while admitting a patient or conducting bedside rounds).
- Cognitive processes that may be 'distributed through time in such a way that the products of earlier events can transform the nature of later

events'[35] (p. 1) (for example, the cognitive actions performed by the medical team about the choice of a treatment plan at admission for a patient with CHF that results in subsequent actions based on the outcome of the treatment implemented).

Distributed cognition takes advantage of the cognitive diversity of individuals which allows, though interaction, the pulling together a variety of cognitive resources that may be needed to accomplish complex tasks. An example from Hutchins[38] is related to the cognitive processes that occur when steering a ship into a harbour. The distributed cognition approach needed to coordinate and analyse this task stems from the interactions among all the different components of the system. This includes individual members of the navigation team with different levels of skills and experience, the environment in which the action is situated and the effect that time has on the sequence and coordination of thinking and performance related to the event. It is the coordination and interaction of the diverse cognitive abilities of each individual that allows successful completion of a challenging task, such as steering a large ship into a harbour. In addition, there is an emphasis on the situated distribution of cognition across individuals, within a context, and over time.

## Situated learning

The third and final theory of social cognition introduced in this chapter is situated learning. Situated learning is characterised by grounding of learning in real experiences of daily living (e.g. situated), creating opportunities for learners to live and learn in the contexts where experiences occur. Knowledge is situational and is the result of a social process and is connected to the social texture, culture and environment in which it takes place.[39,40]

Lave and Wenger[17] emphasise the role of social interactions and participation as key components of the learning process, identifying communities as the ground to share knowledge, reflect and engage in dialogue and practice. Learning is not only situated in a context, but becomes a socio-generative phenomenon that occurs in complex social situations.[17] In other words, social interaction takes a predominant role where the individual becomes part of a community of practice in which the culture and beliefs of the group shape the learning process of newcomers so that the learner moves from a peripheral role in terms of participation towards a more central role and thus from a beginner to a more expert member. This also applies to our ward attending physician and residents in our bedside teaching example, where learning entails participation, is situated at the bedside with a patient with the condition to be learnt and occurs in the social context created by students, residents, patient and attending at the bedside.

Taken further, the individual becomes a potential member of the community, and as he/she continues to engage in the community's educational discourses and activities, he/she will eventually become a more central member of the community. According to the theoretical principles of LPP, learner's participation provides legitimacy and contributes to create a powerful and credible learning position of engagement within the group, creating opportunities for learning. It is by becoming a member and by participation, that learning takes place. Involvement and participation in activities will influence social relations thereby enhancing knowledge and understanding by new group members, allowing them to move to full participation, which when coupled with increased identity and motivation creates learning. For example, the students at the bedside will engage in the discussion about the patient, will ask questions and enhance their understanding about CHF for that particular patient. They will read about the disease and begin practicing manoeuvres to elicit physical findings; in the next session, they may bring to the group new evidence from the literature, bring to the attention of the resident or faculty possible changes in the patient's physical examination and report and interpret pertinent laboratory values or imaging, thus assuming a more credible role within the group. As time progresses, students may begin developing stronger social ties among themselves, not only in the setting of the patient encounter but also outside during informal discussions about other clinical issues or patients in the hospital. They will begin to develop a sense of legitimacy as members of the team, with a greater sense of identity, and develop new motivations to continue to grow within the group moving their participation to a more central position. Through the process of LPP, knowledge can, in fact, be seen as identity as opposed to acquisition of static symbols. This distinction has important implications that we will discuss further in the implications section.

## Examples of applying SCT in healthcare profession education

The components of social cognitive theory serve as a catalyst for a number of potential applications in healthcare profession education: self-efficacy in the setting of health promotion, cognitive apprenticeship as form of participation, situated cognition as a way to diagnose a social situation, distributed cognition in educational methods and in the workplace involving groups and the strategic development of CoPs in medical education. These are discussed as follows:

## Cognitive apprenticeship

Lave and Wenger[17] describe a model where novices gain entry into a community of practice through LPP. As one engages and participates, his/her position in the community becomes more central (increasing responsibility) while the community continues to shape the activity as a whole. From a situated learning perspective, such a cognitive apprenticeship (a term put forth by other theoretical frameworks) is no longer leaning by solely observing the teacher; the novice gains experience by observing and then doing and as proficiency is demonstrated more responsibility within the community is given. Furthermore, the community member learns how to think and recount the job by being engaged in a continuous process of participation that the individual both shapes and is shaped by as they practice within the community. Therefore, in a ward team comprised of students, residents and faculty, the students begin to learn by observing and performing certain limited tasks (much like tailors or butchers[17], refs) and then, as they gain experience and legitimacy in the community, they move to think about patient care with increasingly greater levels of participation as the ward team allows; the individual both shapes and is shaped by their team. Soon, the students find themselves embedded into the social interactions of the team, the culture of the team and the hospital, and further increase their level of participation.[41]

## Self-efficacy

One of the best ways to enhance self-efficacy is performance attainment. For example, the ability of a patient, who had heart surgery for coronary artery disease, to achieve a certain target on a treadmill is a powerful way to enhance self-efficacy via achievement of performance.[42] Vicarious performance[43] can also be a way to enhance self-efficacy yet is believed to be less powerful than independent performance of the activity. Vicarious performance can be used when the patient cannot perform the activity independently – observation of another patient who had a similar heart procedure being able to exercise on a treadmill may be very effective to motivating a patient to achieve this goal for himself. Similarly, a student who has difficulty auscultating a cardiac gallop may benefit from observing the resident do this. In addition, from a self-efficacy argument, the student who has success with taking a history and carrying out a physical examination on his/her own may be more likely to provide a differential diagnosis without prompting from a teacher with subsequent encounters – this continued success and feedback from the ward team could progress to providing management steps for patient care. Such a framework for viewing performance of learners and how we can enhance their progressive independence has implications for the learning environment, which is receiving attention in residency (registrar) education.

Beliefs about personal self-efficacy can affect health promotion and heath behaviours. A high sense of personal efficacy can exert influence over health habits and in particular can help individuals regulate their own motivation and behaviour in order to affect change. The stronger the perceived self-efficacy the greater the achievement in change of health habits and health outcomes in several studies. These beneficial effects have been shown in several areas, including coping with a terminal illness,[44] adherence to immunosuppressive medications in patients with rheumatoid arthritis[45] or self-management of diabetes.[46]

## Communities of practice

A CoPs framework may provide a useful lens to facilitating performance in complex systems such as residency and fellowship education, which are made of many interconnected parts. Green *et al.* describe the effort of an internal medicine community of practice to develop a framework based on ACGME competencies of developmental milestones.[47] In addition, a community of practice can be created to foster research skills in medical students. MacDougal and Riley[48] gathered information from research supervisors about identifying key factors in the creation of a CoP among students involved in research during their undergraduate medical school curriculum. Supervisors reported that connecting students with others and fostering self-efficacy in research skills were critical in initiating students into a CoP, where research skills and the practice of research were the main 'craft' of that community along with the culture, the activities, the social interactions and the environment of that community. Thus, mutual engagement, participation and mutual accountability are essential for the integration of students into such CoPs.

Another application of CoPs relates to the use of technology to support and sustain such CoPs. As stated earlier, LPP is a concept closely related to CoPs, and educators should be familiar with LPP, conveying the notion and meaning of LPP and its relationship with CoP in both live and asynchronous settings. Technology can help in communication and sharing of information to advance practice. Hoadley and Kilner[49] identified four techniques by which technology can support these communities: linking members who share similar practice, providing access to a common repository of information, supporting synchronous and asynchronous conversations within the community and providing the context of shared information resources. For example, educators and students with different levels of experience from different institutions can connect, communicate and learn from each other about shared practices through the use of technology. Technology can help shape the CoP in which knowledge is utilised by groups in shared practices.

It is important for educators to understand and clarify the concept of peripherality to a newly formed group. From an SCT perspective, it is essential that students begin to understand that learning entails are becoming a more central participant of the group, regardless of if the group meets face to face or asynchronously through technology – and engaging is the way to 'evolve in membership'.[17] (p. 53) Additionally, novice learner (new group member) needs to understand that an initial partial participation within group activities does not mean that the individual is disconnected or not engaged in the group. Rather this just represents the beginning process of growing involvement in the community. Educators should foster the concept that learning is in the relationships that are created among people, and hence implement activities that lead group members to move from peripherality to a more central participation. It is also important for educators to underscore that peripherality is a positive term, and it signifies active participation in the learning process. Learners should be made aware that they are relevant and important to the group even though they may feel they are not.

## Assessing authentic social situations

SCTs argue that interactions can be non-linear (they emerge, or evolve, and are dynamic). This raises concerns with using quantitative methodologies and standard statistical methods for SCT healthcare profession research as these assume that the results will approximate a straight line (linearity). For example, designing a bedside rounds 'intervention', where the only outcome assessed is knowledge (via, for example a multiple choice question [MCQ] format) and the only process measure also involves an MCQ (perhaps along the lines of did you enjoy the teaching or did it meet your learning needs), assumes that the other components that go into bedside rounds (the team, their resources, etc.) either do not impact the outcome or do so in a linear means (which could be assessed by a correlation coefficient or a linear regression analysis). What SCT would argue is that while a correlation may (or may not) exist, the investigator is potentially missing out on the use of a lot of potentially meaningful information by simply correlating pre- and post-bedside teaching MCQ performance. Furthermore, the relationship may be other than a straight line, particularly when there are multiple participants and the environment (setting) is variable.

This assessment problem can be addressed by several means. Firstly, using mixed methods approaches (see Chapter 1 for more on this approach). Secondly, consider alternate quantitative methods (non-linear regression, hierarchical linear modelling and structural equation modelling (SEM) to name a few alternatives if one wanted to get a sense of how different variables interact in bedside rounds for the purposes of assessment) and also consider interview or observation data. For example, by interviewing members of the team and/or making observations of the environment, one would glean additional information that may be valuable in determining if bedside rounds improve learning. This approach would also enable the investigator to explore the learning process, which would be missed by simply looking at the presence (or absence) of a linear association. We believe that qualitative methods can be particularly useful as, apart from not assuming linearity, they enable exploration of interactions between participants as well as between participants and the environment.

## Situated cognition as a way to diagnose and treat social situation

Situated cognition provides a potential method to *diagnose* what is potentially going wrong with the teaching or clinical setting. In essence, it provides a different lens or solution to informing what may have gone awry. Returning to our initial scenario, a less than optimal clinical encounter can be dissected using the factors and their component parts. It can also provide a potential way to 'treat' a less than optimal teaching or clinical situation through a number of "what if" scenarios . Returning to our previous examples, this theory can help with 'treating' a number of 'what if' situations through a number of "what if" scenarios. What if the patient did not want medical students in the room during bedside teaching? What if the resident needed to go to continuity clinic? What if the teacher was unable to address a thoughtful question during beside rounds? Situated cognition can also propose a number of solutions to these situations such as proposes other potential means, such as asking the resident (trainee), use of the Internet in the patient's room (environment) or other solutions.

Making situated cognition and its implications explicit to the teacher and other members of the ward team could lead both to considering how the environment impacts performance and how the environment can be potentially altered to effect a more positive outcome. Understanding the potential non-linear interactions can also encourage the teacher and the learner in that a small change in one component of one factor (i.e. encouraging student self-efficacy) could lead to disproportionate positive gains – the trainee becomes more motivated, asks more questions of the teacher during beside rounds, receives more constructive feedback for improvement, and may even enjoy this type of teaching experience more (leading to additional learning gains). From an SCT perspective, such interventions could be expected to lead to large gains in learning and performance.

## Distributed cognition in group learning, technology and decision-making processes

Distributed cognition can be applied to a number of healthcare education topics: learning methods, such as problem-based learning (PBL) where the cognition is distributed among the students of the PBL group; distributed cognition to help better understand the interaction between teachers and/or students and technology; cognitive processes distributed across physicians, nurses, and other staff.

In PBL, cognitive properties of distributed cognition can be found in different steps of the PBL process: the activation of prior knowledge by each individual, the setting of objectives in relation to the problem involves the sharing as well as the coordination and interaction of each individual cognitive property with the context in which they operate. The self-directed study part followed by the report to the group is another activity where the individuals bring to the group their own knowledge and skills and their own interpretations of experiences, which can contribute to create a system of distributed cognition aimed at problem solving.

Because one of the tenets of distributed cognition is that cognition is embedded in the environment and involves the coordination between internal (e.g. attention, memory) and external (e.g. objects, material) structures, technology can play an important role in a distributed cognition approach. For example, the use of Electronic Medical Records (EMR) may be important to foster coordination among team members, create automated checks for errors, share and distribute information, help in the flow of information to develop a system of distributed cognition that may ultimately enhance system-based practice and provide better care for patients. The support of technology can help identify breakdown or problems within a system of practices of an engineering company.[50,51] A similar approach could be used to examine the medical practices of a clinical and educational system (e.g. entire medical school or an intensive care unit).

## Situated knowledge and transfer

As a primary goal of learning is transfer (or application of learning to new situations), we would like to mention some distinctions between SCT and information processing theory. We will not go into great detail about this topic because it is beyond the main scope of this chapter. Studies addressing transfer have repetitively found that what is learnt in one setting may not be transferred to a different situation.[52] For example, what a trainee learns in the classroom may not be transferred to a real life on the job performance (e.g. a lecture on CHF vs a patient presenting with CHF). SCT would argue that transfer requires sufficient overlap between the initial learning situation and the practice situation. This not only entails the 'facts' needed to solve the problem, but also the environment and interactions. This may be in part why transfer has been a vexing problem from the information processing theory perspective.

## Conclusion

Social cognitive theory allows a better understanding of individual and distributed cognitive processes linked with the numerous components provided by the social context. It emphasises the importance of situatedness, or the location of thinking and learning in the specifics of a given event to include culture, the community and interactions with others and the environment.

An incalculable number of events can take place in the bedside encounter that we initially described. The cognition and learning that may occur at the bedside is very difficult to separate from the patient, the bedside environment and the participants. Being familiar with the features of SCT can therefore help educators and their learners gain a better understanding of how to think, teach and learn in such complex environment.

Future research may focus on deepening our understanding of what and how socio-cultural factors play a role in the cognitive processes that affect learning, teaching and performance in the healthcare profession. We have provided some suggestions of future directions in this chapter. We urge the need to view the component parts of the situation and their interactions to understand (and improve) learning, teaching and performance.

---

### Practice points

1 Social cognitive theories (SCTs) propose that learning and performance are social and are influenced by reciprocal interactions between persons, behaviours and environments.

2 Bandura championed SCT with his framework of triadic reciprocality – the interactions between behaviours, personal factors and the environment – which underpins many SCT.

3 A variety of theories can be grouped into SCT. Those examined in this chapter include situated learning, situated cognition and distributed cognition.

4 SCT differ from individual cognitive theories such as information processing theory through emphasising the importance of the environment and social interactions in addition to the individual (e.g. physician).

5 SCT provide a framework for understanding and to study cognitive processes that occur in various social, cultural, material and historical contexts of healthcare profession education nowadays.

---

## References

1 Kahneman, D. (2011) *Thinking, Fast and Slow*. MacmillanISBN 978-1-4299-6935-2.

2 Bandura, A. (1986) The explanatory and predictive scope of self-efficacy theory. *Journal of Clinical and Social Psychology*, **4**, 359–373.

3 Rizzolatti, G. & Craighero, L. (2004) The mirror-neuron system. *Annual Review of Neuroscience*, **27**, 169–192.

4 Eva, K. (2003) On the generality of specificity. *Medical Education*, **37**, 587–588.

5 Eva, K.W., Neville, A.J. & Norman, G.R. (1998) Exploring the etiology of content specificity: factors influencing analogic transfer and problem solving. *Academic Medicine*, **73**, S1–S5.

6 Bandura, A. (1993) Perceived self efficacy in cognitive development and functioning. *Educational Psychologist*, **28**, 117–148.

7 Bandura, A. (1997) *Self-Efficacy: The Exercise of Control*. Freeman, New York.

8 Bandura, A. (2004) Health promotion by social cognitive means. *Health Education & Behavior*, **31**, 143–164.

9 Bandura, A. & Cervone, D. (1983) Self-evaluative and self-efficacy mechanisms governing the motivational effects of goal systems. *Journal of Personality and Social Psychology*, **45**, 1017–1028.

10 Chemers, M.M., Hu, L.T. & Garcia, B.F. (2001) Academic self efficacy and first year college student performance and adjustments. *Journal of Educational Psychology*, **93**, 55.

11 Bandura, A. & Jourden, F.J. (1991) Self-regulatory mechanisms governing the impact of social comparison on complex decision making. *Journal of Personality and Social Psychology*, **60**, 941–951.

12 Bandura, A. & Wood, R.E. (1989) Effect of perceived controllability and performance standards on self-regulation of complex decision making. *Journal of Personality and Social Psychology*, **56**, 805–814.

13 Wood, R. & Bandura, A. (1989) Social cognitive theory of organizational management. *Academy of Management Review*, **14**, 361–384.

14 Bandura, A. (1995) Exercise of personal and collective efficacy in changing societies. In: Bandura, A. (ed), *Self-Efficacy in Changing Societies*. Cambridge University Press, Cambridge, pp. 1–45.

15 Bruner, J. (1990) *Acts of Meaning*. Harvard University Press, Cambridge, MA.

16 Halas, E. (2006) Classical cultural sociology: Florian Znaniecki's impact in a new light. *Journal of Classical Sociology*, **6**, 257–282.

17 Lave, J. & Wenger, E. (1991) *Situated Learning: Legitimate Peripheral Participation*. Cambridge University Press.

18 Wenger, E. (1998) *Communities of Practice: Learning, Meaning, and Identity*. Cambridge University Press, CambridgeISBN 978-0-521-66363-2.

19 Bredo, E. (1994) Reconstructing educational psychology: situated cognition and Deweyian pragmatism. *Educational Psychologist*, **29**, 23–35.

20 Clancey, W.J. (1993) Situated action: a neuropsychological interpretation. Response to Vera and Simon. *Cognitive Science*, **17**, 87–116.

21 Greeno, J.G. (1993) For research to reform education and cognitive science. In: Penner, L.A., Batsche, G.M.,

Knoff, H.M. & Nelson, D.L. (eds), *The challenges in mathematics and science education: psychology's response*. American Psychological Association, Washington, DC, pp. 153–192.

22  Lave, J. (1997) The culture of acquisition and the practice of understanding. In: Kirshner, D. & Whitson, A. (eds), *Situated Cognition: Social, Semiotic and Psychological Perspectives*. Cambridge University Press, New York, NY, pp. 17–36.

23  Young, M.F., Barab, S.A. & Garrett, S. (2000) Agent as detector: an ecological psychology perspective on learning by perceiving-acting systems. In: Jonassen, D. & Land, S.M. (eds), *Theoretical Foundations of Learning Environments*. Earlbaum, Mahwah, NJ, pp. 147–173.

24  Barab, S.A., Cherkes-Julkowski, M., Swenson, R., Garrett, S., Shaw, R.E. & Young, M. (1999) Principles of self-organization: ecologizing the learner-facilitator system. *The Journal of Learning Sciences*, **8**, 349–390.

25  Dewey, J. (1938) *Logic: The Theory of Inquiry*. Henry Holt, New York.

26  Vygotsky, L. (1978) *Mind in Society: The Development of Higher Psychological Processes*. Harvard University Press, Cambridge, MA.

27  Greeno, J.G. (1997) Response: on claims that answer the wrong questions. *Educational Researcher*, **26**, 5–17.

28  Brown, J.S., Collins, A. & Duguid, P. (1989) Situated cognition and the culture of learning. *Educational Researcher*, **18**, 32–42.

29  Young, M.F. (1993) Instructional design for situated learning. *Educational Technology Research and Development*, **41**, 43–53.

30  Whitehead, A.N. (1929) *The aims of education*. Cambridge University Press, Cambridge.

31  Durning, S.J. & Artino, A.R. (2011) Situativity theory: a perspective on how participants and the environment can interact. *Medical Teacher*, **33**, 188–199.

32  Durning, S.J., Artino, A.R., van der Vleuten, C. & Schuwirth, L. (2013) Clarifying assumptions to enhance our understanding and assessment of clinical reasoning. *Academic Medicine*, **88**, 442–448.

33  Durning, S.J., Artino, A.R. Jr,, Pangaro, L., Van der Vleuten, C.P.M. & Schuwirth, L.W.T. (2011) Context and clinical reasoning: understanding the perspective of the expert's voice. *Medical Education*, **45**, 927–938.

34  Durning, S.J., Artino, A.R., Boulet, J., Dorrance, K., van der Vleuten, C. & Schuwirth, L. (2012) The impact of selected contextual factors on experts' clinical reasoning performance. *Advances in Health Science Education*, **17**, 65–79.

35  Hutchins, E. (2000) *Distributed Cognition. International Encyclopedia of the Social and Behavioral Sciences*. Elsevier Science.

36  Hutchins, E. & Klausen, T. (1996) Distributed cognition in an airline cockpit. In: Middleton, D. & Engeström, Y. (eds), *Communication and Cognition at Work*. Cambridge University Press, Cambridge.

37  Hazlehurst, B., McMullen, C.K. & Gorman, P.N. (2007) Distributed cognition in the heart room: how situation awareness arises from coordinated communications in the heart room. *Journal of Biomedical Informatics*, **40**, 539–551.

38  Hutchins, E. (1995) *Cognition in the Wild*. MIT Press, Cambridge, MA.

39  Anderson, J.R., Reder, L.M. & Simon, H.A. (1996) Situated learning and education. *Educational Researcher*, **25**, 5–11.

40  Wilson, A. (1993) The promise of situated cognition. In: Merriam, S.B. (ed), *An Update on Adult Learning Theory*. Jossey-Bass, San Francisco, pp. 71–79.

41  Bleakley, A. (2006) Broadening conception of learning in medical education: the message from team working. *Medical Education*, **40**, 150–157.

42  Bastone, E.C. & Kerns, R.D. (1995) Effects of self-efficacy and perceived social support on recovery-related behaviors after coronary artery bypass graft surgery. *Annals of Behavioral Medicine*, **17**, 324–330.

43  Bandura, A. (1998) Health promotion from the perspective of social cognitive theory. *Psychology and Health*, **13**, 623–649.

44  Beckham, J.C., Burker, E.J., Lytle, B.L., Feldman, M.E. & Costakis, M.J. (1997) Self-efficacy and adjustment in cancer patients: a preliminary report. *Behavioral Medicine*, **23**, 137–142.

45  Brus, H., vandeLaar, M., Taal, E., Rasker, J. & Wiegman, O. (1999) Determinants of compliance with medication in patients with rheumatoid arthritis: the importance of self-efficacy expectations. *Patient Education and Counseling*, **36**, 57–64.

46  Hurley, C.C. & Shea, C.A. (1992) Self-efficacy: strategy for enhancing diabetes self-care. *The Diabetes Educator*, **18**, 146–150.

47  Green, M.L., Aagaard, E.M., Caverzagie, K.J. *et al.* (2009) Charting the road to competence: developmental milestones for internal medicine residency training. *Journal of Graduate Medical Education*, **1**, 5–20.

48  MacDougall, M. & Riley, S.C. (2010) Initiating undergraduate medical students into communities of research practise: what do supervisors recommend? *BMC Medical Education*, **10**, 83.

49  Hoadley, C. & Kilner, P.G. (2005) Using technology to transform communities of practices into knowledge building communities. *SIGGROUP Bulletin*, **25**, 31–40.

50  Rogers, Y. (1992) Ghosts in the network: distributed troubleshooting in a shared working environment. In: J. Turner and R. Kraut (eds), *Proceedings of the Conference on Computer-Supported Cooperative Work*, 346–355. ACM, New York.

51  Rogers, Y. (1993) Coordinating computer-mediated work. *Computer-Supported Cooperative Work*, **1**, 295–315.

52  Mayer, R.E. (1987) The elusive search for teachable aspects of problem solving. In: Glover, J.A. & Ronning, R.R. (eds), *Historical Foundations of Educational Psychology*. Plenum, New York, pp. 327–348.

# 11 Participatory practices at work: Understanding and appraising healthcare students' learning through workplace experiences

*Stephen Billett and Linda Sweet*

*Ben (a third-year medical student) explained his experience of workplace-based learning: 'it's very variable … you go to different wards, different people, it will be very different. … going across the different sort of areas, whether in medicine or surgery; and then within those disciplines you have variability … as to what they expect from you in terms of the learning they give to you'. He identified one discipline rotation, paediatrics, as exemplary: ' … the learning environment, their attitude towards students is very friendly and very supportive and I found that … all the students seem to be happier; all the students want to learn more because of that'. While another discipline rotation, surgery, was much less invitational: they 'didn't "play" well with any of the students, …, no one [students] was very happy to be going in the mornings, they were worried they were going to get shot down for silly things … so during ward rounds you'd sort of be in the background'. However, he goes on to say, there 'are always exceptions. Occasionally you get one who is very good with students, is able to teach and has that passion for teaching. They're the ones that get you through. It's a bit of a strange – it's a very unique kind of dynamic in medicine that I hadn't sort of thought about before'.*

## Introduction

Given the extent of resources directed to healthcare professional education, it is essential to understand how learning to be a healthcare professional arises, so that those education processes can be optimised. In this chapter, one aspect of that learning is given attention: students' learning through healthcare practice, or how students learn in workplaces. Drawing on findings from studies of medical and midwifery students, we outline how these invitational qualities of physical and social circumstances

can be understood in terms of 'affordances' and how learning is dependant in terms of 'engagement' or rather than on how students engage with what is afforded to them. Understanding these practices might help make healthcare students' educational experiences more effective. By the end of this chapter, the reader will be able to:

- Conceptualise learning through work as a relational interdependence of affordances and engagement.
- Evaluate how the social world and its norms, forms and practices influence and is influenced by learning.
- Identify how their and the learning of others in work settings can be understood in terms of affordances and engagements.
- Apply these concepts to curriculum development and educational research.

## Key conceptions, definitions and distinctions

Participatory practices refers to the duality between what is afforded by the social institutions in which individuals participate on the one hand, and how individuals elect to engage in, and learn through those practices.[1] Learners' engagement is premised upon their interest, intentions and capacities, and how they value what is afforded them. What constitutes an affordance is not objective or fixed. Instead, affordances are subject to their projection (i.e. how they are suggested by the social world as norms, form and practices) and the degree to which individuals engage with them. In other words, there is no guarantee that the 'same' invitation to participate is engaged with in the same way by different learners.

*Researching Medical Education*, First Edition. Edited by Jennifer Cleland and Steven J. Durning.
© 2015 John Wiley & Sons, Ltd. Published 2015 by John Wiley & Sons, Ltd.

What is encountered in a healthcare professional educational program may well be construed quite differently, and with distinct kinds of learning arising from them, for different people, depending on factors such as individuals' capacities, subjectivities and agency, all of which shape how people interpret and engage with what they experience (e.g.[1,2]). Those invitations (i.e. affordances) can variously be welcoming and engaging, or restrictive, resisting or excluding individuals' participation. Those experiences perceived to be uninviting can lead students to not participate fully. They might 'hover in the background' or 'go to the library for independent study', while positive invitations can encourage student engagement. What one student might perceive as being helpful supervision, another might view as interference, with both learning different aspects from those experiences accordingly. Similarly, a lack of close supervision might be seen as abandonment by one person, but an opportunity to practice independently by another. Therefore, the perceiving of and engaging with what is afforded is, in part, premised on personal bases and factors. On the other hand, workplaces have particular practices and accordingly afford particular experiences, which individuals must engage with, to enact and sustain those practices and transform them as/when circumstances change.[3]

One reason for emphasising this interdependence, and its relational qualities, is that much of the contemporary conceptualisations about learning and occupations tend to privilege the contributions to learning afforded by the immediate physical and social environment in which students come to think and act, over the contribution of the individual. These have predominated through conceptions such as communities of practice,[4] situated cognition,[5] activity systems[6] and distributed cognition.[7] Such a privileging also has antecedents within early forms of ecological psychology that viewed physical and social circumstances such as hospitals as behavioural settings.[8,9] Behaviour (and learning) in these settings was shaped – and some would suggest – determined by the particular contributions of the environment. However, other perspectives, such as those from cultural psychology,[10] hold that greater reciprocity of contributions is central to understanding processes of human learning and development. There is interdependence between social institutions and the knowledge they generate, and individuals taking up, using and extending this knowledge, thereby sustaining and developing further those institutions. By this we mean that hospitals, for example,

provide a place for occupations such as medicine and midwifery to be enacted, thereby allowing doctors and other healthcare professionals to practice their occupation; develop their competences or capacities further and establish, maintain and develop their occupational identities. Through this enactment, the social practice of medicine is progressed, whereby the practice of medicine is a social action between an individual practitioner and others. In other words, there is interdependence between social institutions and individuals – a relational interdependence between those personal (i.e. participation) and situational factors and contributions. Indeed, the existence and continuity of social institutions (e.g. hospitals) or socially derived practices (e.g. medical work), and how they evolve over time, are premised upon individuals' engagement in remaking and transforming occupational practice through their work. Put simply, what a person learns from a workplace is determined not only by the nature of the workplace but also by the nature of the person. Furthermore, the learning of the person contributes back to the development of that workplace. These factors should not be considered in isolation.

What constitutes medical or midwifery practice (for example) requires the active engagement, remaking and transformation (i.e. change) of that practice which can be brought about by individuals' engagements with them. These processes cannot, and will not be enacted in similar ways by individuals, because what is suggested by the social world is never without ambivalence or lack of clarity, or even uniformly projected.[11] Therefore, how individuals come to construe and construct what they experience is, by degree, the product of individuals' own unique personal histories.[2] Those unique histories arise through the particular sets of experiences that individuals have encountered, and their experiencing of them (i.e. what they have learnt through them). This notion of personal epistemology is described in more detail in Box 11.1 (see also MacMillan, and Mann and Macleod earlier in this book).

For example, when two midwifery students, Mary and Joanne (pseudonyms), faced the impending birth of a baby, their sense-making of the experience varied based on their own personal histories. Mary was a mother herself and had given birth naturally to two babies; she was able to empathise with and support the woman in labour through her painful contractions. She understood the importance and value of the painful contractions for the natural birth process. However, Joanne had never seen or experienced a baby being born, but had experienced severe kidney pain in her life, and hence found herself conflicted by the pain the woman was experiencing. She wanted to provide pain relief as she did not know how to help in other ways. From this affordance, Joanne construed the pain of labour to be an undesirable experience to be overcome through pharmaceutical means. Through these examples of learning in workplace settings, it is possible to see that the concept of participatory practices[12] has been advanced as way of capturing these dual and relational contributions of affordances and engagement.

---

### BOX 11.1   Personal epistemologies

Central to understanding the ways in which individuals engage and learn is the concept of personal epistemologies – the bases and ways by which individuals come to construe and construct knowledge from what they experience.[13] These epistemologies include learners' intentionalities, interests and capacities. There can be no certainty that an experience, which is the product of social suggestions (i.e. norms, forms and practices), will generate a uniform response or outcome from those experiencing it. For instance, in one study, many medical students reported finding the clinical experience with orthopaedic surgeons to be confronting, difficult and personally demeaning.[14] Most reported that it was as if these surgeons wanted to make life difficult for the students, and to dissuade them from considering surgery as a line of specialisation. However, there was one student – a mature female – who, while reporting that the surgical environment could potentially be difficult, noted that not all students were adequately prepared, careful nor considered in their engagement in that environment and with those particular practitioners (the surgeons). Therefore, while there was evidence of a common or potentially objective experience, it was not uniform across the student cohort. This illustrates that it is the interplay between the suggestions of the social world (its affordances) and individuals' engagement with these, which is central to understanding learning in clinical practice.

---

Drawing on interview data from Australian medical and midwifery students, the concept of participatory practice is used to appraise the processes of entering an education program, learning through participating in that program and the kinds of learning arising through clinical experiences. Some of the students' experiences and accounts of the consequences of these experiences for their learning are elaborated in this chapter, interpreted through the lens of participatory practice. We start by outlining the salience of healthcare students learning through clinical work.

## Learning through clinical practice

Healthcare education has always included extensive periods of clinical practice.[15,16] Indeed, practice-based experiences have long been the basis of learning medicine and midwifery within Western traditions. As far back as Hellenic Greece medical students were positioned as assistants who would care for patients[17] and learn through an apprenticeship model.[18] These clinical experiences are not only central to initial preparation of healthcare professionals, but also in assisting them identify the specialisation they would pursue and their preparation for that specialisation.[19]

Most, if not all, of the knowledge required for medicine and midwifery arises from the social world (history, culture, interactions between people, etc.) and how this is manifested in the specific requirements of a particular healthcare setting.[20] Consequently, acquiring this knowledge requires engagement with socially derived sources beyond the individual, such as exposure to and engagement with norms, forms and practices. The norms, forms and practices come via texts, such as policies and practice guidelines; behaviours of experts, other practitioners and students (e.g. how tasks are distributed) and through communication patterns and handover (hand-off) of care. It is the contribution of these norms, forms and practices that can make accessible the occupational knowledge a novice has to acquire via observation, imitation and practice (referred to as mimetic learning,[21]). Much of the explanations about the contributions of norms, forms and practices arise from them being seen as institutional or social facts[22] and derived from disciplines (e.g. medicine or midwifery) whose starting point is the social world and its contributions, and include the particular circumstances (e.g. patients, conditions and facilities) and participatory practices (i.e. activities and interactions). The contributions of social partners, forms and norms that together comprise the suggestions or affordances of the social world are important and essential to explain the experiencing and learning of canonical knowledge (i.e. that knowledge all medical practitioners would be expected to possess). However, it is also important to access the particular circumstances in which this knowledge is practised to understand, and value how it is enacted.

These premises have, more broadly, led to theorising about the contributions to an individual's learning from the particular kinds of activities and interactions provided by educational programs and partners. Hence, considerations of these contributions and how individuals can access and engage with them have become a focus for improving educational practices, and in particular the importance of practice-based experiences.[23,24] This is linked with an increased emphasis on quality assurance throughout healthcare education over the last two decades or so.[25,26]

Workplace-based affordances can comprise the opportunity to engage in practice experiences (e.g. ward rounds, bedside teaching, clinical experiences, meetings with experts and other students) but can also be encouraging or inhibiting of access to the kinds of knowledge required for work. In other words, they can comprise welcoming affordances or conversely efforts to exclude and marginalise learners, and they can play out relationally in person-dependant ways. Individual characteristics such as gender, class and ethnicity may play roles in the opportunities afforded to medical students[27] but other bases of engagement are those associated with how individuals elect to take up the invitation(s) that is afforded them.[14] That engagement might amount variously as wholehearted engagement, or being selective with engagement, or a decision not to participate or to do so in superficial ways to meet the needs of compliance (such as attending a lecture because attendance was compulsory but spending the session checking email).

Wertsch[28] has noted the difference between different types of engagement, which he refers to as mastery and appropriation. 'Mastery', used in this context, refers to mastery of a skill or task without appropriating it into one's professional identity and self (see also chapter by Monrouxe and Rees). In his construct, mastery is a process of engaging superficially to meet the demands of others, while not believing or agreeing that such demands are worthwhile, thereby leading to outcomes (i.e. learning) that are superficial and would not be exercised outside of circumstances of close supervision. Appropriation, on the other hand, is the effortful engagement by individuals, because what is being experienced or suggested is taken to be important and worthwhile. Wertsch's[28] construct

of appropriation refers to acceptance, appropriation and even embodiment of a skill or task into one's professional identity and self. Engagement, which results in appropriation and accepted internalisation by learners, is likely to lead to more focused learning outcomes because it is underpinned by personal commitment. The example of handwashing is illustrative here. The healthcare workers who have appropriated the importance of regular and thorough handwashing are more likely to engage in this task, and in ways not requiring reminders or monitoring. However, workers who do not really believe it are important – who have mastered (but not appropriated) the requirement to wash their hands may be less likely to do so unless they are being prompted and monitored. Therefore, it is individuals who elect whether they engage in mastery or appropriation, based upon what they know, can do and value, with distinct and personally premised consequences for their decision making and learning.

Note that both mastery and appropriation are potentially productive or limiting. An individual might well participate in the mastery of something which is important and worthwhile, even though it may not be evident to the learner at that point in his/her occupational development (e.g. handwashing). Alternatively, a person might engage in the appropriation of knowledge that is flawed and begin to base his/her practice on incorrect assumptions (e.g. handwashing obviates the need for other preventative measures).

These conceptions are now used to illuminate and explain the processes of healthcare students' experiences in clinical settings.

## Investigating healthcare students' participatory practices

The data described and analysed in the following were secured as part of two qualitative projects that captured data about medical and midwifery students' perceptions of their learning experiences and outcomes, and bases for their engagement in their program. Qualitative philosophies, study designs and data collection methods (see chapter by Cleland) were adopted to explore students' motivations, actions and strategies in relation to particular aspects of learning, and to engage with students' narratives to secure validated knowledge of their experiences and learning. Ethical approval for both studies was secured from the host university.

## Case study 1: Medical students' experiences of learning in clinical environments

Medical students completing their third year of a 4-year graduate entry program comprised one study population.[14] In this program, students select one of three models of clinical education for their third of the 4-year program (i.e. 1st clinical year of study). These are: (1) the traditional hospital-based block model, (2) the rural longitudinal integrated curriculum model predominantly in general practice or (3) a hybrid model of these two models. Students progressing through the first and second models were invited to participate in a semi-structured individual face-to-face interview at the end of the year. Of the 13 students consented to take part in the study, 8 informants were in the hospital-based block model and 5 were in the rural longitudinal model.

We present a narrative from one of the medical students (called Sue) who chose to study in the rural longitudinal model and augment these with data from other informants, as a means of presenting and discussing an explanation of the medical students' experiences of learning. The other informants are Jim, a student who chose the teaching hospital-based model of medical education, largely because of family commitments, and Gil, a Canadian student who preferred the longitudinal rural model, but as an international student was excluded from this option, so he undertook the hospital-based block model.

### Clinical experiences and learning

The medical students described their choice of clinical placement model for their third-year program. Sue's preference for her third-year program was to undertake a year-long placement in a rural area, referred to here as Creekland. She was 'absolutely thrilled' to secure this placement. First, she was familiar with the area having undertaken some work experience there at the end of her first year of medical studies, and found working with a rural doctor to be a very positive experience. This earlier, positive experience prompted her to select the year-long program designed to provide students with clinical experiences in regional and rural settings; she concluded that 'it would just be a really good area and the program has been running for 10 years'. Therefore, her response to securing this placement was that this 'would be a really good opportunity'. Evident in this medical education option is a set of institutional arrangements – general practice-based education for one rather than 1 year – afforded to (only some) medical students. Sue did not have to organise, sponsor or fund her way through these experiences. There was a planned provision of educational experiences, as well as accommodation and educational support available locally. Therefore, the institutional affordances were substantial and inviting. Furthermore, Sue demonstrated receptiveness to these affordances. Jim, on the other hand, had had to sell his house to fund his medical studies, and did not want to ask his wife to make the additional sacrifice of moving away from where she was employed to undertake a rural opportunity. Therefore, he had a more restricted set of options – based in the state capital. What was a positive affordance for Sue as a single woman was not possible for Jim with his family commitments. Gil, who was from Canada, also wanted to secure a rural placement. However, as an international student he was ineligible to take up this option due to its funding arrangements.

Sue reported engaging in her new setting enthusiastically (rather than, for example, as somebody who was reluctantly accepting such a placement). She reported engaging actively in and appropriated what she experienced. Her placement or rotation was busy, with each week 'split up into our consulting time in the general practice and sitting with different specialists in the region', either in the local hospital or based in the community. Sue would also be 'on call' one week out of every three and one night every week. Then, there was a formal study day every week focused on problem-based learning, clinical skills teaching and time in the simulation laboratory. There were also tutorials with the general practice supervisor and any available visiting specialists. She had to prepare for this formal teaching and read recent cases in her own time, and hence the typical week was busy, but well organised. Sue also reported engaging with the local community by attending the church service every Sunday morning (which provided her with 'an excellent opportunity to meet people in the community and some of the doctors from my clinic also attended there') and joining the tennis club ('and played for the rest of the summer season, which was a lot of fun'). In this way, she met a range of people from the healthcare community and came to engage in a different way with community members. The duality of participatory practice is evident. On the one hand, there is the intentional provision of experiences for learning, which is supported by institutions, other professionals and her assigned supervisors. On the other hand, there is how Sue has participated intentionally and actively engaging with both the workplace and community. In other circumstances and for other individuals, the affordances may not have been so great, but equally others may have elected not to participate in the ways that Sue did.

The affordances of the rural clinical experience program and Sue's engagement with it provide positive instances of participatory practices. On the one hand, a range of experiences was made available for her, and arrangements were made to organise and promote her engagement and learning. The experiences that she had access to were highly invitational, and structured to ease her taking them up. Sue elected to engage with what was offered to her fully and enthusiastically. Mimetic learning (see earlier) in Sue's case involved the ability to observe and participate (i.e. 'sit in') with GPs and specialists engaging in their practice, following their cases, which is likely to be highly effective for understanding the goals from medical work, and many procedural approaches through which it is undertaken. In particular, in these situations, it would permit the development of goal states (i.e. what outcomes should medical work progress), means of achieving those (e.g. the kind of clinical reasoning that sits behind decision making) and the opportunity for rehearsal of these, which both reinforces and extends what individuals know, can do and value. All of this then leads to considerations of the educational worth of these kinds of experiences.

## The educational worth of clinical experiences

Following from the aforementioned, when asked about the worth of these different experiences, Sue suggested that a lot of the time was very valuable. Her time with her GP supervisor was most noteworthy.

> She's been incredible 'cause … not just having that one-on-one time with the doctor, but also she had a lot of care and consideration that she put into her teaching and it was really important to her that Tracy [another medical student] and I really understood the concepts that we were being taught in our tutorials. (Sue)

These tutorials comprised reading through the PBL cases, and the supervisor would ask us questions about the cases that unfolded.

> She would probe us and test us and get us to do role plays, and ask other peripheral questions and then give us a wealth of wisdom that she had to share [laughs], which was invaluable. She also went to the effort of organising additional tutorials for us before exams so we could cover anything that we would like further revision on with her. But she is just amazing and when we were consulting with her in the clinic she would always run through things very thoroughly and shared little pearls of wisdom with asking histories and clinical examinations and things and test us when we needed to be tested. (Sue)

The quality of what was being afforded by the clinical placement extended to a high level of pro-activity on the part of local practitioners. Sue reported that she and the other student would be called by the hospital staff if there was something unusual occurring; for instance, a patient with a stroke, or by GP obstetricians to attend births or engage with provisions of antenatal care. When pressed, Sue concluded that consulting, in general practice, had been the most continuous way in which she had learnt during clinical placements. She contrasts the difference of experiences between that of sitting in with specialists and working in general practice.

> When we've been attending with the specialists we've taken observatory roles and every now and then depending on who the specialist was they might ask us to, they might say, 'oh this is an interesting sign on the patient, come and have a look' or 'you can come and examine this or that'. But usually that's more of an observatory role in that context. But in the general practice setting the GPs have given us a lot of instruction but then also a lot of room to practice consulting. (Sue)

Thus, after a period of observation, Sue consulted independently, under the supervision of a GP. Sue would relate the patient's history, any examination findings and their conclusions/clinical decision making to the GP, for review and discussion. This model of parallel consulting was central to much of learning over the course of the year's placement.

> So then we would have our own [consulting] room where we would take the patient into the room and take a proper history and then do an examination as far as we could, as much as we thought we needed to examine, and then ring the GP on the phone and let them know that we'd finished. They would come and

see us and come into the room and then they would ask us to report back our history and examination findings and what we thought was going on. (Sue)

Thus, Sue's episodic and authentic experiences placed her in a position where she had to think and act, and consider a range of factors required for clinical reasoning and decision making. This provides an interesting contrast with the experiences reported by Gil and Jim. Jim commented that in the hospital-based program, students are positioned very differently, following consultants around wards and engaging in learning far more passively and remotely. Occasionally, he reported being assigned the task by a consultant (e.g. give the patient some guidance about alcohol or smoking), which is quite different to the experience of full engagement in patient interaction (taking a history and giving counselling, or the entire clinical consideration, reasoning and decision-making process) reported by Sue. For both Jim and Gil, there was less structure to their days. The affordances offered to them depended on:

On who's on the ward and what they get you to do and what their style of teaching is and what they think med students should be doing. There's a big difference. (Gil)

It's kind of luck of the draw. You might see something rare, you might see something random or you might see the same, diabetes 10 times a day. (Jim)

Rogoff and Lave[29] propose that individuals' thinking and acting is structured by the activities they engage in, which thereby influences what is learnt. The episodic and more disengaged processes that Gil and Jim experienced most likely lead to different kinds of outcomes to those achieved by Sue given that activity structures cognition.[29] It is also noteworthy that another study of UK Foundation Year 2 (the first year of full registration) doctors working in hospitals found that, despite having had a lot of clinical experience during their medical training, it was only when they engaged in actual medical tasks, which required understanding and reasoning, that participants realised their knowledge was deficient.[19] In particular, they reported a lack of the kind of foundational knowledge required to reason and make clinical decisions. Only when they were placed in the position of making decisions, did they realise the strengths and limitations of their knowledge.

As noted above, it is most likely that the kind of experiences that Sue was afforded, engaged her in

goal-directed activities (e.g. considering a range of factors through which to identify the patient's condition, and then considerations of what action might be taken). Given that there is no distinction between thinking and acting and learning,[2] the kinds of thinking and acting undertaken and their consequences (i.e. learning) are richly interrelated. Interestingly, the worth of the experiences afforded by the rural programme was understood by students who were unable to engage in it. For example, Jim stated that rural placement students were far more likely to be competent in clinical examinations, because of their regular engagement in these kinds of activities (i.e. regularly seeing patients independently). However, the quality of these learning experiences was not only about what was offered, or afforded, but how ready the individual was to engage with these experiences. For example, Gil reported being involved in a 2-week placement with a GP in a rural community. However, even though he was provided with similar experiences as Sue, he reported them as being a lot less helpful because he was not really ready to engage in those tasks fully due to lack of prior learning or preparedness for practice.

I was involved in the practice and in the little hospital, and I didn't really know anything at all. So I think I didn't get as much out of it as I could of, if I did it later on. They probably would have been the most helpful experience if I'd had it later in the year. (Gil)

Similarly, Jim referred to being in wards where the complexity of patients' cases was often overwhelming, yet where more experienced practitioners assisted his learning:

... the junior doctors were good at pitching things at my level so they'd pick out the important things about the patients. They'd ask me questions with the right expectations so that was good. The chance to see patients in ED and present them that was really helpful. (Jim)

Finally, Sue noted that she 'couldn't quite recognise the patterns early on as to what condition it might be'. However, through repeated practice and feedback provided by the GP across the year, the focus of her questioning and the extent of history-taking and examination went from taking quite a long time and being ill-focussed, to being considerably shorter and more focussed. By the end of the year, her consultation skills had increased significantly. She identified this development not only as a product of practice and feedback, but also of contributions of the problem-based learning approach and other educational experiences, such as tutorials. Therefore, the well-organised, productive and positive affordances of the medical clinic supported her development as a learner, as did her gradual engagement in workplace activities in ways commensurate with her readiness to participate effectively. In other words, there are relational bases for development, between the learners' competence, and what is expected from them and support within workplaces.

What are particularly evident in the data presented here are the differences between the hospital-based and general practice-based models of medical education. Gil and Jim discussed less-meaningful activities than those engaged in by Sue although the exposure or immersion in medical work might be assumed to be greater in the teaching hospital. However, again, more than the provision of a social and physical environment where medical practice is enacted is how the nascent practitioner is able to engage with these suggestions, and the quality of that engagement. For example, it is clear from the data that both the provision of experiences and how Sue elected to engage with them provided an instance of what might be described as productive participatory engagement with the community, which for Sue rendered particularly solid outcomes. The centrality of both sides of participatory practices is evident, illustrating how it is always necessary to consider learners' personal epistemologies and their exercise as shaping the kinds and extent of learning likely to arise. Here, using the narrative example of Sue, that engagement went beyond securing opportune participation to learn as much about medicine in time-effective ways, it also emphasises the importance of engaging fully with the rural community where the medicine is being practised.

## Case study 2: Midwifery students' Continuity of Care Experiences (COCE)

Midwifery students across all years of a 3-year undergraduate program comprised the second study population. In this program, students are required to engage in traditional hospital-based block clinical placements, as well as engage and follow through 20 pregnant women from early pregnancy to post birth, in what is now called Continuity of Care Experience (COCE).

Three first-, five second- and six third-year students participated in focus groups. During the focus groups, students discussed the COCE in relation to learning, and gave rich accounts of participatory practices, affordances and engagement.[30] The focus group discussions were recorded with permission, transcribed verbatim for analysis and coded independently by two researchers, with the other researchers contributing to the development of a coding framework and data interpretation.

Exploration of the midwifery student data shows similar findings in relation to the conceptions of affordances, engagement, sequencing, mastery and appropriation, which are the focus of this chapter. The continuity of care experiences affords students' exposure to real episodes of midwifery practice from the beginning of their 3-year degree program. This is highly motivational for students in first year as it enables them to experience real midwifery practice; 'it's the only time that we are out in the community seeing pregnant and birthing, and mothers with babies'. Students describe the invitational qualities of different clinicians they were exposed to, and the impact of this is highlighted through comments such as 'if you have a nasty midwife you're not going to do anything. It just shuts you down straight away' (first-year student). However, some midwives were recognised for being highly invitational.

> Some of them they stand out of the crowd yeah definitely. Especially if you see the same one after a few weeks like I saw one for a few weeks, few of the visits, and she knew so she targeted me, to ask me 'so remember we did this last time? Now explain it me this time'. Then, next time she had me do it myself and that was with the palpation. (first-year student)

As the COCEs are student-initiated, there is no vetting of cases with which the students engage. As such, they may be exposed to clinical experiences beyond their level of knowledge. For a first year student, even routine tasks, such as the 'paperwork' midwives complete may be unknown. The COCE has limited ability to offer certainty about the sequencing of experiences to which students are exposed, that can lead to a loss of self-confidence and purpose; 'you feel like a bit of a goose when you don't know the basics'.

Midwifery students spoke of the conceptions of mastery and appropriation (see earlier) in their COCE experiences. Some midwifery students described a need 'to understand' and not just 'do things'. The need for a depth of understanding is suggestive of appropriation.

> Seeing this woman go through this experience and going back and looking up things in books. You don't need someone telling you to go and look that up. It's just through trying to understand what's happening. (first-year student)

However, midwifery students were frequently afforded opportunities 'to do' midwifery practices which they had not yet learnt about through the university curriculum. This led them to recognise that they do not have 'the theoretical base at all because we haven't done anything like that yet' (third-year student) but do 'just what the midwife says as we haven't learnt anything about that sort of stuff' (third-year student). These experiences resulted initially in a degree of mastery to do the tasks shown to them, to feel included and have a hands-on role. However, they recognised that style of practice was a form of socially constructed and interrelated.

> That's probably more about working with different midwives and each person you work with has a different approach to how they want you to do things, how things should be done. So you're really at the mercy of not your learning and what we learn at uni, but how each midwife practices throughout that follow through experience. (third-year student)

While there were many positive role models to guide mimetic learning, there were also negative models. However, the midwifery students still found these to be helpful learning experiences.

> We patchwork what will become our practice from all the midwives that we work with and some are great and some are not so great and some we like the things they do and others we think god I would not do that when I'm out there, that's one thing I won't do. (second-year student)

By the second- and third year of study, midwifery students became strategic in structuring their learning experiences through the COCE program. With their increasing knowledge of pregnancy and birth, and the COCE requirements, students became strategic, selecting particular cases (e.g. women not anticipating a surgical birth and/or with rather than who have minimal social problems). These actions minimised their time burden and enabled them to maximise the chances of achieving the goals

for completing course requirements (e.g. attending requisite numbers of appointments, normal births and other care experiences).

> … in the back of your head you're thinking I still need my 40 births so with an obstetrician they're highly likely to have a caesarean or they're not going to let you do the appointment normally, they're not going to let you do as much hands on stuff, so for your own learning [avoid them]. (second-year student)

The particular expectations of public and private maternity care also shaped students' learning experiences. For example, women engaging a private midwife or obstetricians usually expect those professionals to provide their care, positioning midwifery students in observational roles.

What has been discussed above is the salience of providing experiences whose utilities are characterised by their ordering and sequencing in terms of what they provide for students. This is more than designing a helical curriculum, where content and experiences of learning are woven together, developing in pace and complexity as exposure increases. It includes alignment of the learning experiences with students' level of development, including inducting them gradually into decision making and acting as commensurate with their level of development, is critical. When the divide between the readiness of learners and the demands of the situation are too great, the consequences can be unhelpful. When well aligned, they can be highly productive. These kinds of considerations are central to the organisation and enactment of learning experiences: that is the curriculum in all its manifestations.

## Summary

From the accounts presented and discussed above, what constitutes these medical and midwifery students' experiences need to be understood in terms of what they were afforded and how they responded to them (their engagement). These findings suggest that it is important to have distinct considerations of the kinds of experiences that constitute the curriculum of the education program and also of the readiness (i.e. capacities, values and interests) of students. However, to understand the totality of the experiences and how learning arises from them requires a consideration of the interactions between students and affordances in the social world. What has been offered here is a consideration of curriculum as the ordering and enactment of experiences in terms of participatory practices. All this leads to practical considerations about the organisation of the learning experiences, and how these can be strengthened and augmented through pedagogic practices and also the importance of preparing students for, supporting their engagement in, and the helpful reconciliation of what they experience in their practice settings.

These considerations include the following:
- Optimising individuals' access to and engagement in authentic workplace activities based on their readiness to engage and learn productively within them.
- Providing the ability for the students to observe and engage in mimetic processes.
- Followed by the opportunity to practice, refine and hone what has been observed.
- Gauging the students' levels of readiness to participate in practice-based activities and supporting that progressive engagement with close guidance.
- Progressive engagement in tasks of increasing complexity, with an adequate provision for practice and feedback.

## Cautions and limitations

Of course, every approach has its limitations and strengths. In terms of learning through participation in social practices, albeit in the practice or educational setting, there will always be the danger that what is observed, engaged with and practised can lead to the reproduction of inappropriate, dangerous or unhelpful practices. Recent incidents in the United Kingdom (for instance,[31]) demonstrate that when poor practices become the norm, these can easily become replicated across the workforce and over extended periods of time. Yet, even in these situations, those who are learning and participating make decisions about how they progress and when confronted with overt behaviours and practices, may well reject those suggestions. This might be illustrated by seeking employment elsewhere, or reporting incidents, or sticking to one's values (see chapter by Patterson and colleagues). The power of organisational culture has an important influence on outcomes here.

Importantly, much of what is proposed here in terms of participatory practices is that which occurs through the everyday activities within healthcare settings. In other words, things have not changed much since the times of William Osler, who believed strongly that much of medical education occurred

within and through authentic instances of healthcare practice. Here an attempt has been made to explain, elaborate and illustrate the duality, which comprises the process of learning to be a healthcare practitioner through a consideration of participatory practices that are both interdependent and relational.

## Conclusion

Drawing on the theoretical bases of relational interdependence, the participatory practices of affordance and engagement and learning constructs such as mimetic learning and personal epistemologies, we have explored the world of workplace learning in the healthcare professions, using medicine and midwifery as examples. The student experiences presented here may not be a surprise to you; however, we hope to have extended your thinking and consideration of the theories by which individuals learn, and in particular learn in workplaces, from which you may reconsider your understanding and engage in ongoing research. While identifying the influences of participatory practices at work, there is a significant need to consider the pedagogic practices to enhance the learning experience.

---

**Practice points**

- Authentic learning experiences go beyond placing students in work settings; they also need to engage authentically in that practice in an appropriate way depending on their stage of training.
- It is important to consider the entire range of experiences that healthcare students access and how their particular contributions can be effectively utilised in developing healthcare expertise.
- Even the most adept students may need to be assisted in learning how to actively engage with and learn during their practice-based experiences.
- Learners need some occupational capacities (e.g. skills) to be able to effectively engage in workplace tasks and active learning.
- Organising and enacting learning experiences require considering both the kind of activities and interactions, which are on offer (afforded to) learners, and the readiness of the individual learner to engage in.

## Further reading

1 Billett, S. (2014) *Mimetic Learning at Work: Learning in the Circumstances of Practice.* Springer, Dordrecht, The Netherlands.
2 Valsiner, J. (2000) *Culture and Human Development.* Sage Publications, London.
3 Wertsch, J.V. (1998) *Mind as Action.* Oxford University Press, New York.

## References

1 Billett, S. (2001a) Coparticipation at work: affordance and engagement. In: Fenwick, T. (ed), *Sociocultural Perspectives on Learning through Work.* (Vol. 92). Jossey Bass/Wiley, San Francisco.
2 Billett, S. (2009a) Conceptualising learning experiences: contributions and mediations of the social, personal and brute. *Mind, Culture and Activity,* **16**, 32–47.
3 Donald, M. (1991) *Origins of the modern mind: Three stages in the Evolution of Culture and Cognition.* Harvard University Press, Cambridge, Massachusetts.
4 Lave, J. & Wenger, E. (1991) *Situated Learning - Legitimate Peripheral Participation.* Cambridge University Press, Cambridge, UK.
5 Brown, J.S., Collins, A. & Duguid, P. (1989) Situated cognition and the culture of learning. *Educational Researcher,* **18**, 32–34.
6 Engestrom, Y. (1993) Development studies of work as a testbench of activity theory: the case of primary care medical practice. In: Chaiklin, S. & Lave, J. (eds), *Understanding Practice: perspectives on Activity and Context.* Cambridge University Press, Cambridge, UK, pp. 64–103.
7 Salomon, G. (1997) *Distributed Cognitions: Psychological and Educational Considerations.* Cambridge University Press, Cambridge, UK.
8 Barker, R.G. (1968) *Ecological Psychology: Concepts and Methods for Studying the Environment of Human Behaviour.* Stanford University Press, Stanford.
9 Barker, R.G. (1978) *Habitats, Environments and Human Behaviour.* Jossey-Bass Publishers, San Francisco.
10 Valsiner, J. (2000) *Culture and Human Development.* Sage Publications, London.
11 Berger, P.L. & Luckman, T. (1966) *The Social Construction of Reality.* Penguin, Harmondsworth, Middlesex.
12 Billett, S. (2001b) Learning through work: Workplace affordances and individual engagement. *Journal of Workplace Learning,* **13**, 209–214.
13 Billett, S. (2009b) Personal epistemologies, work and learning. *Educational Research Review,* **4**, 210–219.
14 Richards, J., Sweet, L. & Billett, S. (2013) Preparing medical students as agentic learners through enhancing student engagement in clinical education. *Asia-Pacific Journal of Cooperative Education,* **14**, 251–263.
15 Cooke, M., Irby, D. & O'Brien, B.C. (2010) *Educating Physicians: A Call for Reform of Medical School and Residency.* The Carnegie Foundation for the Advancement of Teaching, Washington.
16 Jolly, B. & MacDonald, M.M. (1989) Education for practice: the role of practical experience in undergraduate and general clinical training. *Medical Education,* **23**, 189–195.
17 Lodge, R.C. (1947) *Plato's Theory of Education.* Kegan Paul, Trench, Trubner, London.
18 Dahlen, H.G., Homer, C.S.E., Leap, N. & Tracy, S.K. (2011) From social to surgical: historical perspectives on perineal care during labour and birth. *Women and Birth,* **24**, 105–111.
19 Cleland, J., Leaman, J. & Billett, S. (2014) Developing medical capacities and dispositions through practice-based experiences. In: Harteis, C., Rausch, A. & Seifried, J. (eds), *Discourses on Professional Learning: On the Boundary Between Learning and Working.* Springer, Dordrecht, The Netherlands, pp. 211–219.
20 Phillips, D.J. & Hayes, B.A. (2008) Securing the oral tradition: reflective positioning and professional conversations in midwifery education. *Collegian: Journal of the Royal College of Nursing, Australia,* **15**, 109–114.
21 Billett, S. (2014) *Mimetic Learning at Work: Learning in the Circumstances of Practice.* Springer, Dordrecht, The Netherlands.
22 Searle, J.R. (1995) *The Construction of Social Reality.* Penguin, London.
23 Organisation for Economic Co-operation and Development (2010) *Learning for Jobs.* OECD, Paris.
24 Raizen, S.A. (1991) *Learning and Work: The Research Base. Vocational Education and Training for youth: Towards Coherent Policy and Practice.* OECD, Paris.
25 Davis, N.L., Davis, D.A., Johnson, N.M. *et al.* (2013) Aligning academic continuing medical education with quality improvement: a model for the 21st century. *Academic Medicine,* **88**, 1437–1441.
26 Health Workforce Australia (2012) *Health Workforce 2025 - Doctors, Nurses and Midwives.*
27 Bleakley, A. (2010) Social comparison, peer learning and democracy in medical education. *Medical Teacher,* **32**, 878–879.
28 Wertsch, J.V. (1998) *Mind as Action.* Oxford University Press, New York.
29 Rogoff, B. & Lave, J. (eds) (1984) *Everyday Cognition: Its Development in Social Context.* Harvard University Press, Cambridge, MA.
30 Billett, S., Sweet, L. & Glover, P. (2013) The curriculum and pedagogic properties of practice-based experiences: the case of midwifery students. *Vocations and Learning: Studies in Professional and Vocational Education,* **6**, 237–258.
31 Francis R. (2013). *Report of the Mid Staffordshire NHS Foundation Trust Public Inquiry: Executive Summary (Vol. 947).* TSO Shop

# 12 Theoretical perspectives on *identity*: researching identities in healthcare education

*Lynn V. Monrouxe and Charlotte E. Rees*

'... *during my first late shift ... is really daunting to do late shift or even weekend shift and night shift because you're basically on your own covering three wards or more, you're the first port of call for all the nurses, you have to take all the decisions on your own ... there's only one registrar ... who covers all the medical wards ... I was handed over this patient who was quite unwell during the day ... I was called because the patient's [EWS for recording vital signs] went up to six ... he looked, to be honest, dire. He was struggling to catch any sort of breath, he was already on oxygen and he ... also had end-stage COPD [chronic obstructive pulmonary disease] ... so I quickly called the registrar to tell him about the patient's condition ... I hadn't examined the patient yet because I thought it would be useful to have the ST [speciality trainee] here as soon as possible ... but the registrar told me that I was meant to see a patient before I call him ... I felt unprepared because I wasn't exactly sure what I was meant to do'.*

('Anne', Trainee Doctor, Year 1)

## Introduction

Who we are, who we might become and who we are seen to be are central aspects of our identity. Furthermore, these issues lie at the very heart of *becoming* a healthcare professional.[1,2] But our identity is not a straightforward matter. Firstly, we all develop to varying degrees both primary (gender, race, etc.) and secondary identities (doctor, wife, etc.). Secondly, our identities are not fixed and static; they change both temporally and contextually. Although once developed, primary identities are more resistant to change. Thirdly, there is interplay between our various identities, and in some situations certain identities might be more salient than others (e.g. gender rather than doctor in a situation of sexual harassment in the workplace).[3] Furthermore, researching *identity* is not straightforward: there are a myriad of different theoretical perspectives about what identity comprises, how identities develop and how we might research identities (e.g. individual and developmental, social and contextual and discursive approaches).[4] In this chapter, we aim to provide you with an overview of a range of identity theories alongside a more in-depth exploration of one particular approach: social constructionism. The chapter should provide some understanding of identity theories that will enable you to delve further into the literature with greater confidence. It will also enable you to consider whether any of these theoretical positions appeal to you as an approach to develop within your own research endeavours.

## Overview

When first reading the brief introductory excerpt, taken from a narrative from Anne (pseudonym), a first year junior doctor,[5] we might wonder what it has to do with *identity*. Yet reading it within a social constructionist framework and drawing on the vast amount of linguistic studies available,[6–8] we can see how Anne constructs her identity through her language in her first few weeks of being a trainee doctor. Social constructionism is a grand theory,[9] asserting that knowing in the social world is created through social interaction. This interaction includes our language, our bodies and the social space within which we inhabit and interact (e.g. through our use of materials/artefacts). From this perspective, Anne constructs herself as an anxious novice trainee, not only through *what* she says but also through *how* she narrates (including the tone of her voice, which we attend to when analysing narratives). Thus she asserts that she is 'daunted' at the prospect of night and weekend shifts as this means being responsible for all decisions at those times: as 'the only port of

*Researching Medical Education*, First Edition. Edited by Jennifer Cleland and Steven J. Durning.
© 2015 John Wiley & Sons, Ltd. Published 2015 by John Wiley & Sons, Ltd.

call'. However, in the face of a medical emergency (the patient looked 'dire'), before even seeing the patient herself, she 'quickly' calls her registrar for assistance. Reprimanded for this action, she reveals her nascent doctor-identity through admitting that she did not know what to do. Furthermore, her use of the pronoun *you* (rather than I) at the beginning of her narrative sets up the construction of her own experiences as a *truth*, not just for herself, but for *all* new doctors.

We begin this chapter by outlining some of the many ways that social scientists have approached the subject of identity, linking these with issues of healthcare identity, before going into more detail about the social constructionist approach. To bring more clarity to social constructionism, we provide three examples of how we have utilised it within our own studies employing written, audio and visual qualitative methods.

## Ontology, epistemology, theory and methods in the social sciences

As we have previously argued, medical education can be regarded a social science.[10] Within the social sciences, the construct of identity has received a lot of attention from researchers working across an array of theoretical positions.[4] Before outlining these, it is important to understand that different theoretical perspectives of identity are independent of the research methods utilised. Instead, they depend on differences in ontological (nature of reality) and epistemological (nature of knowledge) assumptions (see Chapter by Cleland in this book for further discussion). Broadly speaking, these assumptions fall under three main perspectives: objectivism, constructionism and subjectivism (see Chapter by MacMillan in this book for further discussion).[11] These, in turn, relate to any macro- and micro-level research theories, methodological approaches and research methods utilised by researchers.

To add another layer of complexity, epistemological positions are not fixed and bounded; rather they comprise 'strong' and 'weak' versions as adopted by different researchers. For example, the phenomenological approach to identity (a qualitative approach) can be deemed as constructionist – identities being created and co-created within social interaction – but often has objectivist (constructivist) undertones in its application, suggesting that identities are represented in the mind (and therefore, individual). Indeed, as Smith

and Sparkes explain, even researchers working with narratives to explore identities do so from a range of different theoretical (and therefore, epistemological) perspectives,[12] from thick individual/thin social-relational (e.g. primarily psychological approaches that consider identity as residing within individual heads) to thick social-relational/thin individual (e.g. primarily sociolinguistic approaches that consider identities as products of language and interaction *between* individuals). Furthermore, researchers themselves do not always clarify (and sometimes understand) their own particular perspectives. Therefore, the muddy waters of identity research are the same as those encountered by many researchers of different foci within the social sciences: each perspective brings with it underlying assumptions in terms of ontology, the role of the researcher and their motivating epistemology and of participants in the research which is often omitted when presenting their work. It is amidst this muddiness that we now outline identity theories reflecting different points along this spectrum before focusing more deeply on the social constructionist perspectives we have utilised in our own research.

## Individual and developmental theories of identity

We begin by outlining three different individualist approaches to identity: identity statuses and related theories; socio-cognitive approaches and narrative approaches.

### Identity statuses and related theories
Marcia's identity statuses theory is a popular developmental theory based on the construct of ego identity within Erikson's ego psychoanalytic theory.[13] Erikson outlined eight stages of ego identity chronologically, suggesting that throughout life we encounter psychosocial crises involving the interplay between our social milieu and ourselves, which are ultimately primarily resolved.[14] During late adolescence, a time when many people go through healthcare education, the psychosocial crisis is that of 'identity versus identity diffusion' as we face the task of relinquishing childhood identities (being *given to*) and instead adopt the adult caregiver role (*giving to* others), reconfiguring childhood identity into the very core of our future identity. While acknowledging the construction of identity within a social setting, it is assumed that identity is an internal (knowable) cognitive structure (suggesting an objectivist ontology).

Marcia began by qualitatively (using the structured 'Identity Status Interview' tool)[13] and quantitatively (using the 'Ego Identity Incomplete Sentence Blank' tool)[13] exploring the two essential criteria identified from within Erikson's theory: *exploration* (or crisis) and *commitment*. Exploration comprises a period of reflection, trying out future identities. Commitment is the degree of personal investment towards a specific course of identity action (e.g. pursuing an occupation) or belief (e.g. personal ideology). Marcia classified individuals into four different identity statuses: *Identity Achievement* (commitment via exploration), *Foreclosure* (commitment with little/no exploration), *Moratorium* (lengthy exploration, commitment struggles) and *Identity Diffusion* (little exploration or commitment).

Decades of research exploring Marcia's identity statuses has found a range of different constructs associated with these positions: for example, Achievers are associated with high levels of self-esteem and reasoning at post-conventional levels (i.e. they consider broader debatable ethical principles and live by their own ethics even if this goes against societal views)[15] and along with Moratoriums they score significantly lower than Foreclosures on measures of authoritarianism.[13] Little work has utilised this theory in healthcare education, often using methods of data collection that differ from the original tools. Findings suggest that preclinical medical students and nursing students could still be classified within the Identity Diffusion group, or at least displaying very tentative professional identities, but later-stage medical students tend to be classified as Achievers or Foreclosures.[16,17]

Marcia's theoretical model has inspired other researchers across the social sciences to consider the *processes through which* we develop our identities. Luyckx *et al.*[18] propose an integrative model, unpacking the concepts of Exploration and Commitment into four interrelated and iterative, identity dimensions. To illustrate this, imagine an adolescent girl. After exploring various future career possibilities by attending events and searching the Internet (*exploration in-breadth*), she decides to become a doctor and go to a medical school (*commitment-making*). However, she does not stop exploring; gathering more specific information (*exploration in-depth*), leading her to develop a growing conviction that this is what she really wants (*strengthening her identification*) or that she cannot see herself as a doctor (*weakening her identification*). If the latter occurs, her search begins again. However, if the former

occurs she continues on towards her medical career (*identification with commitment*).

Using longitudinal questionnaire methods, Schwartz and coworkers demonstrated how commitment-making and exploration in-depth increase linearly over time, demonstrating an upward trend as participants near their transition to work[19]. However, these relationships are not so straightforward as researchers examining identity development at the level of the individual identify substantial differences in trends with personal factors (e.g. conscientiousness) influencing the strength of identification with commitment.[20] Within medical education, the construct of conscientiousness has been linked with professionalism in medical students.[21] By examining identity alongside conscientiousness further, we may be able to understand their interplay longitudinally.

## Social-cognitive approaches

Social-cognitive approaches to identity development consider identity as a cognitive structure within which we encode, organise and comprehend our experiences in relation to our identities (again, these approaches are individual as they assert that identities reside within a person).[22] Thus, the regularities that our brains detect as we experience events become organised into personal constructs (concepts), synthesised into higher order cognitive structures (personal theories).[23] A person's (internal) personal theory of identity is said to contain more than event representations and behaviours; it also includes core values, epistemological assumptions, goals and ideals. On the basis of constructivist epistemological assumptions, our personal theory comprises everything we require to manage and adapt to our daily lives: thus, feedback might signal the need to readjust our theory, illustrating identity as ever-changing.

Within the social-cognitive perspective, different types of processes are used as we engage with, or avoid, identity conflicts and issues: thus it is posited that by the age of 18, we can be classified as different types of 'self-theorists'.[22] Echoing Marcia,[13] the three different orientations are *informational* (an open, informed approach using formal reasoning strategies), *diffuse-avoidant* (avoidance/delaying) and *normative* (inflexible/closed). These identity-processing orientations are thought to function on three levels: *cognitive and behavioural responses* to identity-related issues, *identity-processing strategies* (basic cognitive and behavioural units) and *identity-processing style* (how people typically deal with identity conflicts). It is the latter that has attracted the most research in the social sciences, utilising the *Identity Style Inventory* (ISI)[24] tool to assess social-cognitive processes relevant to identity formation. Conscientiousness, firm goal commitments and values appear to be positively correlated with informational and normative orientations and negatively with the diffuse-avoidant orientation.[22] While there is a plethora of research examining identities from the social-cognitive perspective across a wide range of populations, to our knowledge, none have done so within healthcare education.

### Narrative approaches

We now consider how identity researchers have worked with narratives within an objectivist framework (i.e. thick individual/thin social-relational),[12] where identity is thought to be psychological and an effect of an individual's social world. Despite recognising narratives as constructed in and through social interactions, this perspective privileges the 'inner' world of the individual as conscious decision-makers who reflectively create the possible stories that can be told. Therefore, narratives are portrayed as interior cognitive or psychological structures, rather than as *storied actions*:[7] thereby providing researchers with a window into individuals' internal mental states, identities and authentic lived experiences, including research within the domain of healthcare education.[25–27] Within this framework, it is often assumed that an individual's experience can be 'tapped into' and there is a real 'self', external to the researcher and the methods through which narratives are collected. For example, conducting narrative interviews with medical students during their first year attachments to nurses in hospitals and nursing homes, Helmich *et al.*[25] classified medical students according to the following four 'paradigms' of lived experience: (a) feeling insecure (the burden of fear resulting in avoidance and non-engagement with their new identities); (b) complying (remaining detached, sticking to rules and avoiding critical reflection); (c) developing (engaging in emotional exploration, reflection and personal development) and (d) participating (actively engaging in their own learning to enhance personal and professional development thus enhancing their professional identities). These paradigms closely resemble Marcia's identity status paradigms described earlier, and therefore fit within these personal theories of identity classification.

### Social and contextual approaches

We have so far outlined individualist approaches that conceptualise identities as *personal* attributes or orientations. While acknowledging that personal identities develop within a social world, the following theories are more *social*.

### Social identity and related theories

Unlike the previous section discussing individual/developmental theories underpinned by objectivist perspectives, this section covers theories from a range of perspectives: some with more objectivist positions; others residing within more constructionist philosophical frameworks. Social identity theory (SIT) was the first to theorise a form of identity distinct from a *personal* identity: it focuses on identity at the level of the *group*.[28] SIT suggests that we categorise ourselves into groups (*social categorisation*) and compare other groups to our own (*social identification*). As we are motivated to gain and maintain affirmation within our group identity, we often consider our own positively (*social motivation*). However, social motivation is not wholly about self-enhancement; it is the sense of group distinctiveness that provides us with a meaningful identity. Group identities do not replace or override personal identities: but some situations make our group identity more salient. Developing this idea, *social identity complexity* theory considers four main ways in which we subjectively structure our perception of multiple in-group identities[3]: *Intersection,* bringing together different identities to form an intersecting in-group; *Dominance,* where one group dominates over other group identities; *Compartmentalisation,* where different group identities become salient depending upon the specific context and *Merger,* the combination of all social categories with anyone from any of them being considered part of a person's in-group. Therefore, a male nurse might define his primary social identity as a combination of both gender and profession, regarding only male nurses as the in-group (*intersection*), he might assign primacy to his professional identity, regarding all nurses as in-group members (*dominance*), more than one group identity may be primary and can all be context-dependently activated (e.g. at work or at home: *compartmentalisation*) or his group identifications might combine with in-group identification extending to anyone sharing important social category memberships (*merger*).

Self-categorisation theory, developed from SIT, is a general theory of identity that considers both inter-group and intra-group processes.[29] This theory addresses the issue of when specific identities become salient, issues of social influence, issues around attraction (group or individual) and issues concerning collective behaviour. For example, in terms of considering when specific identities become salient, self-categorisation theory proposes that we have many different group and personal identities at different levels of abstraction. This wide collection available to us (female, sister, mother, doctor and educator) depends on the context: identity is relational and comparative. The same attributes can define group identities (e.g. nursing student, an extrovert and a father) and interpersonal comparative identities (e.g. unlike my sister who is a physiotherapist, an introvert and child-free).

Group identity is undoubtedly an important aspect for healthcare education researchers. The concept of organisational identity and the significance of one's own group (the *in-group*) against other groups (*out-groups*) come to the fore within multi-professional healthcare settings.[30] Indeed, research within healthcare education has utilised SIT to examine a wide range of issues including how inter-professional rivalries and competition limit nurses' engagement within multi-professional teams and the role of identity for students' wellness.[31,32]

## Discursive approaches

Having outlined a few key ideas from social identity theorists coming from an objectivist perspective, we now consider a very different approach to identities, in which assumptions about the nature of mind and causality are rejected. Instead, social constructionism asserts that language and action are central and identities are, therefore, discursively constructed though talk and interaction, rather than being constructed within an individual's cognition. As with all theoretical positions, there are weak and strong versions. Thus, while some theorists believe that there is *nothing beyond the text* (the 'stronger' version) and therefore we cannot lay claim to any psychological basis to identities, others accept a *real world* so that identities are thought to be internalised but inaccessible through any kind of research method (the 'weaker' version). Unlike theoretical approaches to identity found within the individual and developmental theories, thick social and contextual approaches to identities (note, *identities* rather than *identity*) are interested in both 'what' identities are discursively produced and also 'how' they are produced and the broader social/political

meanings of these identities. Rather than laying claim to possessing a 'theory of' identities, they can be classified according to the particular *analytical approach* they adopt (which includes explicit reference to their epistemological and ontological positioning). There are a number of analytical approaches to identities under the broad umbrella of social constructionism, including conversation analysis, discourse analyses, narrative analyses, positioning analysis and intersectionality.[33–36]

As healthcare education researchers, we have found these approaches extremely powerful as they help to visibilise important aspects of the process of *becoming* a healthcare practitioner – of identity *formation*, rather than development – and how through language and social action (talk-in-action), identities of students, healthcare professionals and patients are co-constructed (and sometimes constrained) within healthcare workplace-learning contexts. Our primary method of analysis focuses on *language-in-use* in social interaction to understand how issues such as power impact upon the co-creation of identities *in situ*. Drawing on linguistic research examining how language is used, we can see how personal and professional identities are constructed and co-constructed in-the-moment through language (e.g. directives, questions and pronominal talk), para-language (e.g. laughter), non-verbal communication (e.g. eye gaze) and material use (e.g. use of diagrams).[37] Thus, language is quite simply "the place where culture and 'the social' happen",[36] shedding light onto the ways in which organisational culture is transmitted, appropriated and (sometimes) resisted.

We provide three original examples and interpretations from our own research, purposely selected because they illustrate undergraduate and postgraduate education, medical and healthcare education and different data collection and analysis methods. We begin with our narrative analysis of an undergraduate pharmacy student's intersecting identities constructed as part of a written professionalism dilemma narrative (Example 12.1).[38] We continue with our positioning analysis of a junior doctor's oral narrative recorded as part of a longitudinal audio-diary study (Example 12.2, Box 21.1).[5] Finally, we draw on Goffman's Dramaturgy theory[35] to examine the co-construction of an undergraduate medical student's, general practice (GP) tutor's and a patient's roles and identities through social interaction during a video-recorded observation of a bedside teaching encounter (BTE) (Example 12.3, Box 12.2).[39]

**Example 12.1   Constructing personal and professional identities in professionalism dilemma narratives: intersectionality theory**

Healthcare students develop their professional identities through identifying with their own profession and differentiating themselves from others. Although coming from a different theoretical standpoint to SIT, some research (including healthcare education research) has suggested that students with certain primary identities (e.g. female, lower socio-economic class and non-whites) can underperform at professional schools.[40] However, little is known about the intersectionality of multiple identities in health professional education.[41]

Intersectionality is 'the *interplay* of race, class and gender, often resulting in multiple dimensions of disadvantage' (p. 310: our emphasis).[42] As a theory, intersectionality comprises many different (epistemological and ontological) forms. While some talk about intersecting *categorical* identities (not wholly unlike *social identity complexity* theory outlined earlier[3]), such as gender, race and sexuality,[43] others take a more discursive approach, examining talk to understand how individuals are *recruited to* 'categories', alongside the *subject positions* they choose to adopt in complex interactions.[44]

To demonstrate the utility of this latter approach, we consider how healthcare students construct multiple identities through their narration of professionalism dilemmas: events in which they have witnessed or participated in something they consider unethical.[45] The excerpt comes from a written narrative via an online questionnaire,[38] collected as part of our 10-year programme of professionalism dilemmas research.[46] The pharmacy student is a fourth year, white, female, aged 17–25 years. Her narrative of an event occurring over 12 months previously is fairly typical and includes her construction of her own intersecting personal (gender and age) and professional identities (pharmacy student), along with the patient, locum pharmacist teacher and store manager identities:

1  **What is the gist of your dilemma?** On a Saturday, a *methadone patient turned*
2  *up late* and *so I couldn't give him Saturday's dose but offered him Sunday's* and
3  *got really angry and aggressive*
4  **Where were you and who was present?** There was a counter-assistant who was
5  busy with another customer and *a locum pharmacist who did not help*
6  **What happened?** *He started shouting at me and giving me abuse*
7  **What did you do?** *I tried to calm him down and explain the situation* and *how*
8  *there was nothing else I could do. I offered him Sunday's dose even though I*
9  *didn't have to.* Eventually, he took Sunday's dose and *stormed out the shop,*
10  *making the customers uneasy and uncomfortable*
11  **Why did you do that?** *I gave him the Sunday dose as I didn't want him to go all*
12  *weekend without it. Plus I didn't want him to kick off anymore and I was already*
13  scared.
14  **How do you feel about it now?** I still don't like serving him when he comes to
15  the store even though *he has since apologised when my store manager made him*
16  after *she heard what had happened*
17  **Any other comments about this?** *I feel that if the locum pharmacist had helped*
18  *the situation would have resolved quicker* as I think the patient felt it wasn't my
19  place *to tell him the rules. Also the locum was male and so was the patient, so this*
20  may *have helped as I was just a girl*

She reports her dilemma as being the recipient of verbal abuse from a patient who shouts at her for not providing him with methadone, which is further exacerbated through insufficient supervision from the locum pharmacist who fails to provide her with support during the incident. She describes doing something in the face of this dilemma: she reports simultaneously trying to explain why she could not give the patient his missed dose of methadone and acts to show concern for him by trying to calm him down and offering him Sunday's dose early.

The student constructs the patient primarily as a villain: a drug-user ('methadone patient', line 1) who is unreliable as he turned up late (lines 1 and 2), and is aggressive (lines 3, 6 and 9) and scary (lines 10, 12 and 13). The patient's gender identity is brought to the fore through the narrator's explicit statement about his masculinity: 'the locum was male and so was the patient' (line 19). She constructs herself as the victim: she is blameless (line 2), caring because she offered him Sunday's dose (lines 2, 8, 9, 11 and 12), helpless (line 8) and scared (lines 12 and 13). She alludes to her professional self (line 7). As she places herself in the mind of the patient (lines 18 and 19), the intersection of her multiple identities (a young, female pharmacy student, rather than an older, male pharmacist like the locum) comes to the fore, rendering her as less powerful in the patient's eyes. In doing this, she constructs herself as a young damsel in distress ('I was just a girl', line 20) requiring saving from a *would-be* hero: the locum pharmacist with whom she identifies as a member of her own profession. However, she is not saved by the locum who, like the patient, is constructed as a male (line 19) and negligent (lines 5, 17 and 18). This serves to amplify her own construction as a female victim of two male perpetrators. Finally, a hero emerges after the incident: the female store manager is constructed as assertive and brave in that she later made the patient apologise to the student (lines 15 and 16).

This example illustrates how much identity work goes on, even within a small written narrative; with narrators constructing their own and others' identities and the intersections between them as they retrospectively make sense of difficult professionalism dilemmas involving power and affecting their performance.

### Example 12.2   Trainee doctors' audio-diary narratives of their first months of work: positioning analysis

Developing the idea that identities are constructed through language, we now consider positioning analysis.[33] It has been argued that we construct *situated positions* in which our own sense of self is enacted within normative cultural discourses (e.g. via cultural stereotypes of what it is to be a specific type of person, including what it is to be a certain type of healthcare professional). Positioning analysis seeks to understand cultural discourses and how we align (and misalign) others and ourselves through talk using three levels: (a) How characters are positioned *relationally* via types of actions assigned to them, motivations for assigned actions and character tropes (archetypes) used; (b) The *interactional world* in which narratives are shared and thus are culturally embedded and (c) wider implications of narrators identifying with existing discourses. It is important to remember that the analysis here seeks to understand how identities of both the narrator and other 'characters' in the narrative are *constructed*. No claim to any 'truth' behind these identities is made. Rather, we seek to understand what the implications are for the narrator, for others like them who draw upon similar discourses, and for society.

Here, we present an excerpt (Box 12.1) of one participant's audio-diary taken from our larger study examining preparedness for practice[5] to demonstrate the utility of the research method and of the analytical framework for understanding how identities are narrated, and what this might mean for educators and society in general. At the time of this narrative, Anne (pseudonym) is a Foundation Year 1 doctor (first year since graduating) in post for 6 months. Her narrative is set in a city hospital unit where she has been asked to cover for a colleague on leave.

*Relational positioning (level 1):* Anne positions herself as a helpful (line 1), efficient and capable (lines 9, 20, 21 and 24), caring (lines 16, 23 and 24), understanding and knowledgeable (lines 17 and 18), and professional doctor (lines 22–24). Her use of the possessive pronoun *my* for the nurse (line 4) and patients (lines 23 and 24) suggests that she is at the top of the hierarchy. Nurse 1 (Thursday) is also constructed as helpful (lines 2–4), efficient (line 3) and caring (lines 3 and 4). Both Anne and Nurse 1 stand in stark contrast to Nurse 2 (Friday), who is immediately positioned as being less helpful (lines 4 and 5, 6 and 7, 11 and 12, 21 and 22), lazy (a character trope: lines 5, 6, 7 and 10) and unprofessional (lines 14–17) as she leaves Anne to care for the patients alone. Further, Anne implies a feeling of abandonment when she explains how she collected the equipment to take the patient's bloods herself (a job she had asked the nurse to undertake, lines 11 and 12), further positioning herself as a caring professional. Although a victim of the nurse's unprofessionalism (as the nurse talks about her behind her back, lines 15 and 16), she positions herself as strong, carrying on with her job. It is the patient with a learning disability, who Anne positions as the real victim, with the patient becoming extremely upset as a result of the nurse's poor care (lines 8, 9, 17, 18 and 19). Thus, Anne's altercation with the nurse is portrayed as a professional lapse on the part of the nurse.

*Interactional positioning (level 2):* Anne narrates her event in the context of an audio-diary study examining graduates' preparedness for practice funded by regulators of her profession. Audio-diaries enable participants to set the agenda by handing over decisions about what, when and how much they wish to contribute to the research. Even though physically absent, researchers are ever-present. Interestingly, while none of the research team is involved in teaching or assessing her, she is still motivated to manage our positive impressions of her in the context of this 'preparedness' narrative (lines 29–32).

*Societal positioning (level 3):* Anne's use of the discourses 'the lazy nurse' and 'the patient victim' echoes similar discourses presently found within current media images of healthcare.[47] Further, her use of 'the good doctor' discourse[48] attempts to uphold the status of her profession in the eyes of doctors and society, ignoring issues such as doctors' reluctance to report errors.[49] In positioning these characters as she does, she re-produces and therefore reifies these cultural stereotypes.

Using positioning analysis within this single narrative, we illustrate identity work as Anne narrates a single event experienced as a junior doctor with 6 months' experience. Not only does such positioning shed light onto Anne's professional identity at that snapshot in time but comparisons between this and other narratives at different time points allow for the exploration of Anne's identity formation. Reconsider for a moment Anne's experience in the first few days of being a junior doctor, presented at the beginning of this chapter. Her narrative early on reveals a much less-confident Anne (*'I felt unprepared because I wasn't exactly sure what I was meant to do'*) who refers to patients as 'this' and 'the' and who aligns herself with nurses ('the first port of call for all the nurses') rather than referring to patients and nurses as belonging to her ('my patient', 'my nurse'), as she does 6 months on. Taken together, we see the formation of Anne's professional identity as she shifts over a 6-month period. While there seems a stark contrast between these two narratives, the positions she adopts longitudinally are not necessarily as linear as this example implies.[5] Instead, they depend on both temporal and contextual aspects of events as she moves between feeling unprepared to feeling prepared and back to unprepared again. Ultimately, she narrates a *repertoire* of positions that can be carried forward into other contexts and conversations, thereby making up the *long conversation* she has across her audio-diaries.

---

### BOX 12.1   'I had to do everything on my own': audio-diary of an FY1 Doctor

1 [Thursday] was not very busy *so I was happy to do everything* … I also had *a nice*

2 *nurse … she was ready to measure the patients' calves and do part of the nursing*

3 *jobs* and she was *quite quick with doing observations … Very empathetic towards*

4 *patients* … Friday I had … 10 patients that all came together and *my nurse was less*

5 *helpful.* She would *constantly be on her mobile phone* … When I asked her to help

6 me out with taking bloods or observations, *she would take half an hour or more* before

7 she would do while she was in the treatment room *on her phone or chatting* … I started

8 to get a little bit annoyed … There was a patient that had been *waiting for 2 hours*

9 she had a learning disability … I clerked her in quickly and asked her whether I could do

10 some bloods … *the nurse was not doing anything so I asked her* [to take bloods] while

11 I was seeing to other patients … *She was still in the treatment room while I had*

12 *finished* … *I just collected all the equipment* … and she saw me going to take the blood

13 and then she called me in the treatment room to ask me why … as she was about to do

14 it. I told her that I asked her to do this quite a while ago … she told me that I have a

15 *temper* and was *chatting to all other colleagues and saying that I did not know how*

16 *to speak to nurses* … I then continued to do all my jobs and *caring for the patients* …

17 this was *very unprofessional behaviour* and *patients with learning disabilities*

**18** *tend to not be able to wait for long times … that patient indeed started crying and*

**19** *screaming* because she wanted to go home … I was quite frustrated with the behaviour

**20** of the nurse and *had to do quite a lot of jobs in a limited amount of time* and I also

**21** had *to do two people's job* while *my other colleague [nurse] was not doing*

**22** *anything productive for a patient* … but … it was a good experience … I learnt to *deal*

**23** *with difficult colleagues and with frustration* and *still be as polite and caring to my*

**24** *patients* as possible … *I was able to manage all my patients appropriately.*

### Example 12.3   Understanding the co-construction of identities through workplace learning interactions: dramaturgy analysis

The healthcare workplace is a crucial site for healthcare students' learning of clinical practice. Students learn through their interactions with others (e.g. patients and clinical teachers) and with workplace materials (e.g. diagnostic equipment and computers). Over the past 8 years, we have conducted a programme of observational research in the United Kingdom and Australia of hospital and GP BTEs (i.e. teaching done in the company of patients) during undergraduate medical education.[39,50–52] To illustrate how students, patients and clinical teachers co-construct their personal and professional identities interactionally, we now draw from an exemplar BTE based in a GP setting.[52] We focus on Goffman's Dramaturgy theory,[35] where life is conceptualised *as a stage*, with a director, actors, props and 'non-people' (i.e. people who are talked about as if they are not there) and where people manage each other's impressions with roles and identities being constructed through appearance (e.g. clothing), interaction (e.g. politeness) and material use (e.g. technical equipment).

The scene is a GP surgery in the United Kingdom. Present is a male final year medical student, a female patient in her 50s and a male GP with a longstanding relationship with the patient. The patient attends the practice with a shoulder problem and the GP asks the student to take a brief history, examine the patient and provide a differential diagnosis. The excerpt (Box 12.2) relates to the student's examination of the patient and illustrates the typical roles played by students, patients and doctors across our research programme: the doctor as 'director', the student as 'actor' and the patient as 'prop' and/or 'non-person'. The GP tutor performs the role of a director in several ways as the student examines the patient: he repeatedly interrupts the student with questions (e.g. turn 13), gives numerous verbal directives about how the student should be examining the patient (e.g. turns 3 and 28) and provides tactile directives through physically demonstrating the examination to the student (turn 30, see figure in Box 12.2). The doctor's question-asking and directives construct the student as an actor who performs his role as the actor by complying (e.g. turns 10 and 16). Throughout the examination, the GP and student construct the patient as a non-person by talking about her as if she is not there (turns 5 and 15), referring to her body parts in a depersonalised way (e.g. turn 22) and by affording her no eye contact (here all eye contact is between the student and GP). They also construct her as a prop by giving her verbal directives about how to position her body (e.g. turn 25), and by tactile directives, physically moving parts of her body for her (see figure in Box 12.2). The patient performs this prop role through her compliance with these directives.

In terms of professional identities, the GP tutor and student construct their medical identities though talk, such as asking the patient questions, giving her directives and employing medical talk (e.g. turns 19 and 20) and through their physical appearance (both wear a shirt and tie). The GP's identity as a senior doctor and teacher is constructed through his performance as director as discussed earlier. Even though medical materials are not used here, the GP tutor uses his pen, rather like orchestral conductors use their batons, to repeatedly point at the patient's body parts to direct the student's examination performance. The student's identity as a learner is constructed though his compliant responses to the GP tutor's questions and directives, using polite requests to the patient employing hedges and face-saving pronominal talk (e.g. turn 8). The patient's lay identity is constructed through her limited verbal contribution to the bedside teaching, her being repeatedly touched (and physically positioned) by the GP and student and her physical appearance (casual clothes). Thus, applying Goffman's Dramaturgy theory to a videoed BTE excerpt, we have illustrated how identities and roles are co-constructed moment-to-moment within workplace learning interactions via language, para-language, non-verbal communication, clothing and material use.

## BOX 12.2    Doctor as director, patient as prop, student as actor

1 MD10: (to student) What movements are you going to do first?

2 MS9: first of all passive movements in both sides um so I could ask shoulder abduction

3 MD10: good get her to do active movements first okay

4 MS9: alright yeah

5 MD10: she's going to be in pain …

6 MS9: okay

7 MD10: okay I want you to learn

8 MS9: (to patient) um would it be okay if you can lift your shoulders like that for me

9 FP12: I can go that far

10 MS9: okay so you can't go any higher with the right?

11 FP12: I can but it's very painful

12 MS9: painful okay

13 MD10: (to student) so what movement's that?

14 MS9: slanted shoulder abduction on the right side

15 MD10: yeah so you're going to if you want to do it quickly ask ((patient's name)) to put her hands behind her head

16 MS9: (to doctor) okay (to patient) um could you do that for me? I know it's quite difficult

17 FP12: all the way up?

18 MD10: (to student) what movement is that? What movements are you testing there?

19 MS9: um is it external rotation?

20 MD10: external rotation and abduction

21 MS9: oh right yeah …

22 MD10: (to student) can you move this arm up right up? and you can bring it right up to 180° okay so that's abduction you've got full abduction what other movements are you doing?

23 MS9: um we already did external

24 MD10: well just do it again I didn't see you

25 MS9: (to doctor) okay (to patient) if you can bend your arm like that now if you can move your hand that way so you're going like that (to doctor) so that's external rotation

26 MD10: yeah that's external rotation

27 MS9: and the other way as well that's internal rotation so that's fine

28 MD10: (to student) right (.) do it on the other side now

29 MS9: ((continues examining patient))

30 MD10: *I think I'd probably keep it at a right angle*

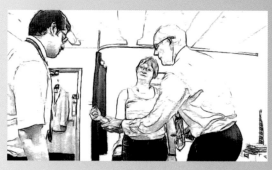

## Conclusion

This chapter introduces the field of identities research within healthcare education. We hope that it brings clarity to the range of theoretical approaches available, making clear the links between theory and methodology in this area of research. We also hope that the examples provided illustrate what can be done within a social constructionist approach, exemplifying different methodologies and methods of data collection and analyses. We hope this chapter enables you to delve into the broad literature with confidence, stimulates your thinking and encourages you to consider research questions and, thereafter, high-quality identities research within healthcare education.

---

**Practice points**

- Identities and the researching of identities matter in healthcare education.

- A range of theoretical approaches from the social sciences can be used to understand identities. These differ in terms of ontological and epistemological perspectives, but are equally valid (depending on research questions) and complementary.[49]

- The breadth of theoretical and methodological approaches, which are potentially suitable for identities research, means it is critical to be clear and explicit about the theoretical and methodological positions underpinning your research, and why.

- Identities can be examined through a range of data collection and analysis methods, including narratives, audio-diaries and video-ethnography.

- 'Joined-up thinking' is crucial: only by engaging with the wider community of identity researchers within healthcare education and across the social sciences can we progress current knowledge through original, rigorous and significant programmatic research.

---

## References

1 Monrouxe, L.V. (2010) Identity, identification and medical education: why should we care? *Medical Education*, **44**, 40–49.

2 Monrouxe, L.V. (2013) Identity, self and medical education. In: Walsh, K. (ed), *Oxford Handbook of Medical Education*. University of Oxford Press, Oxford.

3 Roccas, S. & Brewer, M.B. (2002) Social identity complexity. *Personality and Social Psychology Review*, **6**, 88–106.

4 Schwartz, S.J., Luyckx, K. & Vignoles, V.L. (eds) (2011) *Handbook of Identity Theory and Research*. Springer, London.

5 Monrouxe, L.V., Bullock, A., Cole, J. *et al.* (2014) *How prepared are UK medical graduates for practice? Final report from a programme of research commissioned by the General Medical Council*. General Medical Council. http://www.gmc-uk.org/How_Prepared_are_UK_Medical_Graduates_for_Practice_SUBMITTED_Revised_140614.pdf_58034815.pdf (accessed 6th April 2015).

6 Potter, J. & Wetherell, M. (1987) *Discourse and Social Psychology*. Sage, London.

7 Schiffrin, D. (1994) *Approaches to Discourse: Language as Social Interaction*. Wiley, Oxford.

8 Wetherell, M., Taylor, S. & Yates, S. (eds) (2001) *Discourse Theory and Practice: A Reader*. Sage, London.

9 Rees, C.E. & Monrouxe, L.V. (2010) Theory in medical education research: how do we get there? *Medical Education*, **44**, 334–339.

10 Monrouxe, L.V. & Rees, C.E. (2009) Picking up the gauntlet: constructing medical education as a social science. *Medical Education*, **43**, 196–198.

11 Crotty, M. (1998) *The Foundations of Social Research: Meaning and Perspective in the Research Process*. Sage Publications, London.

12 Smith, B. & Sparkes, A.C. (2008) Contrasting perspectives on narrating selves and identities: an invitation to dialogue. *Qualitative Research*, **8**, 5–35.

13 Kroger, J. & Marcia, J.E. (2011) The identity statuses: origins, meanings, and interpretations. In: Schwartz, S.J., Luyckx, K. & Vignoles, V.L. (eds), *Handbook of identity theory and research*. 1. Springer, New York.

14 Erikson, E.H. (1959) *Identity and The Life Cycle, Volume 1*. International Universities Press, New York.

15 Kohlberg, L. (1981) *Essays on Moral Development, Vol. I: The Philosophy of Moral Development*. Harper & Row, San Francisco, CA.

16 Niemi, P.M., Vainiomaki, P.T. & Murto-Kangas, M. (2003) "My future as a physician" -- professional representations and their background among first-day medical students. *Teaching and Learning in Medicine*, **15**, 31–39.

17 Rimkien, R. & Žydžiūnaitė, V. (2013) Professional Identity Statuses of First-year College Students in General Practice Nursing Programmes: the Case of Lithuania. *Balkan Military Medical Review*, **16**, 79–91.

18 Luyckx, K., Goossens, L., Soenens, B. & Beyers, W. (2006) Identity statuses based upon four rather than two identity dimensions: extending and refining Marcia's paradigm. *Journal of Youth and Adolescence*, **34**, 605–618.

19 Luyckx, K., Schwartz, S.J., Goossens, L. *et al.* (eds) (2011) *Process of Personal Identity Formation and Evaluation*. Springer, New York.

20 Klimstra, T.A., Luyckx, K., Germeijs, V. *et al.* (2012) Personality traits and educational identity formation in late adolescents: longitudinal associations and academic progress. *Journal of Youth and Adolescence*, **41**, 346–361.

21 Chaytor, A., Spence, J., Armstrong, A. & McLachlan, J. (2012) Do students learn to be more conscientious at medical school? *BMC Medical Education*, **12**, 54.

22 Berzonsky, M.D. (2011) A social-cognitive perspective on identity construction. In: Schwartz, S.J., Luyckx, K. & Vignoles, V.L. (eds), *Handbook of Identity Theory and Research*. Springer Science+Business Media, pp. 55–76.

23 Kelly, G.A. (1955) *The Psychology of Personal Constructs*. Norton, New York.

24 Berzonsky MD. 1992. *Identity Style Inventory (ISI-3): Revised Version*. [Unpublished Measure].

25 Helmich, E., Bolhuis, S., Dornan, T., Laan, R. & Koopmans, R. (2012) Entering medical practice for the very first time: emotional talk, meaning and identity development. *Medical Education*, **46**, 1074–1086.

26 Santen, S.A. & Hemphill, R.R. (2011) A window on professionalism in the emergency department through medical student narratives. *Annals of Emergency Medicine*, **58**, 288–294.

27 Clandinin, J., Cave, M.T. & Cave, A. (2011) Narrative reflective practice in medical education for residents: composing shifting identities. *Advances in Medical Education and Practice*, **2**, 1–7.

28 Tajfel, H. (ed) (1978) *Differentiation Between Social Groups: Studies in the Social Psychology of Intergroup Relations*. Academic Press, London.

29 Turner, J., Hogg, M., Oakes, P. *et al.* (1987) *Rediscovering the Social Group: A Self-Categorization Theory*. Blackwell, Oxford and New York.

30 Burford, B., Morrow, G., Morrison, J. *et al.* (2013) Newly qualified doctors' perceptions of informal learning from nurses: implications for interprofessional education and practice. *Journal of Interprofessional Care*, **27**, 394–400.

31 Currie, G., Finn, R. & Martin, G. (2010) Role Transition and the Interaction of Relational and Social Identity: New Nursing Roles in the English NHS. *Organization Studies*, **31**, 941–961.

32 McNeill, K.G., Kerr, A. & Mavor, K.I. (2014) Identity and norms: the role of group membership in medical student wellbeing. *Perspectives on Medical Education*, **3**, 101–112.

33 Georgakopoulou, A. (2013) Building iterativity into positioning analysis: a practice-based approach to small stories and self. *Narrative Inquiry*, **23**, 89–110.

34 Monrouxe, L.V. & Rees, C.E. (2016) Hero, voyeur, judge: understanding medical students' moral identities through professionalism dilemma narratives. In: Mavor, K., Platow, K. & Bizumic, B. (eds), *The Self, Social Identity and Education*. Psychology Press, Hove, UK.

35 Goffman, E. (1959/1990) *The Presentation of Self in Everyday Life*. Doubleday, New York.

36 Wetherell, M. (1998) Positioning and Interpretative Repertoires: Conversation Analysis and Post-Structuralism in Dialogue. *Discourse & Society*, **9**, 387–412.

37 Alvesson, M. & Karreman, D. (2000) Varieties of Discourse: On the Study of Organizations through Discourse Analysis. *Human Relations*, **53**, 1125–1149.

38 Rees, C.E., Monrouxe, L.V. & McDonald, L.A. (2015) My mentor kicked a dying woman's bed … Analysing UK nursing students' 'most memorable' professionalism dilemmas. *Journal of Advanced Nursing*, **71**, 169–80.

39 Monrouxe, L., Rees, C. & Bradley, P. (2009) The construction of patients' involvement in hospital bedside teaching encounters. *Qualitative Health Research*, **19**, 918–930.

40 Costello, C.Y. (2005) *Professional Identity Crisis: Race, Class, Gender and Success at Professional Schools*. Tennessee Vanderbilt University Press, Nashville.

41 Tsouroufli, M., Rees, C.E., Monrouxe, L.V. & Sundaram, V. (2011) Gender, identities and intersectionality in medical education research. *Medical Education*, **45**, 213–216.

42 Macionis, J.J. & Gerber, L.M. (2011) *Sociology*. Pearson Canada, Toronto.

43 Collins, P., Von Anger, H. & Armbriste, A. (2008) Church ladies, good girls, and locas: stigma and the intersection of gender, ethnicity, mental illness, and sexuality in relation to HIV risk. *Social Science & Medicine*, **67**, 389–397.

44 Adams, J. & Padamsee, T. (2001) Signs and Regimes: Rereading Feminist Work on Welfare States. *Social Politics: International Studies in Gender, State and Society*, **8**, 1–23.

45 Christakis, D.A. & Feudtner, C. (1993) Ethics in a short white coat: the ethical dilemmas that medical students confront. *Academic Medicine*, **68**, 249–254.

46 Rees, C.E., Monrouxe, L.V. & Ajjawi, R. (2014) Professionalism in workplace learning: understanding interprofessional dilemmas through healthcare student narratives. In: Jindal-Snape, D. & Hannah, E.F.S. (eds), *Exploring the Dynamics of Personal, Professional and Interprofessional Ethics*. Polity Press, Bristol, pp. 295–310.

47 Wetherall, C. (2012) How to stay afloat. *Nursing Standard*, **26**, 26–27.

48 Monrouxe, L.V. (2009) Negotiating professional identities: dominant and contesting narratives in medical students' longitudinal audio diaries. *Current Narratives*, **1**, 41–59.

49 Roland, M., Rao, S.R., Sibbald, B. *et al.* (2011) Professional values and reported behaviours of doctors in the USA and UK: quantitative survey. *BMJ Quality and Safety*. http://qualitysafety.bmj.com/content/early/2011/02/07/bmjqs.2010.048173.full. doi:10.1136/bmjqs.2010.048173

50 Rees, C.E. & Monrouxe, L.V. (2010) "I should be lucky ha ha ha ha": the construction of power, identity and gender through laughter within medical workplace learning encounters. *Journal of Pragmatics*, **42**, 3384–3399.

51 Rees, C.E., Ajjawi, R. & Monrouxe, L.V. (2013) The construction of power in family medicine bedside teaching: a video observation study. *Medical Education*, **47**, 154–165.

52 Rizan, C., Elsey, C., Lemon, T. *et al.* (2014) Feedback-in-action within bedside teaching encounters: a video ethnographic study. *Medical Education*, **48**, 902–920.

# 13 Health behaviour theories: a conceptual lens to explore behaviour change

*Francois Cilliers, Lambert Schuwirth and Cees van der Vleuten*

*Consider the following scenarios.*

1 *There have been several incidents of unprofessional practice by undergraduate students in your faculty. It appears that the teaching of professionalism is not effective. How would you evaluate and revise the teaching of professionalism so as to change student behaviour?*

2 *There have been longstanding issues with postgraduate teaching in your department. You instituted a system for registrars to give feedback to consultants on their teaching two years ago, but the registrars are increasingly reticent to give feedback, complaining that nothing has changed. When you meet with them, they give disturbing examples of consultants with approaches to teaching that are not helpful and whose behaviour has not changed despite feedback. How do you design an intervention to ensure that consultants respond to feedback from registrars?*

3 *Your medical school has a strong antibiotic stewardship programme and practice guidelines about the use of antibiotics have been widely distributed to practices located around your school. A recent study has revealed that only a small proportion of clinicians are following these guidelines. How would you design a continuing medical education (CME) intervention to enhance the utilisation of guidelines in practice?*

## Introduction

Many of the questions that one may ask as a researcher in healthcare profession education (HPE) have to do with understanding human behaviour with a view to changing that behaviour. Human behaviour is the result of a complex interaction between personal factors and contextual factors, both proximal and distal (Fig. 13.1). Research on human behaviour in HPE needs to identify the various factors at play and explore how they interact. Researchers exploring health behaviour having been trying to do this for many years and provide us with a rich family of theories draw on.[1-3]

## Why health behaviour theories are important to HPE research

Much of educational practice, faculty development and continuing professional education is aimed at changing behaviour, whether of students, faculty or practitioners in the field. To be able to design interventions that are reliably more likely than not to change behaviour, it is necessary to understand *how* intervention I causes outcome O, rather than simply demonstrating *that* I causes O.[4,5] Behavioural science theories have been developed in the field of health behaviour.[6] These health behaviour theories (HBTs) incorporate causal elements that can inform the design of interventions, which should ideally result in more successful interventions than would otherwise be the case.[4,7,8] These theories can be applied in HPE research to inform the development of research questions, to plan interventions to change behaviour and as a framework to interpret and explain observed behaviours and to evaluate interventions.[8,9]

## The origins of the theories

The application of behavioural science theory to health behaviour change dates back to the 1950s. HBT has since evolved into a widely researched set of theories.[2,3] The constructs used in each theory are typically not unique to that theory and the particular set of constructs, and the way they are related in each theory offers a particular perspective on a health behaviour issue (e.g. see Munro *et al.*[10] for a clinical example of the application of multiple theories to a single behavioural issue). Some theories were developed in the first instance to explain behaviour, for example, the theory of planned behaviour, others to guide behavioural interventions, for example, the trans-theoretical model (TTM).[8] There are a wide range of these theories

*Researching Medical Education*, First Edition. Edited by Jennifer Cleland and Steven J. Durning.
© 2015 John Wiley & Sons, Ltd. Published 2015 by John Wiley & Sons, Ltd.

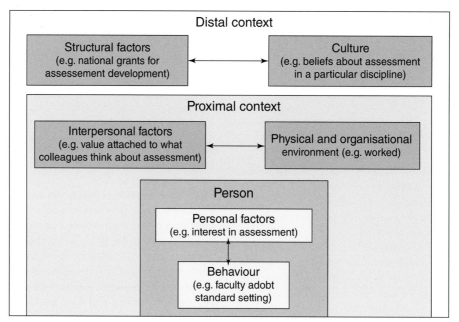

*Figure 13.1* Framework for organising the relationship between factors at various levels that impact on behaviour. For the purposes of illustration, examples are given of how constructs might relate to a theoretical example of a project to research the adoption of standard setting for assessment by faculty. *Source*: Adapted from Eaton *et al.*[1]

focussed at different levels, for example, individual theories, interpersonal theories, organisation level theories and community level theories.[3,11] These theories started finding their way into HPE research in the 1980s (e.g. Montano *et al.*[12]) but it was only after 2000 that increasing – albeit still small – numbers of researchers started turning to these theories.

## Why health behaviour theories?

Theories about human behaviour have been developed in a number of fields. Behavioural science theory traces its roots to work on the psychology of human behaviour. HBTs have traditionally drawn heavily on this, while more recently incorporating insights from sociology. The advantage that these theories offer is that they have been used extensively to understand and to influence human behaviour. There is thus a rich tradition of theory building and applied research to draw on – albeit not in the HPE field – when contemplating the use of any of these theories.

Also dealing with the psychology of human behaviour, but from an industrial psychology perspective, transfer of training theory[13,14] has to do with factors influencing whether people transfer what they learn in a training context to the workplace. This is now being picked up in the higher education[15] and HPE[16,17] literature. Triandis' model

of social behaviour addresses factors such as habit, intention, motivation and facilitating conditions.[18] While this has been used in HPE research, it falls outside of the scope of this chapter. Critical realism[19,20] from sociology offers a sociological perspective on human behaviour in context but is not easily accessible and has not yet permeated the literature[21,22] to the degree that HBT has. Game theory, developed in economics, has to do with decision making in conditions of interaction. Even though it has not been used in HPE as such, there are examples of how game theory has been applied in medical contexts.[23,24]

## Matching theory and approach

HBTs typically focus on the triadic relationship between intra- and interpersonal factors and the behaviour of interest, with or without consideration of the context comprising concentric environmental levels of influence on the behaviour of interest[2,3,8,25] (Fig. 13.1). Four theories about individual behaviour have been selected for the purposes of illustration. Self-regulation perspectives have also been used to explain health behaviour but are covered elsewhere in this volume[26] and will not be addressed here. Social cognitive theory is also used as a HBT[2,27] but is also commonly invoked as a theory of learning (e.g. Mann *et al.*[28]); therefore, even though it has been applied in HPE research (e.g. Jochemsen-van der Leeuw *et al.* [29] and Mann *et al.*[30]), it will not be included here.

For each theory, a brief overview will be given (more detailed descriptions of the theories and their constructs are available in suggested readings at the end of this chapter). For the purposes of illustration, the figure illustrating each theory includes examples of how constructs might relate to a theoretical example of a project to research the adoption of standard setting for assessment by faculty. Actual examples of how the theory has been used in HPE research then follow.

## Theory of reasoned action (TRA), theory of planned behaviour (TPB) and integrated behavioural model (IBM)

These theories represent progressively comprehensive variations on a similar theme. Core constructs (Fig. 13.2) include behavioural intention as moderated by attitudes towards the behaviour, normative beliefs and perceived agency.[31,32] In the integrated behavioural model, additional factors such as knowledge and skills to perform the behaviour, the salience of the behaviour, environmental constraint and habit are also invoked. The TPB is one of the most commonly used theories of the family of HBTs in the context of HPE research.[33]

The issue that concerned Tian and co-workers[34] was how best to evaluate the effectiveness of CME given that, amongst other variables, the design of the CME intervention, the clinical domain and the target audience can vary greatly. The authors contended that the fact that previous studies have been conducted without using a theoretical framework may have resulted in misinterpretation of results and confounded comparison across different studies. The purpose of their study was to develop and validate a survey instrument for evaluation purposes. Similar to the professionalism examples that follow, the focus of CME is on achieving behaviour change, which makes the TPB a suitable conceptual framework.

The selection of a theoretical perspective from which to approach a research project is not straightforward. Something these authors did, which is not that common, is to justify their decision to use the TPB. They compared the use of TPB with Kirkpatrick's evaluation framework and social cognitive theory, highlighting overlaps, before deciding upon their approach. The authors then undertook a rigorous, multistep process to develop their survey

instrument. One step was developing items by operationalising constructs of the TPB – attitudes, beliefs (expectations), perceived norms, perceived behavioural control (self-efficacy) and behavioural intention – in the context of CME. With the exception of the scale about beliefs, the scales that they developed for each construct held up to scrutiny. The authors felt that the decisional balance construct in the TTM (see below) explained their results better than did the TPB for this construct, an illustration of how constructs from different theories can be invoked to explain results.

Not surprisingly, given the behavioural manifestations of professionalism, professionalism has been the subject of several papers using HBTs as a point of departure. The issue that concerned Archer and co-workers[35] was how best to teach professionalism. The problem they identified was that although professionalism is widely taught, medical schools do not have a theoretical framework to inform the design of professionalism teaching and there is little evidence that professionalism is increasing. Because of this, they argue that the teaching of professionalism is often not effective enough to overcome what students discern from the hidden curriculum about professionalism. To change this, they used the TPB as a framework to plan the teaching of professionalism, focussing on the intention to behave professionally as a core issue. They developed a threefold strategy: the teaching of professionalism attitudes (attitude towards the behaviour) must be systematic, prevalent social norms in practice must be studied and addressed where necessary and finally, students' perception of behavioural control should be systematically developed and reinforced.

Rees and Knight[36] explored the assessment of professionalism using the TPB and the IBM. They used this theory because they focussed on the attitudinal component of professionalism, reiterating Hafferty's question: 'Do we want physicians who are professional, or will we settle for physicians who can act in a professional manner?'[36] The challenge in assessing professionalism was highlighted as being the inability to know whether students are undertaking impression management and acting in a certain way due to the contextual demands or whether their behaviour reflects their professional attitudes. Assessing students solely on the basis of their observed performance is not an assessment of their underlying attitudes. The authors point out how environmental factors and the skills and abilities of students will also moderate their behavioural intention. Using the TPB, their suggestions for assessment of professionalism therefore include observation of behaviours, but augmented

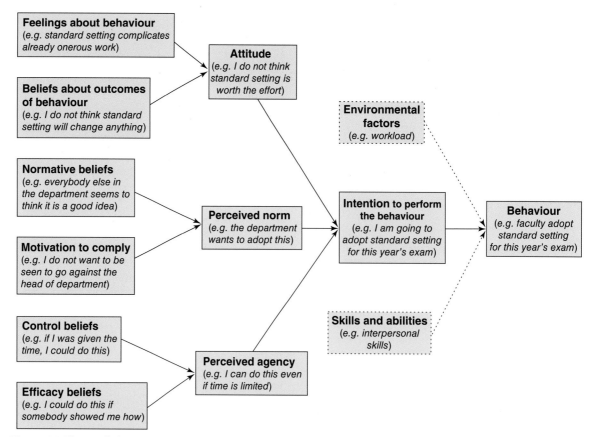

*Figure 13.2* Theory of planned behaviour. Dashed lines illustrate some additional factors included in the integrated behavioural model. *Source*: Adapted from Fishbein and Cappella,[31] Montano and Kasprzyk[32] and Munro *et al.*[10]

by exploration, for example, using narrative or conversation, of personal and contextual factors underlying the observed behaviour.

Although not in the field of HPE, the paper by Alleyne and Phillips[37] warrants a mention as the issue that they address is directly applicable to HPE. The paper deals with the issue of academic dishonesty among students and uses the TPB to conceptualise the study and design the instruments.

These studies all use the TPB as a point of departure, but for quite divergent purposes. One study is concerned with evaluating CME, another with teaching professionalism, a third with the assessment of professionalism and the last with understanding academic dishonesty. What these issues have in common is that they study the manifestation in behaviour of constructs that are 'hidden in the heads' of students or clinicians. The TPB offers an approach to understanding how these constructs interact and manifest, through the formation and enactment of an intention, in (more or less desirable) behaviour. While the nature and manifestation of these hidden constructs always have to be inferred from observed behaviour, basing these inferences

on theoretical assumptions, such as those offered by the TPB, is preferable to making inferences in a conceptual vacuum.

We turn now to a second theory, the health belief model.

## Health belief model (HBM)

The HBM (Fig. 13.3) conceives of individual behaviour as being a result of the interaction between a person's perceptions of a threat to him/herself, beliefs about the behaviour that would obviate that threat and cues to action.[38] The perception of threat has to do with the perception of vulnerability to an outcome and the perceived severity of that outcome. Beliefs about behaviour have to do with the perceived benefits of the behaviour and perceived barriers to performing the behaviour. Self-efficacy has latterly also been incorporated by some as a construct in the model.[8,38]

The HBM has been used to explore decisions about childbearing during residency.[39] This theory was

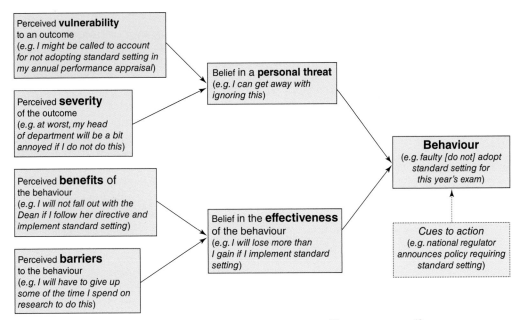

***Figure 13.3*** Health belief model. *Source*: Adapted from Champion and Skinner[38] and Munro *et al.*[10]

deemed appropriate because pregnancy – planning to have children – was framed as a perceived career threat. The model was used as a basis for explaining behaviour and as a framework to design a data collection instrument for a cross-sectional survey. Perceived susceptibility was largely considered to be the susceptibility to adverse career-related outcomes, such as an extended period of training, the inability to get a fellowship position or other adverse effects on the respondent's career. Potentially adverse pregnancy outcomes at a higher childbearing age were also included here. Knowledge about the behaviour was considered to be knowledge about the relationship between age and pregnancy. Cues to action included awareness of certification requirements of medical boards and the leave policies of the residency programme. Using this model, it was demonstrated that two-thirds of the difference between the intention of women and men to have children during residency was mediated by the perceived threat to their career, much of which related to the possibility (threat) of increased residency duration. Given the complexities of human behaviour, a model that explains two-thirds of a difference is impressive.[40–43]

Framing pregnancy as a career threat, researchers were able to identify the magnitude of the possibility of increased residency duration, while also demonstrating that women registrars underestimated their susceptibility to subfertility and involuntary childlessness. The results are of value

for those providing career counselling about residencies, offering the possibility of theory-based gender-differentiated counselling.

We turn now to the TTM. In contrast to the previous two models that aim to explain behaviour, the TTM was developed to guide behavioural interventions.

## Trans-theoretical model (TTM)

The model comprises four sets of constructs (Fig. 13.4): stages of change, processes of change, self-efficacy and decisional balance.[27,44] The model envisions behaviour change as 'a process that unfolds over time through a sequence of stages'[44] until, in some instances, a stage of termination is reached where the new behaviour is entrenched and relapse unlikely. However, progression is neither linear nor inevitable and relapse is contemplated by the model. Using the TTM, interventions aimed at particular processes of change can, for example, be tailored to the different stages of change that groups in the target population find themselves in.

The issue that van der Leeuw and co-workers[45] were interested in was responsiveness to feedback. They explored how and why consultants do or do not adapt their teaching in response to feedback from registrars. The TTM was used to formulate the research question. Deductive analysis of data was then undertaken using a coding framework based on the TTM: for the purposes of coding, the

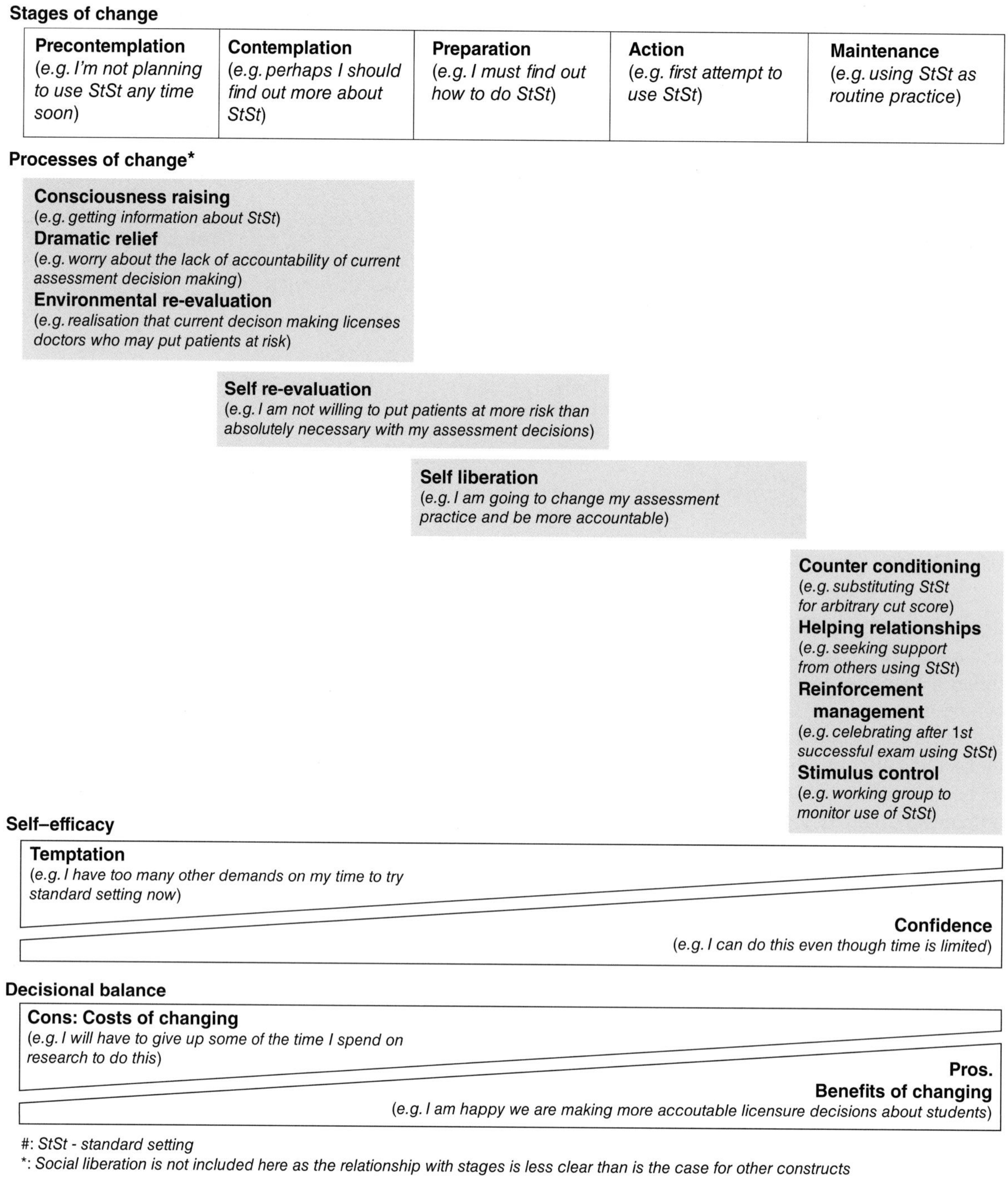

**Stages of change**

| Precontemplation (e.g. I'm not planning to use StSt any time soon) | Contemplation (e.g. perhaps I should find out more about StSt) | Preparation (e.g. I must find out how to do StSt) | Action (e.g. first attempt to use StSt) | Maintenance (e.g. using StSt as routine practice) |
|---|---|---|---|---|

**Processes of change***

**Consciousness raising**
(e.g. getting information about StSt)
**Dramatic relief**
(e.g. worry about the lack of accountability of current assessment decision making)
**Environmental re-evaluation**
(e.g. realisation that current decison making licenses doctors who may put patients at risk)

**Self re-evaluation**
(e.g. I am not willing to put patients at more risk than absolutely necessary with my assessment decisions)

**Self liberation**
(e.g. I am going to change my assessment practice and be more accountable)

**Counter conditioning**
(e.g. substituting StSt for arbitrary cut score)
**Helping relationships**
(e.g. seeking support from others using StSt)
**Reinforcement management**
(e.g. celebrating after 1st successful exam using StSt)
**Stimulus control**
(e.g. working group to monitor use of StSt)

**Self–efficacy**

**Temptation**
(e.g. I have too many other demands on my time to try standard setting now)

**Confidence**
(e.g. I can do this even though time is limited)

**Decisional balance**

**Cons: Costs of changing**
(e.g. I will have to give up some of the time I spend on research to do this)

**Pros.**
**Benefits of changing**
(e.g. I am happy we are making more accoutable licensure decisions about students)

#: StSt - standard setting
*: Social liberation is not included here as the relationship with stages is less clear than is the case for other constructs

**Figure 13.4** Trans-theoretical model (*Source*: after Bartholomew *et al.*,[2] Prochaska *et al.*[44] and Redding *et al.*[27]), approximating the relationship between components of each of the four constructs in the model

researchers composed a version of each component of the four constructs in the TTM applied to the responsiveness of consultants.

The results illustrated how different consultants were at different stages of change, for example, the stage of precontemplation: 'I can imagine that residents perceive me as scary sometimes, but there is not something I can do about it, that's just how it is'; in contrast to the stage of action: 'So after the feedback I started paying attention to my teaching and evaluating situations as learning opportunities for residents. And instead of preparing everything I now let residents think about the case and the possible diagnosis and treatment options. Yes, I involve them more in the decision-making process'.[45] The results also illustrated how the various processes of change and the self-efficacy and decisional balance constructs could be related to where different consultants found themselves in the stages of change. Two factors were found to be associated with progression through the stages of change to the stages of maintenance and termination, that is, the point of having new, established teaching behaviours. These were experiencing negative emotions through not acting on feedback (related to TTM process environmental re-evaluation) and making a strong commitment to change (related to TTM process self-liberation).

This study illustrates nicely how an abstract theory is rigorously operationalised in a specific research context. It also illustrates how theory-based questions for future research arise. One such question is how best to help recipients of feedback deal with negative emotions. The authors suggest the use of facilitated reflection. Vachon and LeBlanc[46] used critical incident analysis to this end and in turn, linked their findings to the TTM by briefly discussing how the use of this approach facilitated the readiness of occupational therapists to change their practice. Another question for researchers is how to induce a strong commitment to change in participants. Interestingly, the researchers did not identify either of these issues as part of an agenda for future research. Nor did they interrogate the implications of the finding that the TTM was a useful framework for understanding the responsiveness of consultants to registrar feedback. Given that the TTM was developed to guide behavioural interventions, it would, for example, have been useful to see a table of implications for the implementation of a feedback system that detailed the type of interventions that could be contemplated at each stage of the behaviour change process.

We turn now to one final example of the application of a specific HBT in HPE research, before examining an example of the eclectic use of constructs from different theories.

## PRECEDE model

The PRECEDE–PROCEED model differs from the previous three theories discussed in that it offers a more comprehensive framework with which to contemplate causal assessment, intervention planning and evaluation together.[47] The PRECEDE model (Predisposing, Reinforcing and Enabling Constructs in Educational/Environmental Diagnosis and Evaluation; Fig. 13.5) was the initial conceptualisation

that was subsequently expanded to develop the PRECEDE–PROCEED model (Policy, Regulatory and Organisational Constructs in Educational and Environmental Development).[47]

Mann and co-workers[28] were concerned broadly with the issue of CME, and more specifically the problem that clinical guidelines were proving insufficient to alter clinical practice. Where Tian *et al.*[34] turned to the TPB, Mann *et al.* used the PRECEDE model to inform the design and evaluation of their intervention. The project was an ambitious, multifactorial intervention aimed at addressing a variety of factors predicted by the model to influence behaviour. The components of the 'determinants' construct of the model were operationalised for the specific intervention, that is, learning how to undertake an effective cholesterol lowering intervention with patients. The evaluation was able to demonstrate how some aspects of the intervention were successful and others not. Having theorised the design of the intervention, the authors were able to speculate on the possible reasons for this and better understand the impact of those facets of the intervention that were successful.

The issue that Gelula and Yudkowsky[48] were trying to address was using faculty development to equip faculty in medicine, dentistry, pharmacy and nursing to teach clinical skills in busy clinical settings. They drew on the PRECEDE model and on Kolb both to design their intervention and interpret their findings. They conceptualised teaching behaviours as part of the lifestyle of clinical teachers. Utilising microteaching, which incorporated interaction with a standardised student and reflective discussion with colleagues based on review of videotaped encounters, they designed a series of three increasingly challenging scenarios about each of three teaching skills, that is, providing feedback to students, brief clinical teaching and asking effective questions. They were able to demonstrate both a commitment to change and subsequent changed behaviour in participants. Using components of the 'determinants' construct of the PRECEDE model, they were able to theoretically situate different components of their intervention. This also provided guidance for future research exploring the relative contribution of the various components to the success of a programme.

These two studies illustrate how theory can be used to guide the design of a comprehensive approach to change the practice of clinicians and clinical teachers, respectively. The resultant interventions were not simple, but were theory-based and both – while resource intensive – were successful in ways that could be related theoretically to

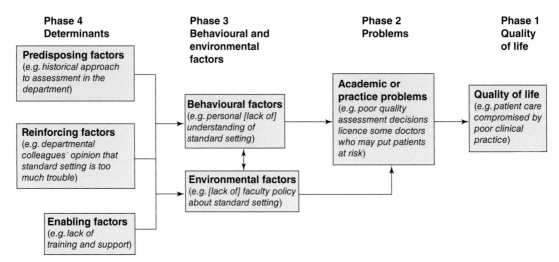

**Figure 13.5** The PRECEDE model. *Source*: After Bartholomew *et al.*[2] and Gielen *et al.*[47]

underlying principles. The PRECEDE model also offers guidance on the design of intervention evaluation that goes beyond the mere documentation of participant satisfaction.

## Eclectic approaches

Any given HBT typically only partially explains a behaviour of interest.[40–43] There is also overlap between HBTs and there have been efforts to highlight similarities in constructs across different HBTs (it is beyond the scope of this chapter to go into this; more information can be obtained from the further readings suggested at the end of this chapter).[4,49–52] Some studies described in this chapter have utilised more than one theory but drawn equally on health behaviour and other theories[28,48] while others have drawn more on one theory than another.[30,34] Other authors have drawn on different theories at different times, for example, van der Leeuw and co-workers drew on the TTM in one study[45] and social cognitive theory in another.[29] As a final example, we now proceed to examine an example of research that did not draw exclusively on any one particular theory.

The issue that Cilliers and co-workers[53,54] were concerned with was the assessment-related learning behaviour of students. The goal of that research programme was originally to devise interventions that used assessment to drive student learning in desirable ways and hence contribute to the creation of powerful learning environments. To their surprise, the researchers discovered that less was known about how assessment drove learning than received wisdom would suggest and, therefore, they adopted a grounded theory approach to explore

medical students' lived experience of summative assessment.

Initial inductive analysis revealed a strong role for various constructs related to motivation and emotion. Developing a grounded theory based on these proved difficult, however, not least because a considerable amount of the data could not be related to these constructs. Serendipitously, one of the group was working in the area of faculty development at the time and exploring HBT as an approach to understanding faculty participation in and utilisation of faculty development. From that emerged the (perhaps retrospectively self-evident!) realisation that student learning behaviours – in this case related to assessment – were nothing other than human behaviour. Given that health behaviour has been extensively researched, HBT was considered a potentially rich source of useful insights. The utilisation of constructs drawn eclectically from different HBTs (Fig. 13.6) resulted in the development of a model that incorporated, but extended beyond, motivation and emotion (see Cilliers *et al.*[9] for a detailed representation of the model).

The model[9,53,54] proposes that for any given student in any given assessment situation, one or more assessment factors result in one or more learning effects and that this relationship is mediated by one or more mechanism factors. The mechanism factors, derived from HBT, lie at the heart of the model. These include impact appraisal, that is, appraisal of impact likelihood and impact magnitude; response appraisal, that is, appraisal of response efficacy, response costs and response value; perceived agency and interpersonal factors, that is, normative beliefs and motivation to comply with those beliefs.

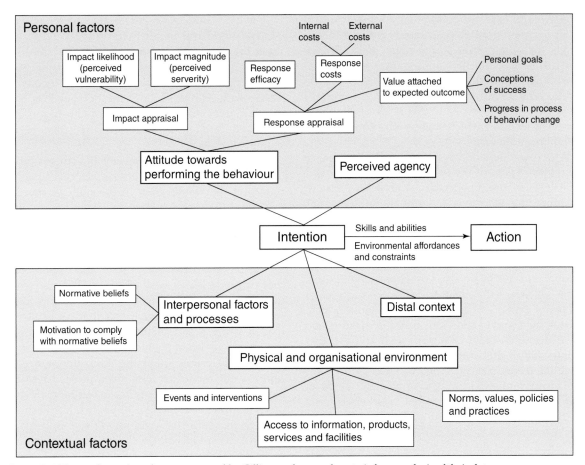

*Figure 13.6* The configuration of constructs used by Cilliers and co-workers to inform analysis of their data.

Illustrative quotes for each of these constructs can be found in Cilliers *et al.*[55]

The proposal of this model has shed new light on the relationship between assessment factors, mechanism factors and learning effects. The research has also opened a range of new avenues for researching the pre-assessment learning effects of assessment, ranging from research necessary to validate the model to the exploration of the relative impact of a large range of assessment factor–mechanism factor–learning effect relationships, some well described in the literature, others less so.

## Practical and research implications of using HBTs

One reason why so many innovations in HPE fail is because of the belief system of teachers and clinicians, which is deeply rooted in their personal experience and professional identity. Therefore, there is often little buy-in for innovations. HBTs may offer an approach to changing those beliefs. So,

what do we learn from these studies? The examples discussed illustrate how HBT has a role to play in illuminating, explaining and changing behaviour in teaching–learning settings, whether campus-based or practice-based. These theories may productively be used to plan studies, to analyse findings and, potentially, to relate findings from different studies. The potential for the latter is limited when comparing studies using different HBTs, though, as the multiple theories overlap only partially as noted above.

Utilisation of a HBT does not imply unquestioning acceptance of the tenets of that theory. There is a reciprocal relationship between research and theory. While a HBT may illuminate the findings of a study, the findings should in turn lend support to or question the contentions of the theory.[9] The studies by Mann *et al.*[28] and Tian *et al.*[34] are examples of studies that found support for some but not all of the constructs of the HBT utilised. Bunge[56] argues that one of the characteristics of genuine science is that important findings pose new problems. The use of theory should generate new avenues for research, but avenues that are conceptually related to and built on prior research. Each study using a theory offers the opportunity to interrogate and advance the theory, to build the validity argument for that theory at one or other level. (Prochaska et al.[7] have proposed a literature-based, hierarchical set of criteria by which to evaluate theories and highlight different levels at which studies may contribute to validating a theory).

When contemplating the use of a HBT, cognisance should be taken of the limitations of the theories. The level of the theory should be noted, that is, whether the theory is individual, interpersonal, organisation or community level[3,11] along with the fact that any particular HBT typically only partially explains a behaviour of interest.[40–43] Equally inasmuch as each theory tends to have its active proponents, HBTs are also not without their critics. One criticism is that the theories tend – to a greater or lesser extent – to assume that behaviour is volitional, the result of conscious decision making, and to discount the role of factors such as habit and emotion; also, that intention and plans will be stable and that the person concerned will necessarily have the means and opportunity to implement whatever course of action they decide on. Another criticism is that some theories tend to ignore the role of the proximal and more distal context, although, as noted earlier, there is an increasing tendency to incorporate these factors into the theories to create integrated models. Critics also charge that there is not always evidence that utilisation of a theory has resulted in meaningful behaviour change.

As discussed earlier in this chapter and elsewhere in this book, theories help inform the development of research questions and for this it is important to select the theoretical lenses well. There is no guidebook or algorithm that will help the researcher in this. Systems theory[57,58] suggests – amongst others – to allow for a sweeping-in phase during which the researcher produces a 'map' of the theoretical world related to his/her domain of interest and proceeds with including theoretical stances until saturation is reached. This is, of course, a judgement call and it typically resembles the saturation of information approach in qualitative methodology – or the efficient diagnostic approach in clinical medicine. If for some time reading including new theories has not shed a fundamental new light on the research, then the researcher can decide to stop including new theories and proceed to matching and selecting the theoretical frameworks that would best illuminate the scientific issue. This decision will again call for a judgement as to which theories will help formulate the clearest research questions and

will help to make most sense of the outcomes of the study. Checkland[57] refers to the boundary decision; basically a 'when enough-is-enough' decision. The studies that have been discussed illustrate how it is not necessary to be wed to one particular theoretical framework. However, once the decision has been made to use a framework, this should be rigorously followed through as illustrated by some of the papers discussed.[28,34,45,48]

Committing to a theory creates of course a pitfall of confirmation bias. The researcher can be led to interpret the results only in the light of the theory used. This is why typically researchers seek to use alternative theoretical frameworks in their discussion or re-analysis of the results. In Cilliers and co-workers'[53] first study, the straightforward behaviouristic theory or stimulus and response did not suffice to make sense of the results. It typically did not produce sufficient data 'fit', that is, there was too much informative text that could not be coded using a simple theoretical model. Instead, when they revisited the literature and selected more helpful HBTs to explain the data, it produced a more valid model of how assessment drives the constructions that students use to self-regulate their own learning. The pivotal difference has been the change in stance between seeing the students as passive receptors of reinforcement and punishment to constructivist agents of their own learning activities.

One final issue to bear in mind when using HBTs is that they are rich and complex, but none of these theories provide a complete explanation of behaviour. Typically, these theories only account for a proportion of the variance of observed behaviour.[40–43] Despite that, HBT offers a theoretical perspective with which to approach complex behavioural challenges in an ordered fashion.

## Conclusion

There are many studies that invoke HBT in passing, few that substantively engage with these theories to inform or understand the work done. Rigorously interrogating and applying these theories has much to offer HPE research, given how much of HPE research is focussed on understanding or trying to change human behaviour. Given the complexity of human behaviour and the relationships that has with environmental variables, HBT has much to offer researchers and to help ensure that small, incremental advances can be conceptually linked to enhance both understanding and practice.

## Practice points

- Health behaviour theory offers an approach to researching human behaviour in a range of teaching–learning contexts.

- There are a range of theories to draw on, each offering a somewhat different perspective on behaviour; therefore, an appropriate type of theory can be selected to match the demands of a range of research questions.

- While HBTs are rich and complex, none of these theories provide a complete explanation of behaviour.

- Researchers wishing to utilise health behaviour theory do not have to draw solely on one theory, especially given the overlap that exists between theories.

- The use of health behaviour theory allows the design of conceptually strong research.

- Different pieces of research based on health behaviour theory can be conceptually linked to build stronger bodies of research on a topic.

## Further reading and key references

Bartholomew, L.K., Parcel, G.S., Kok, G., Gottlieb, N.H. & Fernandez, M.E. (2011) Behavior-oriented theories used in health promotion. In: *Planning Health Promotion Programs: An Intervention Mapping Approach*. Jossey-Bass, San Francisco, pp. 51–112.

Fishbein, M., Triandis, H.C., Kanfer, F.H., Becker, M. & Middlestadt, S.E. (2001) Factors influencing behavior and behavior change. In: Baum, A.S., Revenson, T.A. & Singer, J.E. (eds), *Handbook of Health Psychology*. Lawrence Erlbaum, Mahwah, New Jersey, pp. 3–17.

Fishbein, M. & Yzer, M.C. (2003) Using theory to design effective health behavior interventions. *Communication Theory*, **13**, 164–183.

Gebhardt, W.A. & Maes, S. (2001) Integrating social-psychological frameworks for health behaviour research. *American Journal of Health Behavior*, **25**, 528–536.

Glanz, K. & Bishop, D.B. (2010) The role of behavioral science theory in development and implementation of public health interventions. *Annual Review of Public Health*, **31**, 399–418.

Glanz, K., Rimer, B.K. & Viswanath, K. (eds) (2008) *Health Behavior and Health Education*. Jossey-Bass, San Francisco.

Michie, S., Johnston, M., Abraham, C., Lawton, R., Parker, D. & Walker, A. (2005) Making psychological theory useful for implementing evidence based practice: a consensus approach. *Quality and Safety in Health Care*, **14**, 26–33.

Michie, S., Johnston, M., Francis, J., Hardeman, W. & Eccles, M. (2008) From theory to intervention: mapping theoretically derived behavioural determinants to behaviour change techniques. *Applied Psychology*, **57**, 660–680.

Redding, C.A., Rossi, S., Rossi, R., Velicer, W.F. & Prochaska, O. (2000) Health behavior models. *The International Electronic Journal of Health Education*, **3**, 180–193.

## References

1  Eaton, L., Flisher, A.J. & Aarø, L.E. (2003) Unsafe sexual behaviour in South African youth. *Social Science & Medicine*, **56**, 149–165.

2  Bartholomew, L.K. *et al.* (2011) Behavior-oriented theories used in health promotion. In: *Planning Health Promotion Programs: An Intervention Mapping Approach*. Jossey-Bass, San Francisco, pp. 51–112.

3  Glanz, K., Rimer, B.K. & Viswanath, K. (2008) *Health Behavior and Health Education*. Jossey-Bass, San Francisco.

4  Lippke, S. & Ziegelmann, J.P. (2008) Theory-based health behavior change: developing, testing, and applying theories for evidence-based interventions. *Applied Psychology*, **57**, 698–716.

5  Michie, S., Rothman, A.J. & Sheeran, P. (2007) Current issues and new direction in psychology and health: advancing the science of behavior change. *Psychology & Health*, **22**, 249–253.

6  Rimer, B.K. & Glanz, K. (2005) *Theory at a Glance: A Guide for Health Promotion Practice*. National Cancer Institute, National Institutes of Health, U.S. Department of Health and Human Services, Bethesda, Maryland.

7  Prochaska, J.O., Wright, J.A. & Velicer, W.F. (2008) Evaluating theories of health behavior change: a hierarchy of criteria applied to the transtheoretical model. *Applied Psychology*, **57**, 561–588.

8  Glanz, K. & Bishop, D.B. (2010) The role of behavioral science theory in development and implementation of public health interventions. *Annual Review of Public Health*, **31**, 399–418.

9  Cilliers, F.J., Schuwirth, L.W.T. & van der Vleuten, C.P.M. (2012) Modelling the pre-assessment learning effects of assessment: evidence in the validity chain. *Medical Education*, **46**, 1087–1098.

10  Munro, S. *et al.* (2007) A review of health behaviour theories: how useful are these for developing interventions to promote long-term medication adherence for TB and HIV/AIDS? *BMC Public Health*, **7**, 104.

11  Bartholomew, L.K. *et al.* (2011) *Planning Health Promotion Programs: An Intervention Mapping Approach*, 3rd edn. Jossey-Bass, San Francisco.

12  Montano, D.E. *et al.* (1988) A survey of fourth-year medical students' decisions regarding family practice as a career. *Academic Medicine*, **63**, 830–838.

13  Grossman, R. & Salas, E. (2011) The transfer of training: what really matters. *International Journal of Training and Development*, **15**, 103–120.

14 Blume, B.D. *et al.* (2010) Transfer of training: a meta-analytic review. *Journal of Management*, **36**, 1065–1105.

15 de Rijdt, C. *et al.* (2013) Influencing variables and moderators of transfer of learning to the workplace within the area of staff development in higher education: research review. *Educational Research Review*, **8**, 48–74.

16 van den Eertwegh, V. *et al.* (2013) Learning in context: Identifying gaps in research on the transfer of medical communication skills to the clinical workplace. *Patient Education and Counseling*, **90**, 184–192.

17 Singh, T. *et al.* (2014) Paying attention to intention to transfer in faculty development using the theory of planned behavior. *American Journal of Educational Research*, **2**, 361–365.

18 Winzenberg, T. & Higginbotham, N. (2003) Factors affecting the intention of providers to deliver more effective continuing medical education to general practitioners: a pilot study. *BMC Medical Education*, **3**, 11.

19 Archer, M. *et al.* (1998) *Critical Realism: Essential Readings*. Routledge, London.

20 Danermark, B. (2002) *Explaining Society: Critical Realism in the Social Sciences*. Routledge, Oxford.

21 Quinn, L. (2007) A social realist account of the emergence of a formal academic staff development programme at a South African university. Unpublished PhD Thesis, Centre for Higher Education Research, Teaching and Learning, Faculty of Education. Rhodes University, Grahamstown p. 298.

22 Leibowitz, B. (2014) Conducive environments for the promotion of quality teaching in higher education in South Africa. *Critical Studies in Teaching and Learning*, **2**, 49–73.

23 McFadden, D.W. *et al.* (2012) Game theory: applications for surgeons and the operating room environment. *Surgery*, **152**, 915–922.

24 Tarrant, C., Stokes, T. & Colman, A.M. (2004) Models of the medical consultation: opportunities and limitations of a game theory perspective. *Quality and Safety in Health Care*, **13**, 461–466.

25 Richard, L., Gauvin, L. & Raine, K. (2011) Ecological models revisited: their uses and evolution in health promotion over two decades. *Annual Review of Public Health*, **32**, 307–326.

26 Artino, A. R. *et al.* (2015). Self-regulated learning in healthcare profession education: theoretical perspectives and research methods. *Researching Medical Education*. J. Cleland and S. J. Durning, Wiley.

27 Redding, C.A. *et al.* (2000) Health behavior models. *The International Electronic Journal of Health Education*, **3**, 180–193.

28 Mann, K.V. *et al.* (1997) Increasing physician involvement In cholesterol-lowering practices: The role of knowledge, attitudes and perceptions. *Advances in Health Sciences Education*, **2**, 237–253.

29 Jochemsen-van der Leeuw, H.G.A.R. *et al.* (2013) The attributes of the clinical trainer as a role model: a systematic review. *Academic Medicine*, **88**, 26–34.

30 Mann, K.V. *et al.* (2011) Tensions in informed self-assessment: how the desire for feedback and reticence to collect and use it can conflict. *Academic Medicine*, **86**, 1120–1127.

31 Fishbein, M. & Cappella, J.N. (2006) The role of theory in developing effective health communications. *Journal of Communication*, **56**, S1–S17.

32 Montano, D.E. & Kasprzyk, D. (2008) Theory of reasoned action, theory of planned behavior, and the integrated behavioral model. In: Glanz, K., Rimer, B.K. & Viswanath, K. (eds), *Health Behavior and Health Education: Theory, Research, and Practice*. Jossey-Bass, San Francisco, pp. 67–95.

33 Cleland, J. *et al.* (2007) Using theory to improve communication: designing a communication skills training package for medicine counter assistants. *International Journal of Pharmacy Practice*, **15**, 79–81.

34 Tian, J. *et al.* (2010) The development of a theory-based instrument to evaluate the effectiveness of continuing medical education. *Academic Medicine*, **85**, 1518–1525.

35 Archer, R. *et al.* (2008) The theory of planned behaviour in medical education: a model for integrating professionalism training. *Medical Education*, **42**, 771–777.

36 Rees, C.E. & Knight, L.V. (2007) Viewpoint: the trouble with assessing students' professionalism: theoretical insights from sociocognitive psychology. *Academic Medicine*, **82**, 46–50.

37 Alleyne, P. & Phillips, K. (2011) Exploring academic dishonesty among university students in barbados: an extension to the theory of planned behaviour. *Journal of Academic Ethics*, **9**, 323–338.

38 Champion, V.L. & Skinner, C.S. (2008) The health belief model. In: Glanz, K., Rimer, B.K. & Viswanath, K. (eds), *Health Behavior and Health Education*. Jossey-Bass, San Francisco.

39 Willett, L.L. *et al.* (2010) Do women residents delay childbearing due to perceived career threats? *Academic Medicine*, **85**, 640–646.

40 Sheeran, P. (2002) Intention–behavior relations: a conceptual and empirical review. *European Review of Social Psychology*, **12**, 1–36.

41 Godin, G. *et al.* (2008) Healthcare professionals' intentions and behaviours: a systematic review of studies based on social cognitive theories. *Implementation Science*, **3**, 1–12.

42 Armitage, C.J. & Conner, M. (2001) Efficacy of the theory of planned behaviour: a meta-analytic review. *British Journal of Social Psychology*, **40**, 471–499.

43 Webb, T.L. & Sheeran, P. (2006) Does changing behavioral intentions engender behavior change? A meta-analysis of the experimental evidence. *Psychological Bulletin*, **132**, 249–268.

44 Prochaska, J.O., Redding, C.A. & Evers, K.E. (2008) The transtheoretical model and stages of change. In: Glanz, K., Rimer, B.K. & Viswanath, K. (eds), *Health Behavior and Health Education*. Jossey-Bass, San Francisco.

45 van der Leeuw, R.M. *et al.* (2013) Explaining how faculty members act upon residents' feedback to improve their teaching performance. *Medical Education*, **47**, 1089–1098.

46 Vachon, B. & LeBlanc, J. (2011) Effectiveness of past and current critical incident analysis on reflective learning and practice change. *Medical Education*, **45**, 894–904.

47 Gielen, A.C. *et al.* (2008) Using the PRECEDE-PROCEED model to apply health behaviour theories. In: Glanz, K., Rimer, B.K. & Viswanath, K. (eds), *Health Behavior and Health Education*. Jossey-Bass, San Francisco.

48 Gelula, M.H. & Yudkowsky, R. (2003) Using standardised students in faculty development workshops to improve clinical teaching skills. *Medical Education*, **37**, 621–629.

49 Gebhardt, W.A. & Maes, S. (2001) Integrating social-psychological frameworks for health behavior research. *American Journal of Health Behavior*, **25**, 528–536.

50 Michie, S. *et al.* (2013) The behavior change Technique Taxonomy (v1) of 93 hierarchically clustered techniques: building an international consensus for the reporting of behavior change interventions. *Annals of Behavioral Medicine*, **46**, 81–95.

51 Michie, S. *et al.* (2008) From theory to intervention: mapping theoretically derived behavioural determinants to behaviour change techniques. *Applied Psychology*, **57**, 660–680.

52 Fishbein, M. *et al.* (2001) Factors influencing behavior and behavior change. In: Baum, A.S., Revenson, T.A. & Singer, J.E. (eds), *Handbook of Health Psychology*. Lawrence Erlbaum, Mahwah, New Jersey.

53 Cilliers, F.J. *et al.* (2010) The mechanism of impact of summative assessment on medical students' learning. *Advances in Health Sciences Education*, **15**, 695–715.

54 Cilliers, F.J. *et al.* (2012) A model of the pre-assessment learning effects of summative assessment in medical education. *Advances in Health Sciences Education*, **17**, 39–53.

55 Cilliers, F.J., Schuwirth, L.W.T. & van der Vleuten, C.P.M. (2012) A model of the pre-assessment learning effects of assessment is operational in an undergraduate clinical context. *BMC Medical Education*, **12**, 9.

56 Bunge, M. (2011) Knowledge: genuine and bogus. *Science & Education*, **20**, 411–438.

57 Checkland, P. (1985) From optimizing to learning: a development of systems thinking for the 1990s. *The Journal of the Operational Research Society*, **36**, 757–767.

58 Ulrich, W. (2001) The quest for competence in systemic research and practice. *Systems Research and Behavioral Science*, **18**, 3–28.

# 14 Self-regulated learning in healthcare profession education: theoretical perspectives and research methods

*Anthony R. Artino, Jr., Ryan Brydges and Larry D. Gruppen*

*The world affords people uncountable opportunities to learn many things, but not all opportunities are taken up—people are selective—they self-regulate learning.*
*–Philip Winne (2011)*

## Introduction

Consider Mary, a third year medical student on a surgery rotation. For as long as she can remember, Mary has wanted to become a general surgeon, and her current goal is to learn more about a particular surgical procedure. Mary decides to design her own learning plan: she spends extra time reviewing the literature, practicing her suturing skills and carefully observing the surgical residents. She also sets several short-term goals, such as observing at least five procedures in a week and studying her surgery text at least 2 hours every night. To stay motivated, she rewards herself (e.g. by going out with friends) each time she successfully achieves a set number of her short-terms goals. Whenever she receives feedback from her clinical teachers, she reflects on that input and adapts her learning strategies accordingly. At the end of her surgery clerkship, Mary is at the top of her class and much closer to her goal of beginning surgical residency. By actively regulating her learning activities, Mary bolstered her knowledge and skills in surgery, gained confidence and strengthened her longstanding interest in surgery.

This chapter is about the learning processes of Mary – a highly motivated, self-regulated learner. The purpose of the chapter is to introduce self-regulated learning (SRL) theory to medical education researchers, particularly those who might be interested in applying SRL frameworks to study and improve healthcare profession education. To achieve this purpose, we first provide a broad definition of SRL, followed by a review of the common assumptions that underlie SRL theories. We then discuss in more detail three influential frameworks and describe several research methods to explore SRL in various healthcare profession education contexts. We end with a look into the future of SRL research in medical education.

## Defining self-regulation and self-regulated learning

The study of self-regulation has a long history in the fields of psychology, education and medicine. Broadly speaking, self-regulation can be defined as the processes that individuals use to guide their goal-directed activities by controlling and managing their cognition, affect and behaviour.[1] Simply stated, individuals regulate their thoughts, feelings and actions to achieve their goals. Theories of self-regulation have been used to explain how and why individuals put forth effort to achieve a variety of life goals, from losing weight and quitting smoking to learning to play the guitar and gaining expertise in medicine. As Sitzmann and Ely[1] (p. 421) observed, 'self-regulation enables people to function effectively in their personal lives as well as to acquire the knowledge and skills needed to succeed in higher education and the workforce'. In this way, many scholars believe that self-regulation is an essential component of life success.

SRL is a subset of the broader concept of self-regulation. SRL is a multidimensional construct that includes a number of self-directed *processes* that learners use to turn their mental abilities into academic skill and lasting performance.[2] Thus, SRL is not a mental ability, such as intelligence, nor is it an academic skill, such as reading proficiency; instead it is a set of processes requiring a proactive learner. Viewed this way, learning is not something that happens to individuals who self-regulate, rather it is an activity that individuals initiate, manage and adapt to achieve their goals. In short, self-regulated

*Researching Medical Education*, First Edition. Edited by Jennifer Cleland and Steven J. Durning.
© 2015 John Wiley & Sons, Ltd. Published 2015 by John Wiley & Sons, Ltd.

learners are *active participants* who generate the thoughts, feelings and actions necessary to attain their learning goals.[3]

Notably, SRL is not an all-or-nothing phenomenon. Individuals are self-regulated to the extent that they are cognitively, motivationally and behaviourally involved in their own learning activities.[4] Moreover, individuals self-regulate at varying levels across different contexts. For example, a graduate nursing student, who is part of a research interest group, might engage in much more focused and effortful study during her research methods course compared to a leadership course that she has dreaded for personal reasons.

## Core assumptions and common features of SRL theories

The psychology and education literatures describe many different theories of SRL, all of which propose slightly different features and processes (for a review, see Boekaerts *et al.*,[5] Puustinen and Pulkkinen,[6] Sitzmann and Ely,[1] Zimmerman and Schunk[7]). Despite this theoretical diversity, most models of SRL have in common several core features (see Table 14.1). First, most theories of SRL describe a self-oriented *feedback loop* composed of multiple processes and sub-processes. Self-regulated learners employ these cyclical processes in an effort to monitor the effectiveness of their activities and respond to feedback (both self-generated feedback and feedback from others[7]). Explanations of how learners respond to feedback and which processes and sub-processes are most important differentiate the various theoretical perspectives.

A second common feature of SRL theories relates to *motivation*. That is, most SRL theories address, to some degree, why and how learners choose to use (or *not* use) various learning strategies. Motivation is not only a precursor to self-regulated action, but it can also be considered a beneficial outcome. That is, the consequences of selecting a successful study strategy might be both enhanced skill *and* more intrinsic motivation to engage in the activity in the future.[8] Therefore, clarifying how motivation is enhanced and maintained is fundamental to understanding what differentiates good students from struggling students.

A third common, core feature of most SRL theories is that students have some type of *goal*, criterion or standard against which their academic progress can be compared.[8,9] Using these self-generated goals, learners are able to gauge their progress, determine whether their approach

*Table 14.1* Four core features of SRL theories

| Core feature | Description |
|---|---|
| Feedback loop | Self-regulated learners employ cyclical processes and sub-processes for the purpose of monitoring the effectiveness of their activities and responding to feedback. |
| Motivation | SRL theories address why and how learners choose to self-regulate. |
| Goal setting | Individuals who self-regulate have some type of goal, criterion or standard against which their academic progress can be compared. |
| Self-monitoring | Self-monitoring is the mechanism self-regulated learners use to keep track of how they are doing. |

is working and make appropriate changes. This dynamic approach to learning distinguishes highly self-regulated individuals from their more naïve counterparts.

A fourth common feature of SRL theories is their emphasis on *self-monitoring*. As Cleary *et al.*[10] (p. 467) have described, 'self-monitoring acts as a core feedback mechanism in SRL models because it is through this process that individuals increase their self-awareness and gather the requisite information to effectively evaluate how they performed on a particular task'. Self-monitoring is a mechanism that self-regulated learners use to keep track of how they are doing. A trainee practising a procedure may, for example, track the number of errors he/she makes along with the potential ways he/she might improve. Self-monitoring can also involve more covert monitoring of one's own cognition and cognitive processes through meta-cognition (defined below). Conceptually, accurate self-monitoring improves SRL by helping individuals identify what they know, what they do not know and where they need to focus their efforts to improve future learning and performance.[1]

## Related concepts in medical education

Medical education researchers often fail to make useful distinctions among theoretical frameworks. The result is conceptual confusion, with researchers intentionally or unintentionally blurring important differences among terms and definitions.[11] In medical education, constructs related to SRL include meta-cognition, self-assessment, self-directed learning (SDL) and reflection, to name just a few. Even though it is beyond the scope of this chapter to compare and contrast all of these related constructs, below is a brief discussion of two: meta-cognition and SDL (for a more complete analysis, see Cleary *et al.*,[10] Loyens *et al.*,[11] Lajoie[12]).

The terms meta-cognition and SRL are often used interchangeably, but differ in important ways. Flavell[13] coined 'meta-cognition' as a reference to thinking about one's own thinking. Over the years, the term meta-cognition has been broadened to include the degree to which individuals monitor, control and regulate their own cognitive activities.[14] Models of SRL, by contrast, typically include meta-cognition as just one facet of self-regulation, albeit a central facet. Thus, consideration for meta-cognition and meta-cognitive control strategies is normally incorporated under the broader conceptualisation of SRL.[10]

SDL is another related construct that has received much attention from medical education researchers, who often use SDL interchangeably with SRL. A key difference between the two constructs is that theories of SDL emerged from the adult learning literature whereas theories of SRL developed primarily from the educational psychology literature. Knowles,[15] (p. 18) a well-known adult learning theorist, defined SDL as 'a process in which individuals take the initiative, with or without the help from others, in diagnosing their learning needs, formulating goals, identifying human and material resources, choosing and implementing appropriate learning strategies and evaluating learning outcomes'. This definition has led many medical educators to invoke SDL when describing problem-based learning. Some theorists do not believe that the two concepts are drastically different; for example, Zimmerman and Lebeau[16] (p. 299) noted that definitions of SDL are 'highly similar to what has been termed SRL in the educational psychology literature'. By contrast, others argue that SDL is a much broader concept. Whereas theories of SRL typically characterise the learner, theories of SDL often refer to both the learner and how the learning environment can be designed to facilitate self-direction.[11,17] In sum, although SDL and SRL are closely related ideas, they have emerged from different literatures. What is more, we would argue that SRL has a much richer theoretical and empirical foundation. As such, we encourage medical educators to apply SRL frameworks to research in healthcare profession education in a way that is clear, precise and comprehensive so that other researchers can understand their perspective and build on their work.

## Three influential SRL perspectives

The academic study of SRL and related constructs has been an area of enquiry across a diverse range of research disciplines. From computer engineering to clinical psychology to childhood development, researchers have developed models and theories aimed at clarifying how individuals learn to manage, control and adapt their learning. At present, two of the best resources for in-depth descriptions of those theories are Zimmerman and Schunk's[7] handbook on SRL theoretical perspectives and a recent systematic review and meta-analysis of SRL theories.[1] To cover all of the theories in the depth they deserve, it would span more pages than this textbook. Hence, we only discuss the fundamental principles of three influential theoretical perspectives that represent the continuum from largely cognitive to largely social descriptions of SRL: (1) information processing/control theory, (2) social-cognitive theory and (3) social-constructivist theory.

### Information processing theories of SRL

Information processing theories of SRL evolved from work aimed at developing computer systems in the early 20th century. Called 'control theory' in its primary formulation,[18] contemporary theorists now use information processing to describe their goal of understanding human cognitive functioning as it relates to SRL.[7] Self-regulation is conceptualised as a cyclical process that uses a negative feedback loop to make learners aware of discrepancies between their current state and a goal state.[19] To regulate their learning efficiently and minimise these discrepancies, theorists assert that limited cognitive resources require learners to organise their knowledge into 'chunks' or 'schemas'. Tactics are schemas that learners use to manage information as they learn, and strategies help them coordinate a set of tactics into 'if-then-else' units: IF conditions are met, THEN enact a tactic, ELSE use a different tactic.[19] For example, IF a faculty member uses a term that a student does not understand, THEN she will ask a peer what it means (easy strategy), ELSE she will consult a textbook (more difficult strategy).

One information processing model proposes that SRL consists of three necessary phases, plus a fourth 'optional' phase.[9,20] First, learners process the learning conditions and construct a perception of task expectations.[21] Second, learners build upon their expectations to formulate task goals and the plans they believe will help them accomplish those goals. Third, learners begin their actual work and apply tactics or strategies to their learning situation. The fourth phase occurs if learners believe it is necessary to adapt how their schemas are organised and/or deployed. A learner may realise, for example, that re-reading the textbook multiple times is not a useful tactic for understanding information and may choose to delete that tactic from future strategies aimed at that goal. Central to these phases is 'meta-cognitive monitoring', which Winne[19] describes as the necessary process for identifying whether the discrepancy between current and goal states exists.

In response to criticisms that their models are narrowly cognitive, information processing theorists recently added the social context as an aspect to be considered in Phase 1 of the model.[20] As a part of this shift, researchers have been studying how to use computer systems to 'scaffold' and support self-regulation in ways that help learners shift efficiently from novice to expert.[22] An example of such a system is nStudy, which researchers have developed to provide learners with supports for their SRL while also collecting a repository of 'behavioural traces'. Researchers are data-mining those traces in order to identify useful tactics and strategies from learners' behaviours that they can translate into additional supports (e.g. using how and what learners search in the system to create supportive hints, shortcuts and tutorials).[23] Such efforts have clear application in the study of e-learning modules, which are ever-expanding in healthcare profession education contexts.

## Social-cognitive model of SRL

Evolving from his seminal work on self-efficacy, Bandura's[24] social-cognitive theory has influenced several productive researchers. His key idea of 'reciprocal determinism' is that a learner's behaviour is determined by the interactions between personal factors (i.e. cognitive, affective and biological processes) and environmental factors (i.e. social and physical surroundings). Hence, a change in any of these three systems – behavioural, personal and environmental – will influence the others in a constantly evolving and reciprocal manner.

Social-cognitive theorists encourage researchers to consider the bidirectional transaction between social and cognitive events and depict self-regulatory competence as developing initially from social influences, which eventually shift to self-influences over four non-linear levels.[25] *Observational learning* is the first level, where social influences are strongest and derive from learners watching others perform the task (i.e. task-modelling). Second, learners are in the *emulative level* when they are

able to imitate the observed performance. While learners are internalising observed tasks or strategies, this internalisation relies on exposure to social/environmental cues and thus levels one and two are socially dependent.[26] The third level is called *self-control*, the hallmark being learners' ability to use the acquired skill or strategy independently during performance. While the internalisation process is nearly complete, learners' task representations are still heavily reliant on the observed general pattern of performance.[25] Learners achieve the fourth level when they become *self-regulated* and able to systematically adapt skills and strategies to any changes in personal, behavioural and/or environmental conditions.[26] Key to the social-cognitive model is that, while social influences diminish, they do not disappear with advancing skill acquisition. Thus, a learner who fails to capitalise on feedback available from the social environment may fail to acquire a critical skill needed when self-teaching methods are insufficient.

Researchers have used this model to produce a wealth of evidence on many 'core processes' thought to be enacted during a three-phase self-regulation cycle: forethought, performance and self-reflection (see Fig. 14.1).[27] During forethought, learners will enact self-efficacy and may use their observations of a social model to develop goals and assess value as they prepare to learn.[26] During performance, learners will enact task strategies for learning, such as using self-questioning to compare themselves to social standards and judge progress towards goals. Finally, self-reflection occurs after performance and involves processes such as self-evaluation and learners making causal attributions about the results of their performance (e.g. attributing poor performance to insufficient effort rather than to a limit in one's abilities). Beyond serving as a helpful model for describing and explaining SRL, this cycle has also spawned a methodology called SRL microanalysis (see Cleary *et al.*[28]). In fact, SRL microanalysis has been used increasingly in the healthcare professions to study medical trainees' self-regulation of skills including venipuncture[29] and clinical reasoning skills[30] (see description of SRL microanalysis below).

## Constructivist models of SRL

Constructivism arose from a diverse set of researchers (especially Bartlett, Piaget and Bruner) who believed that learners construct idiosyncratic cognitive schemas, which form the basis for learning and recall. As Paris *et al.*[31] noted, however, a 'second

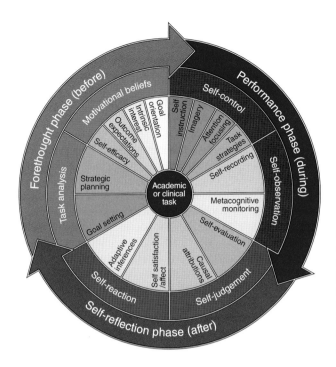

*Figure 14.1* A three-phase, cyclical model of SRL. This model is adapted from Zimmerman,[27] and depicts three sequential phases of SRL: forethought (before), performance (during) and self-reflection (after). The model also shows, within each phase, the sub-processes of SRL. Source: Artino AR, Jones KD. Last Page: Self-regulated learning: A dynamic, cyclical perspective. *Academic Medicine*, 2013; 88: 1048. Reproduced with permission of Wolters Kluwer Health.

wave' of constructivism in the 1990s spurred further theorising, and researchers eventually installed social and cultural influences as key features of how individuals construct theories about themselves and about academic learning.

Under this new model of constructivism, learning is regarded as situated in social and historical contexts, meaning the SRL behaviours and actions to be regulated are malleable and often are shaped by social roles in the learning situation.[31] Research on this process of 'enculturation' has shown that novices learn the practices, values and customs of a community, such as how to behave in the classroom context.[32,33] As learners evolve their identity and sense of group membership, they actively co-construct their self-image and self-regulatory practices with members of the social groups they are joining. Identity tends to be constructed in a personalised way that reflects optimism,[31] though there are instances where the process leads to maladaptive behaviours, such as sheltering one's self-identity by constantly deflecting feedback from others about a deficiency in one's communication skills.

Fundamental to constructivism is the belief that individuals are naturally inclined to construct theories about all facets of their life. Researchers have studied emerging theories about self-competence, education, learning, agency and control and strategies.[31] Learners' beliefs and desires provide the motivation for them to construct certain theories

that they use to justify their behaviours. The relative nature of these theories is key, as they are prone to shift in response to the experiences the learner accrues over time. Hence, the constructivist view situates SRL in the context in which it develops, providing a useful lens for inspecting the multiple individual and social factors that influence how learning is regulated.

Many theories of SRL have emerged from the social-constructivist perspective. Butler and Cartier[34] suggest the need to study the interactions between what individuals bring to a learning context (e.g. beliefs, knowledge, personal theories and cognitive schemas) and features of that specific learning environment. They emphasise that educators and researchers should strive to identify environmental and social supports that will help learners construct the meta-cognitive knowledge and positive self-perceptions required for them to engage in sustained, iterative cycles of goal-directed learning.[35] Expanding these ideas and applying them to collaborative, group learning contexts,[36] suggest that researchers and educators must attend to each individual's 'cognitive angle' (i.e. their cognitions, meta-cognitions and interpretations) as well as the 'situative angle' (i.e. how groups create affordances and constraints for individual and group involvement). According to their model and preliminary evidence, the cognitive and situative angles must be considered jointly to develop a comprehensive model of socially constructed SRL in a given context. Applying such a model would require that researchers study SRL as situated and unique in every different context within which learners work.

## Summary

A common thread across these three theories is that SRL is viewed as a cyclical process that learners are aware of through active self-monitoring processes. A key difference among theories is the source of information used to drive that cycle – information processing theorists believe it is a cognitive negative discrepancy feedback loop, social-cognitivists believe it is self-judgments and causal attributions and socio-constructivists believe it is an analysis of the interaction between social factors and personal theories. Rather than emphasise these divergences, instead we suggest readers consider this brief summary alongside more comprehensive reviews (e.g. Sitzmann and colleagues[1,37]) to see how each theory makes its own unique contribution to a robust overall understanding of SRL. As readers develop their own perspectives on the nature of knowledge, they will find that each theory offers itself as a useful tool for clarifying the different ways that healthcare professionals learn to manage their own learning in the complex training and practice contexts in which education and patient care take place.

## Methods for studying SRL in medical education

The preceding sections provide some guidance for the researcher to identify key constructs in the study of SRL and frameworks for making predictions and hypotheses. However, translating these theoretical questions into research requires careful thought about the methods to be used. Although some methods are closely associated with some theories, there is considerable room (and need) for innovation in designing research studies in educational settings. What follows are descriptions of several methods that have been used to study SRL in healthcare profession education contexts. In addition, Table 14.2 summarises the strengths and weaknesses of each method.

### Questionnaires

Questionnaires and similar self-report methods (e.g. interviews[38,39] and focus groups[40]) account for the majority of studies of SRL. In addition to study-specific questionnaires, several instruments have been proposed for broad use in studying SRL; these include the Student Learning Survey,[41] the Self-Directed Learning Readiness Scale,[42] the Continuous Learning Inventory[43] and the Jefferson Scale of Life-Long Learning. These questionnaires and related methods are frequently used to quantify learner preferences for alternative SRL activities or strategies,[44] clinical situations that stimulate SRL,[45] obstacles and facilitators of SRL[46] and the adoption of innovations into practice.[47] These questionnaires commonly ask respondents to rate the frequency of their behaviours or the intensity of their attitudes or beliefs on Likert-type scales, which may then be aggregated into subscales that measure underlying constructs. Such questionnaires are almost always reports about oneself and are completed in contexts outside of a specific SRL activity. In this way, questionnaires are often used to understand SRL more generally rather than tying facets of SRL to actual learning behaviours.

One example of this methodology is provided by Gruppen *et al.*[48] who used two self-report questionnaires in a repeated-measures design to measure self-assessed diagnostic ability and self-directed study time. This study examined medical students' self-regulation decisions related to the allocation of study time over several patient-presenting complaints representative of problems likely to be encountered on an internal medical clerkship. The specific research question focused on the extent to which these medical students used self-identified strengths and weaknesses in diagnostic skills of these complaints to guide their allocation of study time to each complaint. As used in this study, questionnaires allowed students to report on past behaviours and summarise over multiple events and activities. Ostensibly, their answers were less tied to the peculiarities of a single situation and appeared to generalise across settings that require diagnostic skills. The questionnaires also provided access to learner attitudes and beliefs, though an important limitation of this study is that there were no independent data about their actual behaviours (e.g. the amount of time allocated); the researchers only had the students' self-reports to rely on. We summarise the strengths and limitations of questionnaires in Table 14.2.

### Multiple case studies

A case study is defined as a methodology used to study people, groups or events in order to develop a deep understanding of a phenomenon as it unfolds and is situated in context.[49,50] A comprehensive discussion of case study methods as they apply to research on SRL can be found elsewhere.[51] We provide a brief overview here. Firstly, case studies can

*Table 14.2* Strengths and limitations of three individual methods and one multi-method approach to studying SRL in medical education

|  | Self-report questionnaires | Case studies | SRL microanalysis | Triangulating multiple methods |
|---|---|---|---|---|
| Strengths | – Easy to construct, administer and analyse<br>– Very familiar to learners and requires no special training<br>– Can assess a wide range of variables that are not easily obtained by other methods | – Helps develop hypotheses for further study<br>– Provides rich data<br>– Designed to capture the dynamic, context-specific nature of SRL | – Customisable to specific tasks<br>– Designed to capture the dynamic, context-specific nature of SRL<br>– Assessment is closely linked to theoretical framework, thereby making interpretation easier | – Use of different methods to compensate for each individual methods' bias<br>– Provides rich, detailed data<br>– Designed to capture the dynamic, context-specific nature of SRL |
| Limitations | – Questions may not map accurately to the underlying construct or the learners' experiences<br>– Participants may be prone to recall bias<br>– Less effective at capturing the dynamic, context-specific nature of SRL | – Flexible, iterative nature of data collection and analysis is difficult to master<br>– Relies heavily on researcher's subjective interpretations<br>– Difficult to establish that sampled cases are representative of the phenomenon | – Task-specific protocols are time-consuming to construct, administer and analyse<br>– Data gathered are highly specific to situation and likely do not generalise to other activities<br>– Protocol is somewhat intrusive and may interrupt the natural course of the activity | – Need for expertise in collecting and interpreting data using different methods<br>– Cost and time associated with multiple data sets<br>– Conflicting data from different methods can be difficult to interpret |
| Example HPE studies | Gruppen et al., 2000[48] | Evensen et al., 2001[53] | Artino et al., 2014[30] | Brydges et al., 2013[59] |

be used for many purposes, including describing a phenomenon, exploring cases to generate research questions or for theory-building. Butler[51] describes a case study method, where the research question is central and additional design features are built around it using an iterative, flexible approach. Those additional features include selecting the case (i.e. sampling), collecting data, reducing and interpreting data, warranting assertions and representing findings. Each of these design features are described as fluid and can be returned to and modified as the research project evolves. In choosing cases, for example, case study researchers use 'purposive sampling' to select specific individuals (cases) that will allow them to best answer their research questions.[52]

Evensen et al.[53] used case study methods to investigate first year medical students' SRL within a problem-based medical education curriculum. Specifically, one researcher followed six students during their entire 16-week semester, collecting evidence from various contexts (e.g. PBL sessions, performance assessments), using various techniques (e.g. interviews, observational field notes) and across different time points (i.e. more intensively at first). Therefore, the researchers collected a rich data set for each individual and, rather than pool those data, instead analysed each student as a unique unit of analysis. Ultimately, the authors describe a theory of how the students developed different 'stances' (i.e. proactive, reactive, retroactive, interactive and transactive) that governed their behaviours and use of self-regulation when situated in different learning contexts.

As the aforementioned study shows, case study researchers will draw on multiple data sources in their investigations (e.g. observations, interviews, reports of participants' behaviours, self-reports and performance-based assessments). Having multiple data sources allows researchers to 'triangulate' those sources to develop a robust understanding of the phenomenon under study. As they interpret data and form assertions, researchers often keep an audit trail detailing their rationale for making certain modifications. Originators of the method[50] suggest that researchers might consider each case as an 'independent study', and the analysis of commonalities and discrepancies across cases allows researchers to make coherent assertions about generalisable patterns and theoretical principles that may apply to the particular context under study.[51]

## SRL microanalysis

Microanalysis is a broad term that describes a fine-grained form of assessment that targets an individual's thoughts, feelings and actions as they occur in real time.[54] Microanalytic techniques have been used to study SRL in K-12 students, college undergraduates and medical students.[28] Broadly, the technique targets the cyclical-phase processes of SRL as individuals engage in specific tasks. As an assessment methodology, SRL microanalysis involves making several assumptions about student learning and what is needed to effectively evaluate student performance. A critical assumption of SRL microanalysis is that beliefs, emotions and behaviours are dynamic and fluid and thus will often vary across contexts. This assumption of context specificity suggests that SRL assessment tools should be tailored to specific contexts. Microanalytic approaches address this assumption by including standardised questions about specific self-regulatory processes as trainees engage in authentic learning or performance tasks.

Microanalytic assessments are structured interviews with several distinguishing features. First, microanalytic protocols are administered while learners complete a task that has a clear beginning, middle and end.[54] Second, microanalytic protocols include both close-ended (e.g. Likert-type) and open-ended questions that are customised to the characteristics and demands of the task. This feature distinguishes a microanalytic protocol from a questionnaire that might be used to assess SRL across a variety of settings. To work effectively, SRL microanalytic protocols *must* be customised to the task. Finally, microanalytic assessments are based on SRL theory and are temporally sequenced to coincide with the before, during and after phases of an activity. For example, Zimmerman's[7] three-phase cyclical loop includes forethought, performance and reflection processes. Thus, if one were employing Zimmerman's SRL framework, the microanalytic protocol would be structured such that forethought-phase questions are administered before the task, performance-phase questions are administered during the task and reflection-phase questions are administered after the task. Making direct links between SRL theory, the nature of the task and the assessment approach allows the researcher to generate theoretically grounded interpretations about how SRL processes are initiated and adapted during all phases of a task.

In medical education contexts, the use of SRL microanalysis techniques has only just begun. For example, Artino *et al.*[30] recently used Zimmerman's[7] three-phase cyclical model to create forethought-, performance- and reflection-phase questions (see Fig. 14.1). The authors then asked 71 second year medical students to work through a paper-based, clinical case while administering the SRL microanalysis. Following data collection, the researchers developed a scoring rubric to categorise participants' open-ended responses according to the procedures described by Cleary.[54] The authors found that second year medical students were very much 'novices' when it came to clinical reasoning. That is, no matter their achievement level, these novices did not perform or reflect in very systematic or strategic ways. However, the authors observed differences in how high and low achievers said they approached the task (i.e. their forethought processes). Furthermore, in a follow-up analysis, the authors examined several Likert-type items that assessed students' confidence across several attempts at solving the case. Results from this analysis indicated that students experienced significant declines in both their confidence and meta-cognitive monitoring across several failed attempts to reach a diagnosis. As this study suggests, microanalytic protocols allow researchers to assess fine-grained changes in an individual's thoughts, feelings and actions across several learning or performance cycles. We summarise the strengths and limitations of SRL microanalysis in Table 14.2.

## Triangulating multiple data sources

As indicated in Table 14.2, there is no perfect research method for studying SRL; each method has its own strengths and limitations. One way to address the limitations of any given method is to employ a multi-method approach. The idea is that researchers can be more confident with a given finding if different methods lead to the same result. For example, as prescribed by many case study researchers, much recent work on SRL has focused on cultivating several data sets in an effort to triangulate and produce a refined understanding of SRL as it unfolds in certain contexts. In one such study, Hadwin and colleagues[55] used both 'trace data' and a self-report questionnaire to explore SRL. Trace data (also referred to as audit trails, log files, or dribble files) are logs of an individual's engagement with a computer system that record the sequence of user selections during learning and often include a time-stamped measure of student interactions. In this study,[55] the researchers used a computer program called gStudy to document eight participants' (i.e. cases) behaviours as they learnt. They compared these trace data to the questionnaire data (i.e. 10 items from the Motivated Strategies for Learning Questionnaire[56]) and found that participants' self-reported behaviours did not align well with the events traced in the gStudy system. This misalignment between self-reported behaviour and actual behaviour has been documented many times in educational psychology[57] and cognitive psychology (for a comprehensive review, see Bjork *et al.*[58]).

The performance implications of these misalignments have yet to be fully investigated – hence an area of valuable enquiry is how best to combine and interpret trace data, self-reports and other performance assessments. Recently, one study in the healthcare professions aimed to combine those three data sources.[59] Specifically, the researchers studied novice medical students as they learnt to diagnose simulated heart murmurs. They recorded how trainees sequenced their practice of seven murmurs (behavioural trace), their self-reactions to the learning experience (self-reports) and measured their acquisition and retention of diagnostic accuracy skills (performance measure). While participants' self-reports were positive, their behaviours suggested they did not use consistent learning strategies, which may have had negative implications on their performance of murmur diagnosis.

## Future directions in SRL theory, research and practice

Using SRL theory and the associated methods described here, we believe researchers and practitioners can move the field of healthcare profession education forward. Each of the elements of SRL and the relationships among the elements hold questions that apply to healthcare profession education (e.g. context specificity of SRL and consistency in SRL behaviours over time and place). An example study might entail a comparative analysis of trainees' SRL processes (collected using SRL microanalysis) when trainees are learning communication skills in small groups via role play and standardised patients versus when studying for a cardiovascular exam in large groups using a cardiopulmonary simulator. Such research would help clarify the dynamics of SRL and also might point towards practical interventions for improving the effectiveness and efficiency of learning efforts.

Another line of enquiry involves the development of interventions to improve the SRL process and component skills in healthcare professionals. An example study would be an investigation of trainees' SRL processes as they learn to manage complex virtual patients. The resulting data sets could be mined to identify useful and problematic tactics and strategies that trainees employ. Interventions could subsequently be designed to capitalise on the effective behaviours and provide supports or scaffolds for areas of challenge.

Although SRL has been studied in medical schools and residency training, more work is needed to determine how SRL is enacted in the 'real world' of practice rather than in the temporary and artificial 'laboratory' conditions of medical training. For instance, researchers might use triangulation methods to study practicing physicians' perceptions (via questionnaire), behaviours (via observation data) and clinical competence (via workplace-based assessment). A fundamental question in these settings relates to how more experienced physicians plan, monitor and adapt their learning processes in the midst of very dynamic and complex practice environments, where time-pressures and stressors are likely to be mitigating factors.

Finally, a complementary line of investigation relates to the research methods themselves. Clearly, more innovation is needed to improve how we assess relevant SRL processes. The aforementioned methods represent only few examples. Collaborative work that leads to creative and complementary methods will help us overcome the biases and limitations of current methods as we seek to learn more about SRL in the healthcare professions.

## Conclusion

In summary, we believe that researchers interested in studying the dynamics of learning in the context of healthcare profession education should consider adopting SRL theories and associated methods. Doing so provides a functional lens for examining and interpreting the complex interactions between an individual's thoughts, feelings and actions; the educational environment and the learning and performance outcomes that emerge. Use of this broad perspective will inform medical educators who are looking for ways to support medical trainees' development of necessary knowledge and skills, and will also help trainees develop and capitalise on their SRL capabilities to continuously learn and improve their medical practice.

---

**Practice points**

- Theories of SRL describe the processes that individuals use to optimise their strategic pursuit of personal learning goals.

- Most theories of SRL depict a self-oriented feedback loop composed of multiple processes that individuals use to monitor, control and manage their thoughts, feelings and actions to achieve their learning goals.

- Each SRL theory makes its own unique contribution to a robust understanding of the different ways that healthcare professionals learn to manage their own learning in complex training and practice contexts.

- Many different research methods can be used to study SRL in medical education contexts; three contemporary methods are questionnaires, multiple case studies and microanalysis.

- The best investigations typically employ a combination of methods to capture what individuals think, feel and do in various learning contexts.

---

## References

1 Sitzmann, T. & Ely, K. (2011) A meta-analysis of self-regulated learning in work-related training and educational attainment: what we know and where we need to go. *Psychological Bulletin*, **137**, 421–42. doi:10.1037/a0022777

2 Zimmerman, B.J. (1998) Preface. In: Schunk, D.H. & Zimmerman, B.J. (eds), *Self-Regulated Learning: From Teaching to Self-Reflective Practice*. The Guilford Press, New York, pp. viii–x.

3 Lajoie, S.P. & Azevedo, R. (2006) Teaching and learning in technology-rich environments. In: Alexander, P.A. & Winne, P.H. (eds), *Handbook of Educational Psychology*, 2nd edn. Lawrence Erlbaum Associates, Mahwah, N.J., pp. 803–821.

4 Schunk, D.H. & Ertmer, P.A. (2000) Self-regulation and academic learning: Self-efficacy enhancing interventions. In: Boekaerts, M., Pintrich, P.R. & Zeidner, M. (eds), *Handbook of Self-Regulation*. Academic Press, San Diego, CA, pp. 631–650.

5 Boekaerts, M., Pintrich, P.R. & Zeidner, M. (2000). In: Boekaerts, M., Pintrich, P.R. & Zeidner, M. (eds), *Handbook of Self-Regulation*. Academic Press, San Diego.

6 Puustinen, M. & Pulkkinen, L. (2001) Model of self-regulated learning: A review. *Scandinavian Journal of Educational Research*, **45**, 269–286.

7 Zimmerman, B.J. & Schunk, D.H. (2001). In: Zimmerman, B.J. & Schunk, D.H. (eds), *Self-Regulated Learning and Academic Achievement: Theoretical Perspectives*. Lawrence Erlbaum Associates, Mahwah, N.J..

8 Schunk, D.H. & Zimmerman, B.J. (2008). In: Schunk, D.H. & Zimmerman, B. (eds), *Motivation and Self-Regulated Learning: Theory, Research, and Applications*. Lawrence Erlbaum Associates, New York.

9 Greene, J.A. & Azevedo, R. (2007) A theoretical review of Winne and Hadwin's model of self-regulated learning: new perspectives and directions. *Review of Educational Research*, **77**, 334–372. doi:10.3102/003465430303953

10 Cleary, T.J., Durning, S.J., Gruppen, L., Hemmer, P. & Artino, A. (2013) Self-regulated learning in medical education. In: Walsh, K. (ed), *Oxford Textbook of Medical Education*. Oxford University Press, Oxford, UK, pp. 465–477.

11 Loyens, S., Magda, J. & Rikers, R. (2008) Self-directed learning in problem-based learning and its relationships with self-regulated learning. *Educational Psychology Review*, **20**, 411–427. doi:10.1007/S10648-008-9082-7

12 Lajoie, S.P. (2008) Metacognition, self regulation, and self-regulated learning: a rose by any other name? *Educational Psychology Review*, **20**, 469–475. doi:10.1007/s10648-008-9088-1

13 Flavell, J.H. (1979) Meta-Cognition and cognitive monitoring - new area of cognitive-developmental inquiry. *The American Psychologist*, **34**, 906–911. doi:10.1037/0003-066x.34.10.906

14 Pintrich, P.R., Wolters, C. & Baxter, G. (2000) Assessing metacognition and self-regulated learning. In: Schraw, G. & Impara, J.C. (eds), *Issues in the Measurement of Metacognition*. Buros Institute of Mental Measurements, Lincoln, NI, pp. 43–97.

15 Knowles, M.S. (1975) *Self-Directed Learning: A Guide for Learners and Teachers*. Association Press, New York.

16 Zimmerman, B.J. & Lebeau, R.B. (2000) A commentary on self-directed learning. In: Evensen, D.H. & Hmelo, C.E. (eds), *Problem-Based Learning: A Research Perspective on Learning Interactions*. Lawrence Erlbaum Associates, Mahwah, N.J., pp. 299–313.

17 Brydges, R. & Butler, D. (2012) A reflective analysis of medical education research on self-regulation in learning and practice. *Medical Education*, **46**, 71–9. doi:10.1111/j.1365-2923.2011.04100.x

18 Carver, C.S. & Scheier, M.F. (1990) Origins and functions of positive and negative affect: a control-process view. *Psychological Review*, **97**, 19.

19 Winne, P.H. (2001) Self-regulated learning viewed from models of information processing. In: Zimmerman, D.H. & Schunk, B.J. (eds), *Self-regulated Learning and Academic Achievement: Theoretical Perspectives*. Lawrence Erlbaum Associates, pp. 153–190.

20 Winne, P.H. & Hadwin, A.F. (1998) Studying as self-regulated learning. In: Hacker, D.J. & Dunlosky, J. (eds), *Metacognition in Educational Theory and Practice*.

*The Educational Psychology Series*. Lawrence Erlbaum Associates, Mahwah, NJ, pp. 277–304.

21 Butler, D.L. & Winne, P.H. (1995) Feedback and self-regulated learning: A theoretical synthesis. *Review of Educational Research*, **65**, 245–281 Available at: internal-pdf://3829176425/Butler-1995-Feedback and self-re.pdf.

22 Azevedo, R., Cromley, J.G. & Seibert, D. (2004) Does adaptive scaffolding facilitate students' ability to regulate their learning with hypermedia? *Contemporary Educational Psychology*, **29**, 344–370. doi:10.1016/j.cedpsych.2003.09.002

23 Winne, P.H. & Hadwin, A.F. (2013) nStudy: Tracing and supporting self-regulated learning in the Internet. *International Handbook of Metacognition and Learning Technologies*, 293–308.

24 Bandura, A. (1986) *Social Foundations of Thought and Action: A Social Cognitive Theory*. Prentice-Hall, Englewood Cliffs, NJ.

25 Schunk, D.H. & Zimmerman, B.J. (1997) Social origins of self-regulatory competence. *Educational Psychologist*, **32**, 195–208 Available at: internal-pdf://0304089172/Schunk-1997-Social origins of se.pdf.

26 Schunk, D.H. (2001) Social cognitive theory and self-regulated learning. In: Zimmerman, D.H. & Schunk, B.J. (eds), *Self-regulated Learning and Academic Achievement: Theoretical Perspectives*, pp. 125–152.

27 Zimmerman, B.J. (2000) Attaining self-regulation: A social-cognitive perspective. In: Boekaerts, M., Pintrich, P. & Zeidner, M. (eds), *Handbook of Self-Regulation*. Academic Press, San Diego, CA, pp. 13–39.

28 Cleary, T.J., Callan, G.L. & Zimmerman, B.J. (2012) Assessing self-regulation as a cyclical, context-specific phenomenon: overview and analysis of SRL microanalytic protocols. *Education Research International*, **2012**, 1–19. doi:10.1155/2012/428639

29 Cleary, T.J. & Sandars, J. (2011) Assessing self-regulatory processes during clinical skill performance: a pilot study. *Medical Teacher*, **33**, e368–e374. doi:10.3109/0142159X.2011.577464

30 Artino, A.R., Cleary, T.J., Dong, T., Hemmer, P.A. & Durning, S.J. (2014) Exploring clinical reasoning in novices: a self-regulated learning microanalytic assessment approach. *Medical Education*, **48**, 280–291. doi:10.1111/medu.12303

31 Paris, S.G., Byrnes, J.P. & Paris, A.H. (2001) Constructing theories, identities, and actions of self-regulated learners. In: Zirnmerman, B.J. & Schunk, D.H. (eds), *Self-Regulated Learning and Academic Achievement: Theoretical Perspectives*, 2nd edn, New York. Lawrence Erlbaum Associates, pp. 253–287.

32 Rogoff, B. (1990) *Apprenticeship in Thinking: Cognitive Development in Social Context*. Oxford University Press, New York.

33 Lave, J. (1993) The practice of learning. *Contemporary Learning Theory*, 200.

34 Butler, D.L. & Cartier, S.C. (2004) Promoting effective task interpretation as an important work habit: A key to successful teaching and learning. *Teachers College Record*, **106**, 1729–1758 Available at: http://www.

scopus.com/inward/record.url?eid=2-s2.0-7544219873&partnerID=40&md5=bd157bbb8f34e59bf829040f270349e2.

35 Butler, D.L. & Schnellert, L. (2012) Collaborative inquiry in teacher professional development. *Teaching and Teacher Education*, **28**, 1206–1220 Available at: internal-pdf://1101513929/Butler-2012-Collaborative inquir.pdf.

36 Järvelä, S. & Järvenoja, H. (2011) Socially constructed self-regulated learning and motivation regulation in collaborative learning groups. *Teachers College Record*, **113**, 350–374 Available at: http://www.scopus.com/inward/record.url?eid=2-s2.0-79955459964&partnerID=40&md5=d8eee6af22313b1198f700e6abd57a22.

37 Sitzmann, T., Brown, K.G., Ely, K., Kraiger, K. & Wisher, R.A. (2009) A cyclical model of motivational constructs in web-based courses. *Military Psychology*, **21**, 534–551. doi:10.1080/08995600903206479

38 Watling, C.J. & Lingard, L. (2012) Toward meaningful evaluation of medical trainees: the influence of participants' perceptions of the process. *Advances in Health Sciences Education: Theory and Practice*, **17**, 183–194. doi:10.1007/s10459-010-9223-x

39 Zimmerman, B.J. & Martinez-Pons, M. (1988) Construct validation of a strategy model of student self-regulated learning. *Journal of Education and Psychology*, **80**, 284–290. doi:10.1037//0022-0663.80.3.284

40 Woods, N.N., Mylopoulos, M. & Brydges, R. (2011) Informal self-regulated learning on a surgical rotation: uncovering student experiences in context. *Advances in Health Sciences Education: Theory and Practice*, **16**, 643–653. doi:10.1007/s10459-011-9285-4

41 Hattie, J., Biggs, J. & Purdie, N. (1996) Effects of Learning Skills Interventions on Student Learning: A Meta-Analysis. *Review of Educational Research*, **66**, 99–136.

42 Guglielmino L. M. (1977) *Development of the Self-Directed Learning Readiness Scale*. Unpublished doctoral dissertation, University of Georgia. Dissertation Abstracts International. **38**, 6467.

43 Oddi, L.F. (1986) Development and validation of an instrument to identify self-directed continuing learners. *Adult Education Quarterly*, **36**, 97–107.

44 Li, S.-T.T., Paternniti, D.A., Co, J.P.T. & West, D.C. (2010) Successful self-directed lifelong learning in medicine: a conceptual model derived from qualitative analysis of a national survey of pediatric residents. *Academic Medicine*, **85**, 1229–1236.

45 Wiel, M.W.J., Van den Bossche, P., Janssen, S. & Jossberger, H. (2010) Exploring deliberate practice in medicine: how do physicians learn in the workplace? *Advances in Health Sciences Education*, **16**, 81–95. doi:10.1007/s10459-010-9246-3

46 Green, M. & Ruff, T.R. (2005) Why do residents fail to answer their clinical questions? A qualitative study of barriers to practicing evidence-based medicine. *Academic Medicine*, **80**, 176–182.

47 Mylopoulos, M. & Scardamalia, M. (2008) Doctors' perspectives on their innovations in daily practice: implications for knowledge building in health care. *Medical Education*, **42**, 975–981. doi:10.1111/j.1365-2923.2008.03153.x

48 Gruppen, L.D., White, C.B., Fitzgerald, J.T., Grum, C.M. & Woolliscroft, J.O. (2000) Medical student self-assessment and allocation of learning time. *Academic Medicine*, **75**, 374–379.

49 Stake, R.E. (2013) *Multiple Case Study Analysis*. The Guilford Press, New York, NY

50 Yin, R.K. (2003) *Case Study Research: Design and Methods*. Vol. **5**. Sage Publ Inc., pp. 11.

51 Butler, D. L. (2011). Investigating self-regulated learning using in-depth case studies. In B. J. Zimmerman, & D. H. Schunk (Eds.), Handbook of Self-Regulation of Learning and Performance (pp. 346–360). NY, NY: Routledge.

52 Merriam, S.B. (1998) *Qualitative Research and Case Study Applications in Education*. Jossey-Bass Publishers, San Francisco, CA.

53 Evensen, D.H., Glenn, J. & Salisbury-Glennon, J.D. (2001) A qualitative study of six medical students in a problem-based curriculum: Toward a situated model of self-regulation. *Journal of Educational Psychology*, **93**, 659–676 Available at: internal-pdf://1734575198/Evensen-2001-A qualitative study.pdf.

54 Cleary, T.J. (2011) Emergence of self-regulated learning microanalysis: Historical overview, essential features, and implications for research and practice. In: *Handbook of Self-Regulation of Learning and Performance*. Taylor & Francis, New York.

55 Hadwin, A.F., Winne, P.H., Stockley, D.B., Nesbit, J.C. & Woszczyna, C. (2001) Context moderates students' self-reports about how they study. *Journal of Educational Psychology*, **93**, 477–487. doi:10.1037//O022-0663.93.3.477

56 Pintrich, P.R., Smith, D.A.F., Garcia, T. & Mckeachie, W.J. (1993) Reliability and predictive validity of the motivated strategies for learning questionnaire (Mslq). *Educational and Psychological Measurement*, **53**, 801–813. doi:10.1177/0013164493053003024

57 Winne, P.H., Jamieson-Noel, D.L. & Muis, K. (2002) Methodological issues and advances in researching tactics, strategies, and self-regulated learning. In: Maehr, M.L. & Pintrich, P.R. (eds), *Advances in Motivation and Achievement*. Vol. **12**. JAI, Greenwich, CT, pp. 121–155.

58 Bjork, R.A., Dunlosky, J. & Kornell, N. (2013) Self-regulated learning: beliefs, techniques, and illusions. *Annual Review of Psychology*, **64**, 417–44. doi: 10.1146/annurev-psych-113011-143823

59 Brydges, R., Peets, A., Issenberg, S.B. & Regehr, G. (2013) Divergence in student and educator conceptual structures during auscultation training. *Medical Education*, **47**, 198–209 Available at: internal-pdf://0628175011/Brydges-2013-Divergence in studen.pdf.

# 15 What are values and how can we assess them? Implications for values-based recruitment in healthcare

*Fiona Patterson, Máire Kerrin, Marise Ph. Born, Janneke K. Oostrom and Linda Prescott-Clements*

*'We are clear about the behaviour we expect, and clear about our values' says the Chief Executive of one of the most successful National Health Service (NHS) trusts in the United Kingdom.*

*In July 2013, an independent review into healthcare professionals in the NHS and private healthcare organisations in the United Kingdom was conducted. One of the major themes running through the entire review was the importance of values in healthcare. Of the many healthcare trusts and independent organisations reviewed, the top performers all had one thing in common: their emphasis on values. Conversely, the failure to embed core values into the standards of care expected in healthcare settings has been found to have disastrous consequences. But how do we effectively test them? This chapter examines the evidence base for the effectiveness of a range of selection methods that have the potential to assess values in values-based recruitment. In this chapter, we explore one selection method in detail and provide a review of Situational Judgement Tests (SJTs) as a reliable and valid method for measuring the values that are important in clinical practice, including integrity, caring, empathy and compassion.*

## Introduction

There exists a large body of international research exploring the impact of core values of compassion, empathy, respect and dignity on patients' experience of health and social care services. In the United Kingdom, for example, although the values and behaviours expected of health and social care professionals are preserved in the National Health Service (NHS) Constitution, recent government enquiries[1,2] have highlighted major concerns about the decline in compassionate care within all healthcare roles. Undoubtedly, healthcare education and training can have a major impact on shaping core values, and an important first step is ensuring that the right individuals with the appropriate values are

appointed to any training place or healthcare role. But what are robust selection methods for attracting and selecting students, trainees or employees whose individual values and behaviours align with the desired values in healthcare (delivering compassionate care)?

In this chapter, we explore the latest theoretical developments drawn from the psychology literature on values. The aim of the chapter is to help the readers gain knowledge around a number of key areas relating to the role of values in healthcare recruitment and selection. We then examine the evidence base for a number of selection methods and the strengths of each for use in values-based recruitment. Although there are several selection methods that could be useful in assessing values, we look in detail at situational judgement tests (SJTs). This chapter should give the reader an understanding of (a) what values are, their theoretical underpinnings and how they can be an important addition to recruitment and selection in healthcare; (c) the links between values and factors, such as personality, motivation and behaviours at work and (c) the selection methods that are best used for values-based recruitment in terms of their effectiveness.

## What are values, and how do they link to personality, motivation and behaviours?

In reviewing the evidence base for values-based recruitment, it is important to consider how values are defined in the research literature and explore how they link to other concepts that are often discussed simultaneously (e.g. personality, motivation and behaviours). This is particularly important in a recruitment context as there are implications for the measurement tools available to assess each of these

*Researching Medical Education*, First Edition. Edited by Jennifer Cleland and Steven J. Durning.
© 2015 John Wiley & Sons, Ltd. Published 2015 by John Wiley & Sons, Ltd.

constructs. For example, if one were recruiting for a healthcare role with a view to selecting an individual with certain characteristics that are desirable for that role (e.g. being compassionate and respectful), these would be assessed differently to personality traits such as conscientiousness or agreeableness. Without an understanding of how values and personality are two distinct constructs despite being linked, it will not be possible to accurately assess either of them.

Values are a set of *enduring beliefs* which a person holds about what is good or desirable in life. Each individual holds numerous values (e.g. power, achievement and honesty), and a particular value may be very important to one person but unimportant to another.[3] Whilst values are relatively stable over time, a person's values can change or adapt based on his/her experiences or their environment.[4]

*Values are evaluative* – they guide individuals' judgments about appropriate behaviour both for oneself and others. *Values are also general* – they transcend specific situations, and are relatively stable.[5] In addition, values are ordered by importance, such that one will tend to act according to the more important value when two values are in conflict. For example, consider a person who values hedonism (pursuit of pleasure) more than benevolence (concern for relationships). If forced to choose between a personal hobby and helping a family member, he/she would be more likely to pursue his/her hobby because he/she places greater importance on fulfilling personal desire than on relationships with others.

*Values influence behaviour*, however this relationship is complex and simply holding a value does not necessarily mean that the individual will always behave in a way which is consistent with that value.[5] For example, values such as tradition (respect and commitment to traditional customs and ideas) and stimulation (excitement, novelty and challenge in life) have strong relationships with their related behaviours, such as observing traditional customs and showing modesty, and watching thrillers and doing unconventional things, respectively. In contrast, values such as achievement (personal success through displaying competence) and security (safety, harmony and stability) tend to have weaker correlations with related behaviours, such as studying late into the night before exams despite having already studied well. Thus, in addition to values, there are likely to be other factors that influence a person's behaviour, including knowledge, skills, personality and motivation. The extent to which each of these factors will influence behaviour will vary depending on the given situation.

Until recently, there has been limited understanding of how personality and values are related to one another, much less how they might jointly impact behaviour. Parks and Guay[6,7] provide a detailed review of the personality and values literature in terms of how the constructs are distinct in order to clarify how each relates to motivation and behaviour. We will explain the difference in personality and values in more detail in the following sections. Before doing so, however, we outline the dominant theoretical models in the values literature.

## Theoretical models of values

Schwartz and colleagues have been the dominant researchers in the values domain for much of the last two decades.[8–11] In general, values research has been ascribed to one of two basic models,[12] *'values as preferences'* or *'values as principles'*. Values as preferences are seen as essential attitudes. They indicate the preferences that individuals have for various environments, such as their work environment, and as such can be thought of as 'work values' in this context.[12] Take an individual who values dependability and responsibility at work, for example. They will come to work with a responsible attitude and prefer to work in a manner that is in line with this value; displaying behaviours such as keeping others informed of changes in their schedule or not taking too much time off. In another context, however, the same individual may prefer different values, such as stimulation in his/her free time, or honesty in his/her relationships. Values as principles, often termed 'personal values', are guiding principles regarding how individuals ought to behave. For example, an individual who values honesty believes that all people ought to be honest, while an individual who values achievement believes that people ought to have many accomplishments that will be socially recognised. Research suggests that values as principles (personal values), should more directly impact motivation, because they are general beliefs that one ought to behave a certain way. Parks and Guay[6] define values as *'learned beliefs that serve as guiding principles about how individuals ought to behave'*. While work values (values as preferences) predict vocational choice and job satisfaction, they are narrower in focus than personal values, and thus relate to a narrower range of outcomes. Personal values, however, are predictive of a broad range of behaviours across various life domains.[4,8,13] Because personal values relate to how individuals feel they ought to behave, they have a motivational impact on behaviour in general.

In the context of values-based recruitment – which involves incorporating a method of assessing values into a recruitment process in order to increase the likelihood of selecting individuals with appropriate values for the job role – it is suggested that personal values are as important to consider as work values.

Values are learnt from role models such as parents and teachers, and are passed from generation to generation, and hence there tend to be similarities in values patterns within cultures.[14,15] Values are shaped during adolescence; however, they are generally quite stable in adulthood.[16,17] Nonetheless, because values are learnt initially through social interactions, being exposed to a new social environment can facilitate changes in one's values structure, which is why socialisation efforts can sometimes change the values of newcomers to become more like those of the organisation.[18] Not all employees respond equally to socialisation however, suggesting that some individuals are less willing to make changes in their values structures than others.[19]

Schwartz and colleagues propose a value model that identifies 10 types of basic values, distinguished by the type of motivational goal they express.[5,9,20] Essentially, each of the 10 value types represents an overall goal (such as power or conformity) that has motivational influence over an individual. Each value type is then represented by a number of specific values (e.g. authority and wealth, or politeness and self-discipline) that sit under the umbrella of the overall goal and promote its achievement. For example, if one's primary motivational goal is 'power', defined as *social status or prestige, control or dominance over people or resources*,[9] then actions that express the specific values of authority and wealth will make the achievement of the central goal (power) more likely. Whilst this typology is useful in providing a baseline of human value types that is both universal and comprehensive,[8,9,20] it presents value types as independent entities rather than interconnecting ones. The issue with this is that, in practice, actions taken in the pursuit of one type of value may either complement or compete with that of another type. For example, 'tradition' and 'stimulation' are inherently opposed as one cannot adhere to traditions whilst simultaneously pursuing novelty. Conversely, value types such as 'benevolence' and 'conformity' might complement each other since they are both motivated by a desire to behave in a manner approved of by others. Therefore, a more optimal way of looking at values is from a structural perspective: understanding value systems as a whole and the relations between the types of values. Schwartz[9] proposes a continuum of related motivations, illustrated in Figure 15.1, whereby certain value types share a similar motivational emphasis, and others have opposing motivations.

For example, universalism and benevolence are both concerned with the enhancement of others and transcendence of selfish interests, and as such are positioned adjacent to one another. As the circle continues, all values positioned adjacent to one another have a shared motivational emphasis. Higher-order value types can be seen along the outer circle in Figure 15.1. These broadly illustrate opposing value types through their bipolar arrangement. For example, openness to change and conservation are placed on opposite sides of the continuum since one represents a preference for independent thought and change, whilst the other leans towards self-restriction and preservation of traditions.

## Personality and values

Psychologists agree that the five factor model (FFM) is now a universal template to describe personality.[21,22] The FFM's factors (and examples of the traits comprising each factor) are conscientiousness (responsible, organised and efficient), emotional stability (self-confident, resilient and well-adjusted), extraversion (talkative, ambitious and assertive), agreeableness (friendly, cooperative and loyal) and openness to experience[22,23] (curious, imaginative and open-minded).

Personality, known as *the combination of characteristics or qualities that form an individual's distinctive character*, has been shown to relate to performance, motivation, job satisfaction, leadership and other work outcomes.[24-26] Values and personality both describe components within each individual, and both are believed to impact behaviour, decision making, motivation, attitudes and interpersonal relations. Yet, there are also important differences. Roccas and colleagues[27] refer to *personality* as *enduring dispositions*, and to *values* as *enduring goals*. Whilst personality generally represents the behaviours that come most naturally, values reflect effort (a choice) to behave a certain way. We do not generally think about or choose to be extraverted or introverted. However, there is an element of personal choice involved when we behave consistently with our values. Teachers, for example, may have a naturally introverted personality, and as such, having a job that involves being around large groups of students on a day-to-day basis may not necessarily come naturally or feel the most comfortable thing for them to do. However, if the value 'achievement',

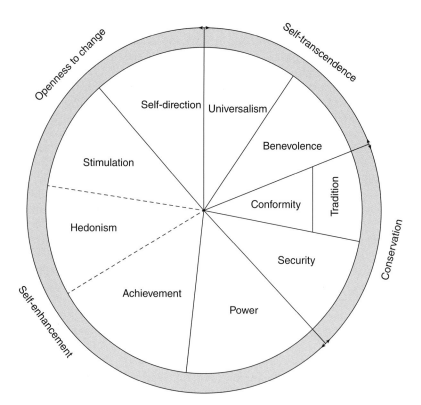

***Figure 15.1*** Model of relations among motivational types of values. Adapted from Schwartz (1994)[9]. Tradition is located outside of conformity due to these two value types sharing a single motivational goal – subordination of self in favour of socially imposed expectations. Competing value types emanate in opposing directions from the centre. Complementary value types sit adjacent to one another.

known as *'personal success through demonstrating competence according to social standards'* is important to them, they may *choose* to be more extraverted because not interacting with students sufficiently may be viewed as a lack of competence.

Values relate to what we believe we ought to do, whereas personality relates to what we naturally tend to do. Personality traits do not conflict with one another (i.e. one can simultaneously express the personality traits of extraversion and conscientiousness), yet values do conflict, as some are pursued at the expense of others.[28]

In spite of theoretical distinctions, separating out behaviour that is caused by personality as opposed to values is difficult in practice. However, personality and values do exhibit different patterns of relationships with different constructs,[27] and a recent meta-analysis[6,29] demonstrates that personality and values are related but separate constructs.

Parks and Guay[6] proposed that *values and personality have different influences on different motivational processes*, where values primarily impact the goals that individuals choose to pursue (*goal content*), while personality traits (especially conscientiousness and emotional stability) primarily impact the amount of effort and persistence that individuals exhibit in pursuit of those goals (*goal striving*).

Parks and Guay's[6,7] model provides a rationale for values contributing incrementally to behaviour (beyond personality). In short, personality generally represents the behaviours that come most naturally; values reflect effort (a choice) to behave a certain way. This is an important distinction when considering assessment tools and measures.

## Theoretical contexts of values

In terms of the context of trainee/employees' values and their impact on the organisation and workforce, a number of theories are discussed in the literature. Whilst many studies report different types of 'fit' theories, representing value congruence between employees and the organisational culture and/or workforce, two other theories that contribute to this area of research are Schneiders' *Attraction-Selection-Attrition* (ASA) theory,[30,31] and *socialisation theories*.[18,32,33]

ASA theory is based on the notion that *'the people make the place'* within organisations.[30] The theory proposes that over a period of time, the values and personalities of individuals working within a particular organisation will become increasingly homogeneous, as individuals are 'attracted' to an organisation with values that they recognise and identify with, are 'selected' by an organisation as a result of value congruence, and where shared values exist are likely to remain within the organisation (conversely, where value congruence is low, 'attrition' will occur). Consequently, it is suggested that it is the people working within the organisation that make the culture.[34]

There have been challenges to the conditions under which some aspects of Schneiders'[30] ASA theory exist. An empirical study by Bilsberry[35] tested the attraction aspect of ASA theory within eight utility organisations in the United Kingdom, concluding that only applicants with familiarity, proximity and previous exposure to an organisation are attracted to it, which is consistent with Schneiders'[30] proposal. However, candidates appeared to select jobs to apply for on the basis of the *type* of role or job, rather than being attracted to the organisation as such. Considering these findings within the context of healthcare, individuals with family members working in healthcare, or those having completed placements as a student may form judgements of organisational values before employment and may be attracted to the organisation (or not) accordingly, as a result of heightened familiarity, proximity and exposure. However, it is also clear that the motivations for individuals' choices regarding which jobs to apply for can be affected by many complex social and personal circumstances, and individuals may be attracted to certain roles and/or organisations for extrinsic rewards, such as job security, social status, and income.[36,37]

Socialisation theories have also been linked to the development of values within an organisation following recruitment.[18,32,33,38] Such theories suggest that although values are relatively stable constructs, upon entering an organisation, individuals' values may change in accordance with those of their immediate work colleagues, and therefore there may be a need to continue to focus on individuals' values throughout employment.[38]

Anderson[39] explored the role of selection and recruitment methods on '*pre-entry socialisation*'. He suggests that selection methods have traditionally been conceived of as neutral predictors of applicant suitability and subsequent role performance.[40,41] However, candidates form impressions of the organisation directly from their experiences in the selection and recruitment processes. For example, selection information (e.g. such as that found on a job description) might convey to candidates that certain values, (e.g. respect) are important for a role in the organisation in question. This would create an expectation that the successful candidate should behave in a way that corresponds to that value

and therefore they will begin to be socialised into that way of thinking and behaving. Anderson and Ostroff[42] propose that selection methods initiate the pre-entry socialisation process and they outline how selection methods vary in their degree of socialisation impact (e.g. information provision). For example, they set out how selection methods convey information to the candidates whether intended to or not by the recruiting organisation. These are important considerations for the values-based recruitment context in terms of understanding the likely impact of chosen selection and recruitment methods on subsequent behaviour in the job.

The effects of both ASA and socialisation theories have been shown to operate simultaneously within organisations,[38] and in the context of wishing to influence culture/values within an organisation, the evidence clearly shows the need for a multi-faceted approach to organisational values beyond recruitment issues alone.[43]

Similarly, '*value internalisation*' and '*behavioural modelling*' are reported as having an impact on an individual's values following employment within an organisation.[34,38,44] For example, if 'creativity' is valued within an organisation and an individual is behaving in a way that is in line with this value over a period of time whilst at work, it will eventually become internalised as part of his/her own value structure. Value internalisation explains the subtle change in an individual's values over time following employment as a result of his/her experiences, and both managers and work colleagues may have a significant impact on new recruits, being powerful role models.[44] This can be positive or negative, depending on whether the values within teams are optimal or suboptimal. Furthermore, managers also influence employees' behaviours through their own actions.

## Value congruence and 'Fit' theories

The concept that the alignment of optimal values between employees within an organisation leads to that organisation operating in a more effective way, has been the driver for several large organisations, such as Disney, Hewlett-Packard and Boeing, to embark on programmes promoting values. Robust evidence that such programmes have had an impact is less prominent, although research demonstrates that individuals are more comfortable working in an environment that is consistent with their own values.[45]

*Value congruence* is often the measurable construct representing the extent to which an individual's values are similar to those of the organisation in which he/she works. This measure is used to define the level of 'fit' an individual has with the organisation, its culture (values) or that of the other employees within it. In an attempt to investigate the dynamics of value congruence, a number of types of 'fit' have been described in the research literature.[46] A detailed review of the relationships between different types of fit, both in terms of *'direct'* (i.e. perceived fit) and 'indirect' fit, can be found elsewhere.[34,47,48]

## Impact of value congruence on job satisfaction, organisational commitment and turnover

A key objective of this chapter is to explore the evidence base underpinning the effectiveness of values-based recruitment and how this relates to important outcomes, especially demonstrating care and compassion towards patients. However, the majority of the existing literature describes the impact of value congruence on other outcomes (largely from the employee perspective), such as job satisfaction and employee turnover, with very little research focusing on job performance or specific behavioural outcomes. When an individual's values closely match those of the organisation (as defined by co-workers or supervisors), he/she reports a significant increase in job satisfaction, and satisfaction with the organisation.[14,47,49,50] Perceived congruence between employee and organisational values are also positively associated with satisfaction, and negatively associated with intent to leave and attrition.[14,49,50]

In terms of an individual's *commitment* to an organisation, his/her perception of the degree of similarity between the organisational values and his/her own values is key.[45,51] *Affective* (where an individual is emotionally attached to an organisation), *normative* (where an individual has feelings of obligation towards an organisation) and *continuance* commitment (where an individual is committed as a result of accumulating investments in the organisation) are each predicted by different clusters of values, with 'humanity' values (defined in this study as courtesy, consideration, cooperation, fairness, forgiveness and integrity) being most associated with affective commitment to an organisation.[45]

Few studies explored the impact of value congruence on organisational performance outcomes; however, a case example from Salford Royal NHS Foundation Trust in the United Kingdom points to the conclusion that having a clear set of values shared by every employee can result in higher performance and staff satisfaction.[2] Conversely, Ostroff *et al.*[34] reported that value incongruence was likely to lead to frustration, difficulty in working effectively with others and a lack of role clarity from the perspective of the employee.

## Selection methods for values-based recruitment: the research evidence

The diversity of measurement tools claiming to be of use for values-based recruitment is noteworthy, and hence generalisation of findings is problematic.[14] Some studies have been criticised for using a unilateral measure for values, since values are known to be complex constructs – as we hope is clear from earlier in this chapter. Some researchers suggest that a more appropriate approach for measurement tools would be to focus on 'clusters' of related values rather than using an overall value hierarchy.[45] For example, focusing on measuring a cluster of values that includes 'helpful', 'honest' and 'responsible', which are all related as they can be said to fall under the umbrella of 'universalism', may be more appropriate than simply measuring 'universalism' alone. Van Vianen[48] questions whether measurement tools for values should be included during recruitment, as there is arguably little evidence that values are related to job performance. This is a criticism often directed at values-based recruitment; however, research around values and P-O fit has illustrated that it is an important contributor to long-term outcomes, such as performance.[52,53] Van Vianen[48] further argues that measurement tools for values in a selection process values may be 'fakeable'. This issue is considered as we review and explore further the measurement tools and the criteria to evaluate their effectiveness in this context.

Over several decades, many different selection methods have been reviewed by researchers across many different occupations.[54–57] As such, there is now a large volume of research evidence examining the effectiveness of different selection methods as predictors of job performance across many occupational groups. Historically, there has been a great emphasis on identifying which methods are the most reliable and valid. However, current research also advocates including analyses of selection system design, in terms of how best to combine selection methods. For example, when there are high volumes of applicants, recruiters must decide on which combination of selection methods are best used at early stage; aptitude tests are more often used at an early screening stage whereas interviews are more typically used at final-stage selection.

The vast majority of research literature available in a healthcare context focuses on selection for medicine and dentistry, and here the focus has largely been on pre-entry recruitment for medical/dental school admissions. For example, a systematic search and review of the evidence base for selection methods in both undergraduate and postgraduate medical education has recently been undertaken.[58] It included a review of all the main selection methods, such as *interviews, references/referee's reports, CVs, application forms, personal statements, autobiographical submissions, personality tests, SJTs* and *selection/assessment centres*. Most of these methods have been used in practice in medical selection for some years (e.g. personal statements, CVs, structured interviewing and Multiple Mini Interviews (MMIs)). Others, such as selection centres and SJTs,[59,60] have substantial evidence of use and effectiveness in other occupations but are relatively recent applications in the field of medical education. The paper presents data on the relative strength of the research evidence underlying the quality of each of these methods as well as their findings to scope a future research agenda and to inform future practice. Importantly for this chapter, the evidence suggests that some selection methods will be more effective as part of values-based recruitment. The next section explores case material with the aim of providing practical illustration and theoretical underpinnings of a selection method's effectiveness.

## Applying the theory: case material evaluating selection methods for values-based recruitment

In applying theory to practice, in this section, we explore case material regarding the application of SJTs as a values-based recruitment tool, for several reasons. First, in reviewing selection methods, there is good evidence of SJT effectiveness compared to several other tools.[59,61] Second, there are interesting theoretical developments emerging in relation to the construct validity of SJTs that is relevant to values-based recruitment. Here we explore the evidence base for SJTs as a selection methodology for values-based recruitment, using a range of practical examples, followed by a summary of key theoretical developments and reflections on practice.

### SJTs: A selection methodology for values-based recruitment

An international review of selection practices for the healthcare professions[62] explored whether SJTs may be a valid and reliable method for assessing a broad range of important non-academic attributes for high-volume selection. To what extent can an SJT measure values that are important in clinical practice, such as integrity, caring, empathy and compassion? A summary of the evidence in relation to values-based recruitment is presented in this section.

SJTs are a measurement methodology rather than a single style of test presentation, that is, there is no single type of SJT; they can be constructed differently using different formats depending on the requirement of the role. SJTs are designed to assess an applicant's judgement regarding situations encountered in the workplace (or in education settings), targeting professional attributes rather than knowledge.[63]

In an SJT, applicants are presented with written or video-based depictions of hypothetical scenarios and asked to identify an appropriate response from a list of alternatives. A variety of response formats can be used and these are typically classified into one of two formats: knowledge-based (i.e. *what is the best option*) or behavioural tendency (i.e. *what would you most likely do*).[64] See Table 15.1 for example SJT items and response formats.

SJTs are typically scored by comparing applicants' responses to a pre-determined scoring key agreed by subject matter experts. As a selection tool, SJTs are growing in popularity because they have useful levels of face, content and predictive validity, and scenarios used in SJTs are typically derived from job analysis studies.[65–69]

SJTs are an established method of selection for use in high-volume selection for many occupational groups, and they can be used to reliably select for a range of professional attributes. Although there are other selection methods which can be used to select for these attributes, such as panel interviews and personality questionnaires, SJTs offer significant advantages over these methods. For example, panel interviews are often criticised for their potential to be biased or for their lack of standardisation[70] whilst personality tests offer lower face validity and are less acceptable to candidates as a selection tool.[71] By contrast, SJTs offer a standardised method of objectively assessing a broad range of attributes for large numbers of applicants, whilst being face valid to candidates since scenarios used in SJTs are based on job-relevant situations.[72] SJTs can also be used in settings where applicants have no prior job-specific experience (e.g. at entry to medical school[73]). Indeed, there is good evidence to show that SJTs are a useful methodology to evaluate a range of professional attributes for selection into medicine and dentistry.[74] Long-term studies have shown an SJT measuring empathy,

*Table 15.1* Example situational judgement tests items and response formats

| SJT item using a multiple response format | SJT item using a ranking response format | Three SJT questions nested in one scenario using a rating response format |
| --- | --- | --- |
| *You review a patient on the surgical ward who has had an appendicectomy done earlier on in the day. You write a prescription for strong painkillers. The staff nurse challenges your decision & refuses to give the medication to the patient.* | *You are reviewing a routine drug chart for a patient with rheumatoid arthritis during an overnight shift. You notice that your consultant has inappropriately prescribed methotrexate 7.5mg daily instead of weekly.* | *A consultation is taking place between a senior doctor and a patient; a medical student is observing. The senior doctor tells the patient that he requires some blood tests to rule out a terminal disease. The senior doctor is called away urgently, leaving the medical student alone with the patient. The patient tells the student that he is worried he is going to die and asks the student what the blood tests will show.* |
| **Choose the THREE most appropriate actions to take in this situation.** | **Rank in order the following actions in response to this situation** (1= Most appropriate; 5= Least appropriate). | **How appropriate are each of the following responses by the medical student in this situation?** |
| (A) Instruct the nurse to give the medication to the patient<br>(B) Discuss with the nurse why she disagrees with the prescription<br>(C) Ask a senior colleague for advice<br>(D) Complete a clinical incident form<br>(E) Cancel the prescription on the nurse's advice<br>(F) Arrange to speak to the nurse later to discuss your working relationship<br>(G) Write in the medical notes that the nurse has declined to give the medication<br>(H) Review the case again | (A) Ask the nurses if the consultant has made any other drug errors recently<br>(B) Correct the prescription to 7.5mg weekly<br>(C) Leave the prescription unchanged until the consultant ward round the following morning<br>(D) Phone the consultant at home to ask about changing the prescription<br>(E) Inform the patient of the error | (Q1) Explain to the patient that he is unable to comment on what the tests will show as he is a medical student<br>(Q2) Acknowledge the patient's concerns and ask whether he would like them to be raised with the senior doctor<br>(Q3) Tell the patient that he should not worry and that it is unlikely that he will die |

integrity and resilience (used to select candidates applying for training in UK general practice) to be the best single predictor of subsequent job performance and licensing outcomes compared to other selection methods.[75,76] An SJT has been used successfully to measure applicants' interpersonal awareness in medical and dental school admissions in Belgium.[77] SJTs are also less susceptible to group differences than other selection tools (Box 15.1).[78]

## Key theoretical developments and reflections on practice

In summary, research suggests that certain selection methods are effective for VBR (e.g. SJTs and structured interviews) whereas others are not (e.g. personal statements and CVs). While this conclusion is drawn from the wider evidence base on effective selection method design, there are also some important theoretical developments in this area that can contribute to understanding why certain methods work better.

To explain why SJTs are often correlated with measures of personality traits, Motowidlo, Hooper and Jackson[79] developed the implicit trait policy (ITP) theory. According to the ITP theory, SJTs measure ITPs and general experience (and, depending on job level, specific job knowledge). ITPs are beliefs about the *costs/benefits of expressing certain traits* (which guides behaviour). Thus, implicit trait policies are an individual's judgement about the relative cost/benefits of expressing certain traits in certain situations (and so are related to trait *expression* rather than traits, per se). For example, making a judgement that generally being agreeable in a situation (e.g. towards a patient, a colleague or a supervisor) might be a more successful strategy in dealing with the situation than being disagreeable. In this way, SJTs measure the procedural awareness about what is effective behaviour in a given situation and this is likely to be linked to an individual's values.

Like values, it is thought that ITPs are shaped by experiences in fundamental socialisation processes, such as parental modelling during childhood. This may teach the utility of, for example; *agreeable expressions*, that is, helping others in need or turning the other cheek; or *disagreeable expressions*, that is, showing selfish preoccupation with one's own interests or advancing ones own interests

## BOX 15.1    Practical Example of Developing an SJT for Values-Based Recruitment in healthcare

### Context

*Every year, nearly 8000 final year medical students apply for junior doctor posts in the UK's Foundation Programme. The 2-year programme is a requirement for all medical graduates wishing to work as doctors in the United Kingdom. Competition into the programme is intensifying due to the expansion of UK medical schools and the ever-increasing number of international applications.*

*The Department of Health recommended that an SJT was implemented to assess professional attributes, judgement and employability for a Foundation Programme post and to replace the open-ended competency-based application questions previously used. The SJT presents applicants with scenarios they are likely to encounter as a Foundation Year 1 (F1) doctor and asks how they would react in these situations. Their responses are scored against a pre-determined key defined by subject matter experts. The SJT ensures candidates selected have the aptitude and values required of a successful doctor.*

### Key issues and how these were addressed

*In order to understand and define the attributes required to be successful in the role, a job analysis of the F1 doctor role was undertaken. A person specification was developed based on this analysis. Each year, educational supervisors, clinical supervisors and other Foundation Programme experts contribute to the development of new test questions based on the person specification. These questions are further reviewed, including input from Foundation doctors to ensure that the hypothetical situations are realistic and appropriate. From the job analysis, five target domains were identified to be assessed in the SJT and each item is designed to measure one of these. The five target domains are outlined in Table 15.2 along with examples of the kinds of scenarios, which might be included under each.*

### Outcomes and evaluation

*The SJT has been in operational use since 2013, and to date approximately 16,000 medical school graduates have completed the test with results informing their allocation to Foundation Programme places alongside a measure of educational attainment. Each year the SJT is subject to full psychometric analysis, and the results consistently show that the SJT is a reliable, valid and appropriate method for foundation selection. Applicant reactions to the test have been positive, with the majority of students indicating that the content of the test seems fair, relevant*

*to the Foundation Programme and appropriate for their level. Work is currently underway to assess the predictive validity of the SJT, comparing performance on the test with performance on the foundation programme. This will examine the extent to which the SJT is able to predict a doctor's attitude and values in the job.*

*Table 15.2* SJT target domains and example SJT scenarios

| | |
|---|---|
| Commitment to Professionalism | E.g. Issues of confidentiality such as hearing a colleague talking about a patient outside of work |
| Coping with Pressure | E.g. Dealing with confrontation such as an angry relative |
| Effective Communication | E.g. Gathering information and communicating intentions to other colleagues |
| Patient Focus | E.g. Taking into account a patient's views/concerns |
| Working Effectively as Part of a Team | E.g. Recognising and valuing the skills and knowledge of colleagues, when faced with a disagreement about a patient's care |

Note: These domain areas have been clearly mapped to the NHS constitutional values of working together for patients, respect and dignity, commitment to quality of care, compassion, improving lives, everyone counts.

at another person's expense. Having entered University in early adulthood, the challenge of educational supervisors is to teach students the utility of effective behaviour in the role of nurse or doctor. This socialisation is tutored during supervised clinical practice at University, regarding effective behaviour by a clinician in any given situation.

Whilst personality generally represents the behaviours that come most naturally, values reflect effort (motivational goals) and a choice to behave a certain way.[6,7] Here, we argue that an individual also has procedural awareness about the costs/benefits of taking certain courses of action (as measured in an SJT), which also guides behaviour. In a given situation, we may choose to 'treat others with respect' for example. Therefore, it is likely that SJTs can be constructed to measure aspects of an individual's values since SJTs measure implicit trait policies. SJTs are not measures of ethical values per se, but more measures of an individual's awareness about what is effective behaviour in work-relevant contexts, for important interpersonal domains.

Our chapter focuses on an analysis of the theory behind SJTs, although it is important to note that this is just one selection method that could prove useful in values-based recruitment.[58] 'Personality assessments, alongside structured interviews, may also prove a useful method to explore values in recruitment and further research is warranted in this area to examine the issues'.

## Where next?

This chapter has explored (1) what values are, their theoretical underpinnings and how they can be an important addition to recruitment and selection in healthcare; (2) the links between values and factors such as personality, motivation and behaviours at work and (3) the selection methods that are best used for values-based recruitment in terms of their effectiveness, and why some methods are more appropriate for values-based recruitment than others. Therefore, how can the content of this chapter inform research? What needs to be done in terms of VBR in healthcare education? And how can the information in this chapter be applied in practice?

In terms of research, existing evidence suggests that an important part of the VBR agenda is being able to identify employees who will deliver high quality and safe care; however, there is currently a significant gap in the literature with regard to how values can be accurately measured specifically within a healthcare context. Whilst this chapter has examined the effectiveness of a number of selection methods for measuring values, this area remains a fruitful avenue for future research. Research more generally has shown emerging theory development in some selection methods. For example, the theory underlying SJTs suggests that they measure implicit trait policies,[73] which are likely to be linked to an individual's values. SJTs therefore show promise as a potential way to measure values in healthcare recruitment. In addition, this chapter has highlighted the importance of understanding what exactly constitutes a 'value' and how it differs from other similar constructs, such as personality. This has implications for both future research, as whilst there is extensive theory exploring personality generally, there is no extensive research examining personality, and values. More systematic long-term validation studies are needed to explore the extent to which SJTs correlate with subsequent behaviour in clinical practice. Further research is required regarding construct validity in an attempt

to uncover how SJTs might be best used to assess values. Ranking-based SJT response formats (as opposed to rating formats) might be optimal to measure values as research shows values relate to goal choice. Since medicine is practiced across the globe, using the theory presented in this chapter, the potential role of cross-cultural differences in values should be explored as an important next step.

Finally, the research evidence supports the promotion of values-based recruitment as only one part of embedding values in an organisation given individuals recruited into an organisation with optimal values for the delivery of high quality, competent and compassionate care, may be at risk of changing practice through either socialisation (value internalisation) or attrition, if placed within teams where suboptimal values are evident. This indicates a clear need for a multifaceted approach to developing and researching organisational values beyond recruitment issues alone.

## Summary and conclusions

There is a complex relationship between values and other psychological attributes such as personality, ability and motivation. This means assessing and measuring values during recruitment is challenging and less straightforward than assessing abilities and skills.

Some selection methods are effective for values-based recruitment (e.g. SJTs and MMIs), whereas others are not (e.g. personal statements and CVs), and it is important to continue to develop our understanding of the theory underpinning the effectiveness of such methods. This field of research is still emerging within the field of medical education and there are many areas for further study.

---

**Practice points**

- Personality and values are distinct – personality refers to enduring dispositions, while values refer to enduring goals.

- There are links between values and factors such as personality, motivation and behaviours at work, hence the importance of measuring values at the point of recruitment.

- A particularly promising approach to measuring a variety of non-academic attributes beyond clinical knowledge including values, which are especially relevant to medical education, training and practice, is SJTs.

- While there is increasing evidence of SJT effectiveness compared to several other selection tools in terms of accurately measuring values within a healthcare context, this is an area ripe for further research.
- Moreover, values-based recruitment is only one part of embedding values in a healthcare context: there is a need for a multifaceted approach to developing and researching organisational values beyond recruitment alone.

## Acknowledgements

We gratefully acknowledge support from Maria St Ledger and Sarah Stott in the literature searches and helping in the preparation of the final manuscript.

## References and bibliography

1 Francis R. (2013). *Report of the Mid Staffordshire NHS Foundation Trust Public Inquiry: Executive Summary (Vol. 947). TSO Shop*

2 Cavendish, C. (2013) *An Independent Review into Healthcare Assistants and Support Workers in the NHS and Social Care Settings*. Department of Health, London.

3 Schwartz, S.H. (2012) An overview of the Schwartz theory of basic values. *Online Readings in Psychology and Culture*, **2**.

4 Rokeach, M. (1973) *The Nature of Human Values*. Free Press, New York.

5 Bardi, A. & Schwartz, S.H. (2003) Values and behavior: Strength and structure of relations. *Personality and Social Psychology Bulletin*, **29**, 1207–1220.

6 Parks, L. & Guay, R.P. (2009) Personality, values, and motivation. *Personality and Individual Differences*, **47**, 675–684.

7 Parks, L. & Guay, R.P. (2012) Can personal values predict performance? Evidence in an academic setting. *Applied Psychology: An International Review*, **61**, 149–173.

8 Schwartz, S.H. (1992) Universals in the content and structure of values: Theoretical advances and empirical tests in 20 countries. In: Zanna, M.P. (ed), *Advances in Experimental Social Psychology*. Academic Press, San Diego, CA, pp. 1–65.

9 Schwartz, S.H. (1994) Are there universal aspects in the structure and contents of human values? *Journal of Social Issues*, **50**, 19–45.

10 Schwartz, S.H. & Bilsky, W. (1987) Toward a psychological structure of human values. *Journal of Personality and Social Psychology*, **53**, 550–562.

11 Schwartz, S.H. & Bilsky, W. (1990) Toward a theory of the universal content and structure of values: Extensions and cross-cultural replications. *Journal of Personality and Social Psychology*, **58**, 878.

12 Ravlin, E.C. & Meglino, B.M. (1987a) Issues in work values measurement. In: Preston, L. (ed), *Research in Corporate Social Performance and Policy*. Vol. **9**. JAI Press Inc., pp. 153–183.

13 Locke, E.A. (1997) The motivation to work: What we know. In: Maehr, M.L. & Pintrick, P.R. (eds), *Advances in Motivation and Achievement*. Vol. **10**. JAI Press Inc., pp. 375–412.

14 Meglino, B.M. & Ravlin, E.C. (1998) Individual values in organisations: concepts, controversies, and research. *Journal of Management*, **24**, 351–389.

15 Oishi, S., Schimmack, U., Diener, E. & Suh, E. (1998) The measurement of values and individualism–collectivism. *Personality and Social Psychology Bulletin*, **24**, 1177–1189.

16 Kapes, J.T. & Strickler, R.E. (1975) A longitudinal study of change in work values between 9th and 12th grades. *Journal of Vocational Behavior*, **6**, 81–93.

17 Rokeach, M. (1972) *Beliefs, Attitudes, and Values: A Theory of Organization and Change*. Jossey-Bass Inc., San Francisco, CA.

18 Cable, D.M. & Parsons, C.K. (2001) Socialisation tactics and person-organisation fit. *Personnel Psychology*, **54**, 1–23.

19 Weiss, H.M. (1978) Social learning of work values in organizations. *Journal of Applied Psychology*, **63**, 711–718.

20 Schwartz, S.H. & Bardi, A. (2001) Value hierarchies across cultures taking a similarities perspective. *Journal of Cross-Cultural Psychology*, **32**, 268–290.

21 McCrae, R.R. & Costa, P.T. Jr., (1997) Personality trait structure as a human universal. *American Psychologist*, **52**, 509–516.

22 Mount, M.K. & Barrick, M.R. (2002) *The Personal Characteristics Inventory Manual*. The Wonderlic Corporation, Libertyville, IL.

23 Goldberg, L.R. (1992) The development of markers for the Big-Five Factor structure. *Psychological Assessment*, **4**, 26–42.

24 Judge, T.A., Heller, D. & Mount, M.K. (2002) Five-factor model of personality and job satisfaction: a meta-analysis. *Journal of Applied Psychology*, **87**, 530.

25 Motowidlo, S.J., Borman, W.C. & Schmidt, M.J. (1997) A theory of individual differences in task and contextual performance. *Human Performance*, **10**, 71–83.

26 Schmidt, F.L. & Hunter, J.E. (1983) Individual differences in productivity: An empirical test of estimates derived from studies of selection procedure utility. *Journal of Applied Psychology*, **68**, 407.

27 Roccas, S., Sagiv, L., Schwartz, S.H. & Knafo, A. (2002) The Big Five personality factors and personal values. *Personality and Social Psychology Bulletin*, **28**, 789–801.

28 Williams, R. & Pons, H. (2001) *Cultura y sociedad, 1780-1950: De Coleridge a Orwell*. Nueva Visión.

29 Parks L. (2007). Personality and values: A meta-analysis. Paper presented at the *annual conference for the society of industrial and organizational psychology*, New York.

30  Schneider, B. (1987) The people make the place. *Personnel Psychology*, **40**, 437–453.

31  Schneider, B., Goldstein, H.W. & Smith, D.B. (1995) The ASA framework: an update. *Personnel Psychology*, **48**, 474–773.

32  Bauer, T.N., Morrison, E.W. & Callister, R.R. (1998) Organizational socialization: A review and directions for future research. *Research in Personnel and Human Resources Management*, **16**, 149–214.

33  Chao, G.T., O'Leary-Kelly, A.M., Wolf, S., Klein, H.J. & Gardner, P.D. (1994) Organisational socialisation: Its context and consequences. *Journal of Applied Psychology*, **79**, 730–743.

34  Ostroff, C., Yuhyung, S. & Kinicki, A.J. (2005) Multiple perspectives of congruence: relationships between value congruence and employee attitude. *Journal of Organisational Behaviour*, **26**, 591–623.

35  Bilsberry, J. (2007) Attracting for values: an empirical study of ASA's attraction proposition. *Journal of Managerial Psychology*, **22**, 132–149.

36  Hollup, O. (2012) Nurses in Mauritius motivated by extrinsic rewards: A qualitative study of factors determining recruitment and career choices. *International Journal of Nursing Studies*, **49**, 1291–1298.

37  Arnold, J., Coombs, C., Wilkinson, A., Loan-Clarke, J., Park, J. & Preston, D. (2003) Corporate images of the United Kingdom National Health Service: Implications for the recruitment and retention of nursing and allied health profession staff. *Corporate Reputation Review*, **6**, 223–238.

38  De Cooman, R., De Gieter, S., Pepermans, R. *et al.* (2009) Person-organisation fit: Testing socialisation and attraction-selection-attrition hypotheses. *Journal of Vocational Behaviour*, **74**, 102–107.

39  Anderson, N., Born, M. & Cunningham-Snell, N. (2001) Recruitment and selection: Applicant perspectives and outcomes. In: Anderson, N. (ed), *Handbook of Industrial Work and Organizational Psychology*. Sage, London, pp. 200–218.

40  Guion, R.M. (1998) *Assessment, Measurement, and Prediction for Personnel Selection*. Erlbaum, Mawah, NJ.

41  Schmidt, F.L., Ones, D.S. & Hunter, J.E. (1992) Personnel selection. *Annual Review of Psychology*, **43**, 627–670.

42  Anderson, N. & Ostroff, C. (1997) Selection as socialization. In: *International Handbook of Selection and Assessment*. John Wiley, London, pp. 413–440.

43  Rapping, J.A. (2009) You can't build on shakvey ground: laying the foundation for indigent defense reform through values-based recruitment, training and mentoring. *Harvard Law and Policy Review*.

44  Maierhofer, N.I., Griffin, M.A. & Sheehan, M. (2000) Linking manager values and behaviour with employee values and behaviour: A study of values and safety in the hairdressing industry. *Journal of Occupational Health Psychology*, **5**, 417–427.

45  Finegan, J.E. (2000) The impact of person and organisational values on organisational commitment. *Journal of Occupational and Organisational Psychology*, **73**, 149–169.

46  Ostroff, C. & Zhan, Y. (2012) Person–environment fit in the selection process. In: Schmidt, N. (ed), *The Oxford Handbook of Personnel Selection and Assessment*. Oxford University Press.

47  Kristof-Brown, A.L., Jansen, K.J. & Colbert, A.E. (2002) A policy-capturing study of the simultaneous effects of fit with jobs, groups and organisations. *Journal of Applied Psychology*, **87**, 985–993.

48  Van Vianen, A.E.M. (2000) Person-organisation fit: The match between newcomers' and recruiters preferences for organisational cultures. *Personnel Psychology*, **53**, 113–149.

49  Amos, E.A. & Weathington, B.L. (2008) An analysis of the relation between employee-organisation value congruence and employee attitudes. *Journal of Psychology*, **142**, 615–631.

50  Verquer, M.L., Beehr, T.A. & Wagner, S.H. (2003) A meta-analysis of relations between Person-Organisation fit and work attitudes. *Journal of Vocational Behaviour*, **63**, 473–489.

51  Hoffman, B.J. & Woehr, D.J. (2005) A quantitative review of the relationship between person-organisation fit and behavioural outcomes. *Journal of Vocational Behaviour*, **68**, 389–399.

52  Kristof, A.L. (1996) Person-organization fit: An integrative review of its conceptualizations, measurement, and implications. *Personnel Psychology*, **49**, 1–49.

53  Tziner, A. (1987) Congruency issue retested using Fineman's achievement climate notion. *Journal of Social Behavior and Personality*, **2**, 63–78.

54  Campion, M.A., Palmer, D.K. & Campion, J.E. (1997) A review of structure in the selection interview. *Personnel Psychology*, **50**, 655–702.

55  Lievens, F. & Thornton, G.C. (2005) Assessment centres: recent developments in practice and research. In: Evers, A., Smit-Voskuijl, O. & Anderson, N. (eds), *Handbook of Personnel Selection*. Blackwell, Oxford, pp. 243–264.

56  Ryan, A.M. & Ployhart, R.E. (2014) A century of selection. *Annual Review of Psychology*, **65**, 20.1–20.25.

57  Salgado, J.F. & Anderson, N. (2002) Cognitive and GMA testing in the European Community: Issues and evidence. *Human Performance*, **15**, 75–96.

58  Patterson, F., Knight, A. *et al* (2016) A systematic review of selection methods. *In press Medical Education*.

59  McDaniel, M.A., Hartman, N.S., Whetzel, D.L. & Grubb, W.L. III, (2007) Situational judgment tests, response instructions, and validity: A meta-analysis. *Personnel Psychology*, **60**, 63–91.

60  Weekley, J.A. & Ployhart, R.E. (2006) *Situational Judgment Tests: Theory, Management, and Application*. Erlbaum, Mahwah, NJ.

61  Patterson, F., Prescott-Clements, L., Zibarras, L., Edwards, H., Kerrin, M. & Cousans, F. (2015under review) Recruiting for values in healthcare: a preliminary review of the evidence. *Advances in Healthcare Sciences*, 1–23.

62  Prideaux, D., Roberts, C., Eva, K. *et al.* (2011) Assessment for selection for the health care professions and

specialty training: Consensus statement and recommendations from the Ottawa 2010 Conference. *Medical Teacher*, **33**, 215–223.

63 Cleland J, Dowell J, McLachlan J, Nicholson S & Patterson F. (2012) *Identifying best practice in the selection of medical students.* Research report to the General Medical Council http://www.gmc-uk.org/Identifying_best_practice_in_the_selection_of_medical_students.pdf_51119804.pdf

64 McDaniel, M.A. & Nguyen, N.T. (2001) Situational judgment tests: A review of practice and constructs assessed. *International Journal of Selection and Assessment*, **9**, 103–113.

65 Christian, M., Edwards, B. & Bradley, J. (2010) Situational judgement tests: constructs assessed and a meta-analysis of their criterion-related validities. *Personnel Psychology*, **63**, 83–117.

66 Lievens, F., Peeters, H. & Schollaert, E. (2008) Situational judgment tests: a review of recent research. *Personnel Review*, **37**, 426–441.

67 Motowidlo, S.J., Dunnette, M.D. & Carter, G.W. (1990) An alternative selection procedure: The low-fidelity simulation. *Journal of Applied Psychology*, **75**, 640–647.

68 Patterson, F., Baron, H., Carr, V., Lane, P. & Plint, S. (2009) Evaluation of three short-listing methodologies for selection into postgraduate training: the case of General Practice in the UK. *Medical Education*, **43**, 50–57.

69 Whetzel, D., McDaniel, M. & Nguyen, N. (2008) Subgroup differences in situational judgment test performance: A meta-analysis. *Human Performance*, **21**, 291–309.

70 McDaniel, M.A., Whetzel, D.L., Schmidt, F.L. *et al.* (1994) The validity of employment interviews: A comprehensive review and meta-analysis. *Journal of Applied Psychology*, **79**, 599–616.

71 Steiner, D.D. & Gilliland, S.W. (1996) Fairness reactions to personnel selection techniques in France and the United States. *Journal of Applied Psychology*, **81**, 134–141.

72 Weekley, J.A. & Ployhart, R.E. (2013) *Situational Judgment Tests: Theory, Measurement, and Application.* Psychology Press.

73 Motowidlo, S.J. & Beier, M.E. (2010) Differentiating specific job knowledge from implicit trait policies in procedural knowledge measured by a situational judgment test. *Journal of Applied Psychology*, **95**, 321–333.

74 Patterson, F., Ashworth, V., Zibarras, L., Coan, P., Kerrin, M. & O'Neill, P. (2012) Evaluations of situational judgement tests to assess non-academic attributes in selection. *Medical Education*, **46**, 850–868.

75 Lievens, F. & Patterson, F. (2011) The validity and incremental validity of knowledge tests, low-fidelity simulations, and high-fidelity simulations for predicting job performance in advanced-level high-stakes selection. *Journal of Applied Psychology*, **96**, 927–940.

76 Patterson, F., Lievens, F., Kerrin, M., Munro, N. & Irish, B. (2013) The predictive validity of selection for entry into postgraduate training in general practice: evidence from three longitudinal studies. *British Journal of General Practice*, **63**, 734–741.

77 Lievens, F. (2013) Adjusting medical school admission: assessing interpersonal skills using situational judgement tests. *Medical Education*, **47**, 182–189.

78 Clevenger, J., Pereira, G.M., Wiechmann, D., Schmitt, N. & Harvey, V.S. (2001) Incremental validity of situational judgment tests. *Journal of Applied Psychology*, **86**, 410–417.

79 Motowidlo, S.J., Hooper, A.C. & Jackson, H.L. (2006) Implicit policies about relations between personality traits and behavioral effectiveness in situational judgment items. *Journal of Applied Psychology*, **91**, 749–761.

# 16 Emotions and learning: cognitive theoretical and methodological approaches to studying the influence of emotions on learning

*Meghan McConnell and Kevin Eva*

*A second year family medicine resident is at the end of a busy shift that involved five vaginal deliveries and two Caesarian sections. At 0500h, a young woman is admitted; her labour is precipitous, she is fully dilated and is pushing on arrival. Initial foetal heart tones are reassuring but as the vertex becomes visible, there is a deep deceleration with poor recovery. With the next contraction, there is another deceleration without recovery. Alone, the resident decides to try the 'Mighty-Vac', a skill she has done under the watchful eye of the senior obstetrical resident on two other occasions. After the first pull, the handle snaps off. The nurse reports the foetal heart as 60 beats per minute. The resident quickly applies forceps, checks their position and delivers the baby's head with two pulls. However, three loops of the umbilical cord are wrapped tightly around the baby's neck and there is thick meconium. The baby is suctioned on the perineum, delivered and while being transferred to the resuscitation cart, begins to wail to everyone's relief.*

## Introduction

This example illustrates the wide range of emotions that can impact healthcare professional trainees. The resident hoped for success, was fearful of failure and felt relief and pride after successfully completing the procedure. These emotions have the potential to strongly influence trainees' learning, motivation, critical thinking, identity development and life-long learning[1]. Having a better understanding of how emotions influence various learning and transfer processes will not only help students respond flexibly to different educational settings but will also enable educators deliberately plan their efforts to take advantage of these processes.

To understand the influence of emotions on the training and assessment of clinicians, medical educators need to have a strong grasp of the methods and theories underlying emotion research. Cognitive psychologists have a rich history of studying the way in which emotions influence how information is processed within learning environments, how it is organised and retrieved from memory and how it is used to make decisions and inform learners' behaviours and actions[1,2].

In this chapter, we use research within cognitive psychology to (a) highlight some of the theoretical approaches used to explain how emotions modulate learning, (b) describe several methodologies that can be used to elicit and assess emotions in various educational environments and (c) identify outstanding research questions regarding the impact of emotions on the training of healthcare professionals. It is our aim that this chapter will not only improve readers' understanding of the role of emotions in training, assessment and performance of clinicians, but will also serve as a reference guide for healthcare professional education researchers embarking on emotion research (see practice points).

## Defining the terms

As the medical education community begins to recognise the importance of emotions within the context of learning, it is important for researchers to use consistent conceptualisations and operationalisations of relevant phenomena, including affect, mood and emotion[3] (see Table 16.1).

Affect refers to a broad, inclusive neurophysiological state that typically involves simple, non-reflective feelings[4]. People are continuously in an affective state, although its nature and intensity varies over time. Examples of affect include pleasure, tension, calmness and tiredness. In this way, affect is an umbrella term that includes not only moods and emotions, but constructs such as feelings, beliefs, preferences, evaluations and attitudes.

*Researching Medical Education*, First Edition. Edited by Jennifer Cleland and Steven J. Durning.
© 2015 John Wiley & Sons, Ltd. Published 2015 by John Wiley & Sons, Ltd.

*Table 16.1* Definitions of affect, mood and emotion

| Term | Definition | Example |
|---|---|---|
| Affect | A neurophysiological state interpreted as a simple, non-reflective feeling | Pleasure, displeasure, tension, calmness, energy and tiredness |
| Mood | A free-floating affective state that can last for hours, days or weeks and is not associated with a specific object or event | Waking up in an irritable mood, feeling content for no specific reason |
| Emotion | Psychophysiological changes that occur in response to a given object or event, including behavioural reactions (e.g. actions such as approach or avoidance), expressive responses (e.g. facial and/or vocal expressions), physiological reactions (e.g. neuronal or hormonal) and cognitive appraisals (e.g. subjective evaluations of the situation) | Being irritable in response to an argument, being elated due to a positive performance. |

Moods typically refer to free-floating affective states that can last for hours, days or weeks and are not associated with a specific object or event[5]. For example, one may wake up in an irritable mood, a state that could vary in duration and is not linked to a specific event, object or person.

Emotions, in contrast, are associated with a specific event or moment, real or imagined, that can take place in the past, present or future[3]. Examples include being happy about a positive diagnostic outcome, or fearful about an upcoming clinical rotation with a particularly difficult supervisor. Within cognitive psychology, emotions are further defined as a series of psychophysiological changes that occur in response to a given object or event. These changes include behavioural reactions (e.g. approach or avoidance), expressive responses (e.g. facial and/or vocal expressions), physiological reactions (e.g. neuronal or hormonal) and cognitive appraisals (e.g. subjective evaluations of the situation)[6]. In this way, learners in different emotional states are expected to respond differently to a given educational event. For example, after receiving constructive feedback on a performance evaluation, a learner who is feeling particularly anxious may avoid the preceptor (a behavioural response), become rather quiet (a vocal expression), feel like his heart is racing (a physiological reaction) and perceive the event as quite negative (a cognitive appraisal of the situation).

## Conceptual foundations

### The structure of emotion

Two broad approaches can be used to classify emotion research: the discrete approach and the dimensional approach.

Researchers espousing *dimensional approaches* view emotions as entities that share a set of underlying dimensions. By way of analogy, specific labels can be put on individual colours, but the spectrum of colours can be defined more succinctly through dimensions of brightness, hue and saturation[7]. The most common dimensional model of emotion, the circumplex model, posits that emotions are defined based on their valence (positive vs negative) and their level of physiological arousal or activation (high vs low)[8]. In this way, valence and arousal are thought to be orthogonal, bipolar dimensions that enable one to quantify different emotional states.

Others have argued that these dimensions are too simplistic to account for the heterogeneous nature of affect[7,9]. For example, Fontaine *et al.*[7] analysed 24 emotional terms in three European cultures and found that four dimensions were needed to adequately distinguish among these terms – valence, activation, potency-control (e.g. feelings of power or weakness, which differentiate feelings of anger and contempt from feelings of shame and despair) and novelty-unpredictability (e.g. reactions to unexpected events, whereby feelings such as surprise and fear are distinguished from most other emotions). Lövheim[9], on the other hand, espoused a three-dimensional model, termed the 'cube model of affect', whereby affective states are quantified as a function of three main monoamine neurotransmitters: serotonin, dopamine and noradrenaline.

The debate over the number and nature of the underlying dimensions of affective states is ongoing as researchers have found that different emotions within the same dimensional space can have different effects[10,11]. These researchers have argued for a *discrete states approach*, whereby each emotion is considered to be unique[7,12]. Discrete models of emotion present each emotional state with unique behavioural and cognitive manifestations, somatic and visceral symptoms, expressive behaviours (e.g. facial, postural and vocal expressions), coping responses and so forth. For example, the emotion of anxiety is associated with the presence of an 'uncertain, existential threat'[13]; limited attention to peripheral details and avoidance strategies (e.g. specific attention- and action-related biases)[14]; increased respiratory rate, heart rate and cardiovascular output (e.g. unique visceral and somatic symptoms)[15] and tense facial, postural and vocal expressions (e.g. expressive behaviours)[16].

While discrete approaches emphasise the unique aspects of different emotions, it is also clear that some emotions closely resemble one another (e.g. shame and guilt, terror and fear, envy and jealousy). Thus, in a variant of the distinct states approach, several researchers have attempted to compose categories of emotions, whereby members of each category closely resemble one another. For example, the category of 'anger' may include rage, wrath and annoyance. The manifestations (behavioural, cognitive, physiological, expressive, etc.) of these emotions are thought to be similar to one another, but different from emotions belonging to other categories, such as those defined by love (e.g. adoration, compassion, affection and tenderness) or fear (e.g. horror, fright, panic and terror)[3]. Whether this revision of the discrete states approach blurs the boundaries between it and dimensional approaches or whether some categories simply reflect the existence of synonyms within common language remains to be seen. For now, the best recommendation that can be made for researchers is to make a deliberate choice regarding which model seems most appropriate given the questions and context under study.

### Incidental versus integral emotions

Because emotions are thought to arise in response to a specific object or event, they can also be conceptualised based on the focal cause (or source) of the emotion and its relevance to the task at hand. *Incidental* emotions are derived from a source that is unrelated to the task. For example, if one is trying to study the Krebs cycle, incidental emotions can include anger caused by an earlier confrontation with a colleague or frustration caused by an intermittent Internet connection. In contrast, *integral* affective states are directly related to the task – the excitement that arises when a trainee correctly diagnoses a challenging case, or the trepidation that arises the first time a resident intubates a patient without the assistance of a senior physician. In these examples, the affective state is induced by the event, and thus, is integral to the learning experience.

There is evidence that both integral and incidental emotions influence the judgments and choices people make[10,17]. It is reasonable to suspect, however, that incidental and integral affective states can have differential effects on learning, thereby providing further cause to carefully distinguish between sources of emotions. For example, in a review of the literature on the relationship between stress and performance, LeBlanc[18] suggests that when the task being performed is integrally related to the source of stress (e.g. resuscitating a patient), attention will be focused towards the task itself, and performance may be enhanced; however, if the source of stress is incidental to the task being performed (e.g. loud noises and disruptive team members), then attention will be focused away from the task and towards the source of the stress, which should have detrimental effects on performance. Thus, whether or not emotions are induced by the learning event should modulate their influence on learning, knowledge retention and knowledge transfer.

### Theoretical approaches

Several theories have been developed to explain the relationship between emotion and cognition. The affect-as-information model[19] posits that emotional responses provide physiological and experiential information, and this information subsequently guides individuals' responses to various situations. According to this theory, emotional responses to a particular judgment, object or event signal the overall value (e.g. pleasant/unpleasant and desirable/undesirable) and importance (e.g. urgent/not urgent and important/unimportant) of the situation. Imagine a paramedic treating a critically injured child. In such a case, feelings of anxiety indicate that the stakes are high, that there are significant threats to the child's well-being and that time is of the essence[20]. In this way, the affect-as-information account would argue that emotions influence learning by prioritising certain information within the learning environment. This is very much a dimensional approach in that the information gleaned from emotions is a function of valence (e.g. value) and arousal (e.g. importance).

In contrast, researchers adopting a discrete states approach to studying emotions have emphasised the importance of cognitive appraisals in defining different emotional states. Appraisal theorists posit that emotional experiences are the result of how individuals interpret, or *appraise*, a given object, event or situation[12,21]. According to appraisal theories, emotions result from the interpretation of ongoing events and situations[21]; the same situation can produce different emotions in different people based on their appraisal (or interpretation) of the situation. Imagine an instance where a trainee is being harshly criticised by his/her supervisor for making a mistake that could have had severe consequences for a patient. How the trainee responds depends on how he/she interprets the situation.

The trainee may respond with anger if he/she believes the criticism is misplaced because others are to blame or he/she may maintain positive emotions if he/she believes he/she did the best one could, given the situational demands. Appraisals are important because they mediate the impact of situational factors and can be targeted by educational interventions intended to foster positive emotional development[22].

More recently, the control-value theory of emotions was developed to understand the role that emotions play in academic or achievement settings[22]. This theory distinguishes between two types of emotions: activity emotions pertaining to ongoing achievement-related actions and outcome emotions pertaining to the results of these activities[23]. Activity emotions include excitement at the chance to learn something new, or anger about a challenging assignment; outcome-related emotions include the joy and pride experienced when academic goals are met[22]. This theory argues that both activity- and outcome-based achievement emotions and the appraisals that accompany them influence learners' academic engagement and performance.

Because the control-value theory was developed specifically to examine emotions in achievement settings, it is particularly useful in understanding the effects of emotions on motivation, learning and performance.[24]

## Mechanisms of action

Within cognitive psychology, emotions have been the subject of considerable theoretical and empirical research over the past several decades. Emotions are thought to influence learning and performance along five general routes: cognitive resources, strategies of learning and problem-solving, memory, self-regulation and interest/motivation[25].

### Cognitive resources
Emotions influence the distribution of cognitive resources within working memory. Resource allocation models[26] posit that emotions unrelated to ongoing learning activities (incidental emotions) will consume working memory resources and reduce the cognitive resources available for task demands. This reduction in available cognitive resources will in turn impact performance negatively[27,28]. For example, a student who is anxious about an upcoming licensure examination or is saddened by the death of a patient will have fewer cognitive resources available to devote to current learning demands. Fraser and colleagues[29] recently

examined the relationship between emotion, cognitive load and diagnostic performance during simulation training and found that (a) cognitive load was highest when trainees reported high levels of 'invigoration' and low levels of 'tranquility' and (b) trainees' ability to accurately diagnose a trained murmur decreased as cognitive load increased. These results are among the first within medical education to demonstrate the impact of emotion and cognitive load on performance.

Most studies in this area, however, have focused predominantly on incidental emotions, whereby participants' emotions are measured (or manipulated) before completing a 'neutral' task. When emotions are integral to the task demand (e.g. responding to emotional words or images), emotions have been shown to facilitate working memory performance[30], particularly in arousing situations[31]. These results suggest that incidental and integral emotions have differential effects on working memory, and consequently, on learning and performance.

### Strategies of learning and problem-solving
Emotions modulate an individual's use of 'cognitive shortcuts', including schemata, attributes, heuristics, stereotypes and rules of thumb. Negative moods are associated with the use of systematic, analytical processes while positive emotions are associated with more creative ways of solving problems[32]. These findings suggest that positive emotions promote the use of flexible learning strategies, such as elaboration and organisation of learning materials, while negative emotions can facilitate the use of more rigid strategies, such as simple rehearsal[33,34]. In this way, emotions influence the way in which learners think during educational activities.

### Memory
Highly emotional experiences tend to be well remembered. In general, (a) negative events are more likely to be recalled than positive events[35] and (b) arousing experiences are more easily remembered than less-arousing experiences[36]. When emotions are linked to a specific learning experience, trainees may remember the information gained from the learning event in more detail than non-emotional experiences. However, such emotionally enhanced memory may not be beneficial in cases where emotions are 'carried over' from prior experiences (e.g. are incidental to the current task). For example, imagine a situation in which Janet, a senior internal medicine resident, misdiagnosed an anaphylactoid reaction as a worsening of a patient's asthma. Janet experienced severe

anxiety, regret and guilt over the event. Several weeks later, a 30-year-old male was admitted onto the internal medicine service with asthma complicated by pneumonia. He was given antibiotics, but 24 hours later, his wheezing became worse and he was having difficulty breathing. Upon hearing this, Janet became incredibly anxious and feared she had made another mistake. In this case, the emotions of the initial event were transferred to a novel situation. These relived emotional experiences can have important influences on how the resident deals with her new patient.

## Self-regulation

In educational settings, students must plan, monitor and evaluate their knowledge to adapt their learning strategies to task demands and learning goals[34]. Researchers have shown that emotional states can influence self-regulatory processes: positive, arousing emotions, such as enjoyment of learning, promote self-regulation, while negative emotions, such as anxiety or shame, facilitate reliance on external guidance to recognise learning needs[22,34]. Furthermore, research has shown that emotions influence the extent to which individuals monitor and revise educational goals. Richard and Diefendorff[37] found that participants in positive moods are more likely to report higher academic goals (e.g. grades strived for on the next test), while those in negative moods tend to have lower goals. The authors theorised that positive emotions signal to the individual that the likelihood of success is high, whereas negative emotions suggest that the likelihood of success is low.

## Interest and motivation

Finally, emotions can impact students' learning and performance by inducing and sustaining interest in learning material[38]. Individual interest is defined as an enduring predisposition to attend to certain stimuli, events and objects and is associated with positive emotions and increased learning[39]. For example, a medical student with an interest in obstetrics will seek out opportunities to engage in associated activities, and such engagement will ideally lead to emotions such as enjoyment or excitement as he expands his knowledge. Situational interest is generated by specific environmental stimuli, such as the way educational tasks are organised and presented. Researchers have argued that situational interest is particularly important when dealing with learners who have no pre-existing individual interests in the pedagogical activities[38,39]. Positive emotions in academic settings, such as enjoyment, can lead to greater motivation to engage in learning activities; negative

emotions, on the other hand, such as hopelessness and boredom, can have detrimental effects on motivation[34]. Empirical research has shown that interest-based learning has many benefits, including promotion of self-regulated learning and enhanced learning outcomes[38,39].

Together, these findings demonstrate that emotions influence a variety of cognitive processes involved in learning that should be relevant in medical education. More research is needed to determine the extent to which these findings can be generalised from cognitive psychology laboratories to real-world educational environments. As such, the next section of this chapter will outline common strategies for exploring the influence of emotion on learning.

## Inducing and measuring emotions

Researchers interested in studying emotions experimentally have typically treated affective states both as an independent variable, whereby emotions are manipulated to determine their impact on various phenomena and an outcome variable, whereby emotions are measured using self-reports, facial or vocal expressions and autonomic or central nervous system activation.

### Emotion induction tactics

A number of experimental emotion induction procedures have been developed to provoke transient affective states that theoretically mimic emotions arising in natural situations[40]. These manipulations are most often incidental emotion interventions rather than integral.

#### Films

One of the most common emotion induction procedures is the use of films or film fragments[41,42]. These stimuli have several desirable properties, including being readily standardised, involving no deception, having high degree of ecological validity and being dynamic rather than static[41].

#### Music

Music has been used to induce emotions in a wide variety of experiments, both alone and combined with other stimuli[43]. In such studies, participants listen to a mood-suggestive piece of music after being instructed to try and feel the emotive state expressed. Interestingly, while films have been shown to elicit discrete emotional states[44], research suggests that music may be better suited to manipulate valence and arousal rather than specific emotions[44].

### Self-referential methods

Two other commonly used mood induction procedures include the Velten method and the autobiographical recall procedure. In the Velten method, participants read 60 self-referential statements and try to feel the emotion described by the statements[45]. This procedure uses a dimensional approach to emotions (e.g. participants in a positive/aroused condition read statements such as 'This is great, I feel really good, I am elated about things'). While numerous researchers have used the Velten statements in mood induction studies, there are inconsistencies in the literature regarding the effectiveness of the method[46,47].

During the autobiographical recall procedure, participants are asked to recall one or more emotional life events. For example, individuals may be asked to recall and write about a situation where they felt angry, happy, serene, sad and so on. Autobiographical recall has been associated experimentally with changes in both arousal and valence. [48,49]

### Challenges associated with investigating emotions

Emotion researchers are often presented with methodological and ethical challenges when designing and conducting experiments. The aforementioned emotion induction procedures are typically used to study incidental emotions, as emotions are induced separately from the experimental task. For such incidental mood inductions to work, researchers have argued that participants should be unaware that their emotions are being manipulated or measured. Otherwise, participants try to correct for potential affective biases[50]. As such, mood inductions are typically framed as a separate study that is unrelated to the primary task.

In this way, investigating the influences of emotions on learning and performance often requires some form of deception, thereby making it impossible to provide fully informed consent. As a result, it is important, first of all, to not utilise manipulations that are too extreme in order to minimise the likelihood of risk to participants. Further, it is essential that emotion researchers fully debrief participants after completion of the study, particularly in cases where participants are induced to experience negative emotional states. It is clearly unethical to create emotions such as anger, fear, sadness or shame without attempting to dissipate such emotions upon completion of the learning experience.

## Measuring and assessing emotions

Assessing emotions, especially in real-world situations, is a complex, daunting task, but techniques exist to measure both dimensions of emotions and discrete emotional states. This chapter distinguishes between non-verbal measures and self-report measures of emotion.

### Non-verbal measures

Non-verbal instruments include those that assess either expressive or physiological changes that accompany emotions. Expressive aspects of emotion include facial, vocal and postural changes. Facial expressions are a key component of emotion, and studies have shown moderate-to-strong correlations between facial expressions and subjective experiences[51,52]. A number of observer-based systems have been developed to measure facial expression, including the Facial Action Coding System (FACS)[53–55]. An advantage of non-verbal instruments is that they are not language dependent and, therefore, can be used across different cultures.

Like facial expression instruments, patterns of vocal cues have been linked to emotions[56], including average pitch, changes in pitch, intensity, speaking rate, voice quality and articulation. Unfortunately, links to discrete emotional states have proven to be challenging[57].

Physiological components of emotions involve changes in the autonomic nervous system (ANS) and can be measured using a variety of techniques, such as blood pressure responses, heart rate, skin responses and hormonal changes[15]. However, there is still substantial debate among researchers as to whether the relationship between emotions and ANS activation is best understood using dimensional[58] or discrete[59] models of emotions. The variability of individuals' emotional response patterns, across both emotional dimensions and discrete states, is likely due, in part, to the variability in emotion induction procedures across experiments[60].

### Self-report measures

While expressive and behavioural components of emotions can be measured in a variety of ways, the assessment of the experiential component of emotion is arguably the most important (given it is the definition of the actual experience). However, such measurements can be considerably more challenging than non-verbal measures of emotions. There exists a wide range of self-report scales, all of which claim to measure different aspects of emotions. As such, emotion researchers are faced with the challenge of choosing the most appropriate self-report

*Table 16.2* Commonly used self-report measures of emotions

| Measure | Construct | Description |
| --- | --- | --- |
| Feeling scale (FS) [61] | Dimensional approach (valence only) | • Single-item scale<br>• 11-point bipolar scale ranging from −5 to +5, with anchors at all odd integers<br>• Ranges from 'Very Bad' (−5) to 'Neutral' (0) to 'Very Good' (+5)<br>• Typically used in conjunction with Felt Arousal Scale (see below) |
| Felt arousal scale (FAS)[62] | Dimensional approach (arousal only) | • Single-item scale<br>• 6-point bipolar scale, with anchors only present at 1 ('Low Arousal') and 6 ('High Arousal').<br>• Typically used in with Feeling Scale (see above) |
| Circular mood scale (CMS)[63] | Dimensional approach (valence and arousal) | • Single-item scale<br>• Measures arousal and valence.<br>• Consists of a circle surrounded by eight emotional states (clockwise from top *active/attentive, euphoric/elated, happy/friendly, calm/relaxed, uninvolved/inactive, bored/sluggish, unhappy/grouchy and alarmed/angry*). |
| Positive affect and negative affect scale (PANAS)[64] | Dimensional approach (positive vs negative affect) | • Consists of 20 adjectives, 10 representing positive affect (now called positive activation) and 10 representing negative affect (now called negative activation).<br>• Each adjective uses a 5-point scale that ranges from 'Very slightly/Not at All' to 'Extremely' |
| Activation deactivation adjective checklist (AD ACL)[65] | Dimensional approach | • Consists of 20 adjectives<br>• Measures energy, tiredness, tension and calmness<br>• 4-point response scale, ranging from 'definitely feels', 'slightly feels', 'cannot decide' and 'definitely do not feel'. |
| Four-dimension mood scale (4DMS)[66] | Dimensional approach | • Measures positive energy, tiredness, negative arousal and relaxation.<br>*Or*<br>• Energetic arousal and tense arousal |
| Profile of mood states (POMS)[67] | Discrete approach | • Measures six distinct states: fatigue-inertia, vigour-activity, tension-anxiety, depression-dejection, anger-hostility and confusion-bewilderment.<br>• Consists of 65 adjectives, each with a 5-point Likert scale. |
| Achievement emotion scale (AEQ)[68] | Discrete approach | • Specific to academic settings<br>• Based on Pekrun's (2006) control-value theory of achievement emotions.<br>• Measures enjoyment, hope, pride, relief, anger, anxiety, shame, hopelessness and boredom<br>• Consists of 24 items using a 5-point Likert scale (1 = completely disagree, 5 = completely agree). |

measures, and the decision to use one scale over another is often not well understood or justified.

Choosing the appropriate measure from the vast number of self-report tools requires a firm understanding of the underlying theoretical perspectives that preceded this section. At the most basic level is whether the researcher is interested in emotional dimensions (e.g. valence and arousal) or discrete emotional states (e.g. anger and excitement). Table 16.2 highlights some of the most commonly used self-report measures. For an excellent review, see Ekkekakis[3].

## Recommendations for future research

As alluded to at the beginning of this chapter, medical school is saturated with emotional experiences, and as such, understanding the role emotions play in learning and performance has important implications for medical educators. Traditionally, emotions and reason have been viewed as processes that oppose one another, the assumption being that affective processes reduce rationality, cloud judgement and distort reasoning. By viewing emotions as the antithesis of logic and reason, some medical educators have contributed to a culture that implicitly or explicitly encourages students to detach themselves from clinical experiences. This attitude of 'detached concern' and the importance of emotional neutrality may have substantial impacts on how trainees acquire and apply clinical knowledge in complex environments.

While most medical educators recognise the omnipresence of emotions, little research has been conducted to identify when and how emotions influence learning and practice within clinical settings[69,70]. By understanding how emotions influence learning and performance, medical educators will be better able to develop more accurate pedagogical interventions aimed at various aspects of training. The following are general areas of exploration within medical education that may benefit from incorporating emotion research.

### The development of expertise
According to current models of clinical decision making, clinical reasoning occurs through two modes: System 1, which is fast, automatic, intuitive and energy-efficient, and System 2, which is slow, controlled, deliberative and energy intensive. These two reasoning systems have been thoroughly researched in a variety of different contexts and settings[71]. While the distinction appears analogous to the emotional vs. rational dichotomy, they are far from synonymous distinctions and little has been said about the influence of emotion on these two modes of processing. Some research has suggested that clinical expertise amounts to having many diagnostic strategies available to facilitate problem-solving[72]. While novices tend to rely on analytic reasoning[73], highly experienced individuals are more likely to rely on non-analytic reasoning[74]. Studies of performance differences across novices and experts, however, have not controlled for differences in emotion between groups. It is plausible that novice clinicians are more likely to feel anxious when making diagnoses, especially in an educational setting where their accuracy is being judged. On the other hand, experienced physicians may be less likely to feel anxious given the routine nature of many of their activities (though there is good reason to believe that even they feel

anxious in formal assessment settings). Differences in emotional valence and arousal may magnify any differences in diagnostic accuracy. As such, the influence of emotions in the development of clinical expertise, confidence and professional identity is an important area for future research.

### The self-regulated learner
Medical professionals are required to continuously monitor their current knowledge state to identify potential gaps in clinical and/or professional skills, abilities or knowledge that may impact patient safety. In this way, effective self-regulated learning is critical not only during medical training, but throughout the entirety of one's medical career[75]. Because self-regulated learners need to be aware of how emotions influence their learning process,[76] training physicians to be aware of how their emotions may bias perceptions, interpretations and actions may prove beneficial.

Emotions tend to be heightened for learners during early clinical experiences[70,77]. As McNaughton[74] eloquently states, 'under great pressure to prove themselves worthy of entering the profession, students are afraid to admit that they have uncomfortable feelings about patients or procedures and hide these feelings behind a cloak of competence' (p. 75). Clinical educators must play an active role in developing emotionally cognizant, self-regulated learners by helping them reflect upon their emotions and understand how affective states may influence learning and performance. Faculty members need to facilitate and encourage discussions of the various emotional states faced by trainees. Importantly, these discussions should not be limited to negative emotions, such as anger, grief, shame and sadness, but should also highlight the positive emotions that accompany medical training, such as pride, excitement and compassion. Considerable research has demonstrated the importance of emotions in developing efficacious therapeutic relationships between patients and clinicians[78,79], but little research has examined the potential educational benefits of training medical faculty to be more aware of learners' emotions.

### Educating healthy physicians
To date, most of the literature on emotion in medical education has focused on negative emotions. This focus is justified given that medical students and residents report high levels of stress, depression, intimidation and harassment during training[80]. When asked about emotional experiences during training, the majority of physicians are able to list a variety of negative emotional events. Because of

the high prevalence of stress and burnout among healthcare professionals, it is worthwhile for medical educators to try to foster positive emotional experiences in trainees. For example, research has shown that positive emotions foster psychological resiliency and reduce the detrimental impact of negative emotional experiences and stress on mental and physical well-being[81]. Such findings suggest that positive emotions are a crucial building block for psychological resiliency. To what extent these findings transfer to medical education remains to be seen.

## Summary

The primary goal of this chapter was to introduce medical educators to several theoretical and methodological approaches to emotion research. While there have been substantial strides made in understanding how emotions influence learning and performance in higher education[1], less research has examined how emotions influence medical trainees' acquisition and application of knowledge and skills in clinical settings. To paraphrase Artino and Durning[82], for medical education to advance, it is necessary to broaden what we consider important and begin to explore the role of emotion in learning. Researchers need to examine emotions within medical education settings to understand any number of issues ranging from fundamental learning processes through resilience in medical school to continuing professional development and self-regulated maintenance of competence. Through such research, medical educators can use the link between emotions and learning to determine whether, when and how teachers might modulate emotional environments to optimise learning.

---

### Practice points

Emotions play a major, but often underappreciated, role in learning and knowledge transfer. Before conducting emotion research, it is important to consider the following:

- Define your construct. Are you interested in emotions or moods? Do you want to examine integral or incidental affect?

- Model your construct. Are you conceptualising affective phenomena using a dimensional or discrete approach?

- Weigh your options for measuring and/or manipulating emotions. Do any of the strategies

outlined in the 'Inducing and Measuring Emotions' section of this chapter seem particularly appropriate given the context in which your study is taking place?

These points should be considered in order because the definition and model selected should determine the most appropriate methods to both induce and measure affective states.

---

## References

1 Schutz, P.A. & Pekrun, R. (eds) (2007) *Emotions in Education.* Academic Press, San Diego, CA.

2 Fontaine, J.J.R., Scherer, K.R. & Soriano, C. (eds) (2013) *Components of Emotional Meaning: A Sourcebook.* Oxford University Press, Oxford, UK.

3 Ekkekakis, P. (2013) *The Measurement of Affect, Mood, and Emotion: A Guide for Health-Behavioral Research.* Cambridge University Press, New York.

4 Gray, E.K. & Watson, D. (2007) Assessing positive and negative affect via self-report. In: Coan, J.A. & Allen, J.J.B. (eds), *Handbook of Emotion Elicitation and Assessment.* Oxford University Press, New York, pp. 171–183.

5 Oatley, K., Keltner, D. & Jenkins, J.M. (2006) *Understanding emotions,* 2nd edn. Blackwell, Malden, MA.

6 Scherer, K.R. (2005) What are emotions? And how can they be measured? *Social Science Information*, **44**, 695–729.

7 Fontaine, J.J.R., Scherer, K.R., Roesche, E.B. & Ellsworth, P.C. (2007) The world of emotions is not two-dimensional. *Psychological Science*, **18**, 1050–1057.

8 Russell, J.A. (1980) A circumplex model of affect. *Journal of Personality and Social Psychology*, **39**, 1161.

9 Lövheim, H. (2012) A new three-dimensional model for emotions and monoamine neurotransmitters. *Medical Hypotheses*, **78**, 341–348.

10 Lerner, J.S. & Keltner, D. (2000) Beyond valence: Toward a model of emotion-specific influences on judgment and choice. *Cognition and Emotion*, **14**, 473–493.

11 Lerner, J.S. & Keltner, D. (2001) Fear, anger, and risk. *Journal of Personality and Social Psychology*, **81**, 146–159.

12 Siemer, M., Mauss, I. & Gross, J.J. (2007) Same situation – different emotions: How appraisals shape our emotions. *Emotion*, **7**, 592–600.

13 Lazarus, R.S. (1991) *Emotion and Adaptation.* Oxford University Press, New York.

14 Eysenck, M.W., Derakshan, N., Santos, R. & Calvo, M.G. (2007) Anxiety and cognitive performance: Attentional control theory. *Emotion*, **7**, 336–353.

15 Kreibig, S.D. (2010) Autonomic system activity in emotion: A review. *Biological Psychology*, **84**, 394–421.

16 Banse, R. & Scherer, K.R. (1996) Acoustic profiles in vocal emotion expression. *Journal of Personality and Social Psychology*, **70**, 614–636.

17  Townsend, E. & Campbell, S. (2004) Psychological determinants of willingness to taste and purchase genetically modified food. *Risk Analysis*, **24**, 1385–1393.

18  LeBlanc, V.R. (2009) The effects of acute stress on performance: Implications for health professions education. *Academic Medicine*, **84**, 25–33.

19  Clore, G.L. & Storbeck, J. (2006) Affect as information about liking, efficacy, and importance. In: Forgas, J. (ed), *Affect in Social Thinking and Behavior*. Psychology press, New York, NY, pp. 123–142.

20  LeBlanc, V.R., McConnell, M.M. & Monteiro, S.D. (2015) Predictable chaos: A review of the effects of emotions on attention, memory, and decision making. *Advances in Health Sciences Education Theory Practice*, **20**, 265–282.

21  Ellsworth, P.C. & Scherer, K.R. (2009) Appraisal processes in emotion. In: Davidson, R.J., Scherer, K.R. & Goldsmith, H. (eds), *Handbook of Affective Sciences*. Oxford University Press, Oxford, pp. 572–595.

22  Pekrun, R. (2006) The control-value theory of achievement emotions: Assumptions, corollaries, and implications for educational research and practice. *Educational Psychology Review*, **18**, 315–341.

23  Pekrun, R., Elliot, A.J. & Maier, M.A. (2006) Achievement goals and discrete achievement emotions: A theoretical model and prospective test. *Journal of Educational Psychology*, **98**, 583–597.

24  Artino, A.R., Holmboe, E.S. & Durning, S.J. (2012) Can achievement emotions be used to better understanding motivation, learning, and performance in medical education? *Medical Teacher*, **34**, 240–244.

25  Schunk, D.H., Pintrich, P.R. & Meece, J.L. (2008) *Motivation in education: Theory, research, and applications*, 3rd edn. Upper Saddle River, NJ, Pearson Education Inc.

26  Ellis, H.C. & Ashbrook, P.W. (1988) Resource allocation model of the effect of depressed mood states on memory. In: Fiedler, K. & Forgas, J. (eds), *Affect, Cognition and Social Behavior*. Hogrefe International, Toronto, pp. 25–43.

27  Ashcraft, M.H. & Kirk, E.P. (2001) The relationships among working memory, math anxiety, and performance. *Journal of Experimental Psychology: General*, **130**, 224–237.

28  Shackman, A.J., Sarinopoulos, I., Maxwell, J.S., Pizzagalli, D.A., Lavric, A. & Davidson, R.J. (2006) Anxiety selectively disrupts visuospatial working memory. *Emotion*, **6**, 40–61.

29  Fraser, K., Ma, I., Teteris, E., Baxter, H., Wright, B. & McLaughlin, K. (2012) Emotion, cognitive load and learning outcomes during simulation training. *Medical Education*, **46**, 1055–1062.

30  Linderstrom, J.R. & Bohlin, G. (2011) Emotion processing facilitates working memory performance. *Cognition and Emotion*, **25**, 1196–1204.

31  Lee, T.H., Itti, L. & Mather, M. (2012) Evidence for arousal-biased competition in perceptional learning. *Frontiers in Psychology*, **3**, 1–9.

32  Bolte, A. & Goschke, T. (2010) Thinking and emotion: Affective modulation of cognitive processing modes. In: Glatzeder, B.M., Goel, V. & Müller, A. (eds), *Towards a Theory of Thinking: Building Blocks for a Conceptual Framework*. Springer-Verlag, Berlin, pp. 261–277.

33  Pekrun, R., Frenzel, A.C., Goetz, T. & Perry, R.P. (2007) The control-value theory of achievement emotions: An integrative approach to emotions in education. In: Schutz, P.A. & Pekrun, R. (eds), *Emotion in Education*. Academic Press, Burlington, MA, pp. 13–36.

34  Pekrun, R., Goetz, T., Titz, W. & Perry, R.P. (2002) Academic emotions in self-regulated learning and achievement: A program of quantitative and qualitative research. *Educational Psychologist*, **37**, 91–106.

35  Humphreys, L., Underwood, G. & Chapman, P. (2010) Enhanced memory for emotional pictures: A product of increased attention to affective stimuli? *European Journal of Cognitive Psychology*, **22**, 1235–1247.

36  Otani, H., Libkuman, T.M., Widner, R.L. & Graves, E.I. (2007) Memory for emotionally arousing stimuli: A comparison of younger and older adults. *Journal of General Psychology*, **134**, 23–42.

37  Richard, E.M. & Dienfendorff, J.M. (2011) Self-regulation during a single performance episode: Mood-as-information in the absence of formal feedback. *Organizational Behavior and Human Decision Processes*, **115**, 99–110.

38  Ainley, M., Hidi, S. & Berndorff, D. (2002) Interest, learning, and the psychological processes that mediate their relationship. *Journal of Educational Psychology*, **94**, 545–561.

39  Rotgans, J.I. & Schmidt, H.G. (2011) Situational interest and academic achievement in the active-learning classroom. *Learning and Instruction*, **21**, 58–67.

40  Baños, R.M., Liaño, V., Botella, C., Alcañiz, M., Guerrero, B. & Rey, B. (2006) Changing induced moods via virtual reality. In: Ploug, T., Hasle, P. & Oinas-Kukkonen, H. (eds), *Persuasive Technology*. Springer, Berlin Heidelberg, pp. 7–15.

41  Gross, J.J. & Levenson, R.W. (1995) Emotion elicitation using films. *Cognition and Emotion*, **9**, 87–108.

42  Rottenberg, J., Ray, R.D. & Gross, J.D. (2007) Emotion elicitations using films. In: Coan, J.A. & Allen, J.J.B. (eds), *Handbook of Emotion Elicitation and Assessment*. Oxford University Press, New York, pp. 9–29.

43  Västfjäll, D. (2002) Emotion induction through music. A review of the musical mood induction procedure. *Musicae Scientiae*, **5**, 173–211.

44  Kreutz, G., Ott, U., Teichmann, D., Osawa, P. & Vaitl, D. (2008) Using music to induce emotions: Influences of musical preference and absorption. *Psychology of Music*, **36**, 101–126.

45  Velten, E. (1968) A laboratory task for induction of mood states. *Behaviour Research and Therapy*, **6**, 473–482.

46  Jennings, P.D., McGinnis, D., Lovejoy, S. & Stirling, J. (2000) Valence and arousal ratings for Velten mood induction statements. *Motivation and Emotion*, **24**, 285–297.

47  Westermann, R., Spies, K., Stahl, G. & Hesse, F.W. (1996) Relative effectiveness and validity of mood induction procedures: A meta-analysis. *European Journal of Social Psychology*, **26**, 557–580.

48  Baker, R.C. & Gutterfreund, D.G. (1993) The effects of written autobiographical recollection induction

procedures on mood. *Journal of Clinical Psychology*, **49**, 563–568.

49 Jallais, C. & Gilet, A.L. (2010) Inducing changes in arousal and valence: Comparison of two mood induction procedures. *Behavior Research Methods*, **42**, 318–325.

50 Gasper, K. & Clore, G.L. (2000) Do you have to pay attention to your feelings to be influenced by them? *Personality and Social Psychology Bulletin*, **26**, 698–711.

51 Bonanno, G.A. & Keltner, D. (2004) The coherence of emotion systems: Comparing "online" measures of appraisal and facial expression, and self-report. *Cognition and Emotion*, **18**, 431–444.

52 Mauss, I.B., Wilhelm, F.H. & Gross, J.J. (2004) Is there less to social anxiety than meets the eye? Emotion experience, expression, and bodily responding. *Cognition and Emotion*, **18**, 631–662.

53 Cohn, J.F. & Kanade, T. (2007) Use of automated facial image analysis for measurement of emotion expression. In: Coan, J.A. & Allen, J.B. (eds), *Handbook of Emotion Elicitation and Assessment*. Oxford University Press, Oxford, pp. 222–281.

54 Keltner, D., Ekman, P., Gonzaga, G.C. & Beer, J. (2009) Facial expression of emotion. In: Davidson, R.J., Scherer, K.R. & Goldsmith, H. (eds), *Handbook of Affective Sciences*. Oxford University Press, Oxford, pp. 415–432.

55 Ekman, P., Friesen, W.V. & Hager, J.C. (2002) *Facial Action Coding System*. Salt Lake City, UT, Research Nexus.

56 Scherer, K.R., Johnstone, T. & Klasmeyer, G. (2009) Vocal expression of emotion. In: Davidson, R.J., Scherer, K.R. & Goldsmith, H. (eds), *Handbook of Affective Sciences*. Oxford University Press, Oxford, pp. 433–456.

57 Backorowski, J. & Owren, M.J. (2003) Sounds of emotion: Production and perception of affect-related vocal acoustics. *Annals of the New York Academy of Sciences*, **1000**, 244–265.

58 Feldman, B.L. (2006) Are emotions natural kinds? *Perspectives on Psychological Science*, **1**, 28–58.

59 Levenson, R.W. (2009) Autonomic specificity and emotion. In: Davidson, R.J., Scherer, K.R. & Goldsmith, H. (eds), *Handbook of Affective Sciences*. Oxford University Press, Oxford, pp. 212–224.

60 Stemmler, G. (2009) Methodological considerations in the psychophysiological study of emotion. In: Davidson, R.J., Scherer, K.R. & Goldsmith, H. (eds), *Handbook of Affective Sciences*. Vol. **2009**. Oxford University Press, Oxford, pp. 225–255.

61 Hardy, C.J. & Rejeski, W.J. (1989) Not what but how one feels: The measurement of affect during exercise. *Journal of Sport and Exercise Psychology*, **11**, 304–317.

62 Svebak, S. & Murgatroyd, S. (1985) Meta-motivational dominance: A multi-method validation of reversal theory constructs. *Journal of Personality and Social Psychology*, **48**, 107–116.

63 Jacob, R.G., Simons, A.D., Manuck, S.B., Rohay, J.M., Waldstein, S. & Gatsonis, C. (1989) The circular mood scale: A new technique of measuring ambulatory mood. *Journal of Psychopathology and Behavioural Assessment*, **11**, 153–173.

64 Watson, D., Clark, L.A. & Tellegen, A. (1988) Development and validation of brief measures of positive and negative affect: The PANAS scales. *Journal of Personality and Social Psychology*, **54**, 1063–1070.

65 Thayer, R.E. (1989) *The biopsychology of mood and arousal*. Oxford University Press, New York.

66 Gregg, V.H. & Shepherd, A.J. (2009) Factor structure of scores on the state version of the Four Dimension Mood Scale. *Educational and Psychological Measurement*, **69**, 146–156.

67 McNair, D.M., Lorr, M. & Droppleman, L.F. (1971) *Profile of Mood States (POMS) Manual*. San Diego, CA, Educational and Industrial Testing Service.

68 Pekrun, R., Goetz, T., Frenzel, A.C., Barchfeld, P. & Perry, R.P. (2011) Measuring emotions in students' learning and performance: The achievement emotions questionnaire (AEQ). *Contemporary Educational Psychology*, **36**, 36–48.

69 Artino, A.R. (2013) When I say … .emotion in medical education. *Medical Education*, **47**, 1062–1063.

70 McNaughton, N. (2013) Discourse(s) of emotion within medical education: the ever-present absence. *Medical Education*, **47**, 71–79.

71 Evans, J.S.B. (2008) Dual-processing accounts of reasoning, judgment, and social cognition. *Annual Review of Psychology*, **59**, 255–278.

72 Eva, K.W. (2005) What every teacher needs to know about clinical reasoning. *Medical Education*, **39**, 98–106.

73 Ark, T.K., Brooks, L.R. & Eva, K.W. (2006) Giving learners the best of both worlds: Do clinical teachers need to guard against teaching pattern recognition to novices? *Academic Medicine*, **81**, 405–409.

74 Eva, K.W. (2002) The aging physician: Changes in cognitive processing and their impact on medical practice. *Academic Medicine*, **77**, S1–S6.

75 Borrell-Carrió, F. & Epstein, R. (2004) Preventing errors in clinical practice: A call for self-awareness. *Annals of Family Medicine*, **2**, 310–316.

76 Boekaerts, M., Pintrich, P.R. & Zeidner, M. (2000) *Handbook of self-regulation*. Academic Press, San Diego, CA.

77 Ofri, D. (2013) *What doctors feel: How emotions affect the practice of medicine*. Beacon Press, Boston.

78 Marcum, J.A. (2013) The role of emotions in clinical reasoning and decision making. *Journal of Medicine and Philosophy*, **38**, 501–519.

79 Weng, H.C., Chen, H.C., Lu, K. & Hung, S.Y. (2008) Doctors' emotional intelligence and the patient-doctor relationship. *Medical Education*, **42**, 703–711.

80 Dhalin, M., Joneborg, N. & Runeson, B. (2005) Stress and depression among medical students: A cross-sectional study. *Medical Education*, **39**, 594–604.

81 Ong, A.D., Bergeman, C.S., Bisconti, T.L. & Wallance, K.A. (2006) Psychological resilience, positive emotions, and successful adaptation to stress in later life. *Personality Processes and Individual Differences*, **91**, 730–749.

82 Artino, A.R. & Durning, S.J. (2011) It's time to explore the role of emotion in medical students' learning. *Academic Medicine*, **86**, 275.

# 17 Research on instructional design in the health sciences: from taxonomies of learning to whole-task models

*Jeroen J. G. van Merrienboer and Diana H. J. M. Dolmans*

*Inez Delores became the educational director of an undergraduate programme in the health sciences about one year ago. Now, she is confronted for the first time with the results of the regular annual programme evaluation. Students seem to be quite satisfied with the quality of their teachers and courses. That is good news. Yet, what worries her is the common complaint of students that they experience the whole programme as a rather disconnected set of topics and courses, with implicit relationships between them and unclear relevance to their future profession. Moreover, both graduated students and workplace supervisors report difficulties with applying the acquired knowledge and skills at the workplace. Inez wonders if action needs to be taken, and if so, what she could do about the situation.*

## Introduction

This situation is representative for the kinds of problems that are studied in the field of instructional design. This field of study aims to develop evidence-informed guidelines and models for the design of instruction, ranging from the design of particular instructional materials, via lessons and courses, to complete curricula. It covers the entire continuum of education; thus, in healthcare profession education, it includes undergraduate and graduate programmes as well as continuous medical education. The guidelines and models developed in the field of instructional design help educators in the health sciences to make instruction more effective, efficient and attractive. Effectiveness relates not only to learning outcomes but also to translational outcomes such as safer patient care and better patient outcomes. Efficiency relates to optimising the balance between outcomes and investments in terms of time, effort and money. And attractiveness relates to increasing students' motivation to learn.

For example, the above-mentioned complaint of the students that they experienced their programme as a disconnected set of topics and courses prompted the initial interest in 'integrative goals'[1]. Such goals are frequently encountered when instruction must reach beyond a single lesson or course; for example, when professional competencies or complex skills are taught. This shift towards integrative goals had important consequences for research on instructional design: 'Whole tasks' rather than distinct learning goals became the basis for the design and development of educational programmes.

The main aim of this chapter is to discuss research themes that are pertinent to the field of instructional design. First, a brief description will be provided about the ADDIE model that characterises the main phases in instructional design: Analysis, Design, Development, Implementation and Evaluation. Second, for the analysis phase, how research is moving away from taxonomies of learning towards cognitive task analysis will be described. Third, for the design and development phases, the main research themes for the specification of 'whole' learning tasks and the use of media are described. Fourth, for the implementation and evaluation phases, research on how whole-task models affect the preparation of stakeholders and the quality culture in educational organisations is described. The chapter ends with a summary of the main conclusions and future research directions.

## The ADDIE model

Figure 17.1 presents the five phases in the ADDIE model[2]: (a) the analysis of fixed conditions and desired learning outcomes, (b) the design of instructional strategies, (c) the development of instructional materials, (d) the implementation of the developed instruction in the educational

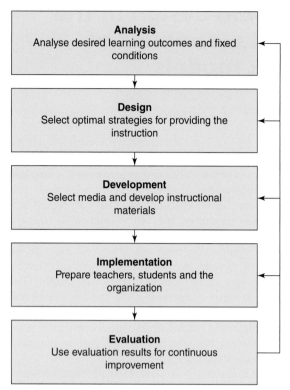

*Figure 17.1* The ADDIE model.

organisation and (e) its evaluation aimed at continuous improvement. Though the model appears to be linear with predefined phases or steps that must always be taken in the same order, it does not have to be followed rigidly. The model may be repeatedly used to develop related units of instruction, phases may be skipped because particular information is already available, or later phases may provide inputs that make it necessary to reconsider earlier phases. It is thus best seen as a project management tool that helps instructional designers to think about the different activities that must be conducted.

In the analysis phase of the ADDIE model, the focus is on the analysis of fixed conditions and desired learning outcomes. With regard to fixed conditions, analyses pertain to the analysis of the *context* (availability of equipment, time and money, culture, setting such as school or work organisation;[3]), the analysis of the *target group* (prior knowledge, general schooling, age, learning styles, handicaps;[4]) and the analysis of *tasks* and *subject matter* (tools and objects required, conditions for performance, risks). Traditionally, desired learning outcomes are expressed as learning goals, but as indicated above, they increasingly take the form of 'integrative goals' such as complex skills or professional competencies

(e.g. the CanMeds competencies;[5]). For example, Inez Delores from our example cited above might decide to describe the final attainment levels that must be reached by her students, no longer as lists of learning goals but in terms of professional competencies, because these might provide a better basis for integrating the curriculum and preparing the students for the workplace.

In the design phase, instructional strategies are selected that best help to reach the desired outcomes, given the fixed conditions. The basic idea is that both desired outcomes and fixed conditions determine the optimal instructional strategies to select. For example, if the desired outcome is memorising the names of the bones in the hand, rehearsal with the use of mnemonics is a suitable strategy, but if the desired outcome is reattaching a finger following a traumatic injury, guided practice with feedback on a wide variety of scenarios is a more suitable strategy. Furthermore, the use of high-fidelity simulation, that is, simulation that mimics the real working environment to a very high degree, might be a suitable strategy for teaching a complex surgical skill if there is sufficient equipment or money available, but if there is no equipment or money available, guided on-the-job learning might be more suitable. Inez Delores might, for instance, come to the conclusion that the current curriculum does not provide enough practice opportunities for the development of professional competencies, and decide to make more use of simulation-based learning in the future curriculum.

In the development phase, the focus is on the selection of suitable media and the actual construction of instructional materials. For example, when it is impossible to organise face-to-face meetings because target learners live in different countries and/or different time zones, online forms of education may be used. Or when practising particular skills at the workplace is out of the question due to safety issues, simulation-based training may be offered. Furthermore, specific design guidelines exist for different media, such as instructional texts[6], slides for lectures[7], multimedia materials such as animations and dynamic representations[8], e-learning applications[9], simulations and serious games[10] and so forth. In our example, Inez Delores may decide to develop role plays with simulated patients and clinical scenarios for simulation-based practice and ask the teachers in her programme to construct these learning tasks and include them in their courses.

In the implementation phase, the focus is on the introduction of the newly developed instruction in the setting in which it will be used and on supporting the actual use of the instructional materials. First, it pertains to strategies for preparing teachers and staff, ranging from short teacher-training programmes for teaching a newly developed course to complete faculty development programmes preparing them for a change from a traditional discipline-based curriculum to, for example, a whole-task curriculum. Second, it pertains to strategies for preparing students. Third, for larger design projects, it may pertain to preparing or changing the educational organisation in such a way that it best sustains the newly developed instruction. Inez Delores may, for instance, quickly find out that it is necessary to start renovations of the building in order to create spaces where students can meet simulated patients and work on simulation-based scenarios. Furthermore, she might decide to offer a training programme on simulation-based teaching to her staff and form multidisciplinary teams that would be responsible for organising the role plays and running the scenarios.

Finally, in the evaluation phase, a process of quality management is needed to continuously evaluate and improve the instruction. Here, it is critical that not only student satisfaction but also whether applied instructional strategies are apt to reach the desired outcomes given the fixed conditions (context, target group, etc.) are taken into account. In order to evaluate whether the goals of the instruction have been met, all relevant stakeholders (students, teachers, management, future employers, etc.) need to be involved. A good system of evaluation is continuous, improvement-oriented and must be embedded in a well-developed quality culture. For this reason, Inez Delores might decide to get rid of the existing evaluation system, which only gathers data on student satisfaction at the level of courses and teachers, and introduce a new evaluation system that also gathers data on student progress throughout the curriculum and on how well they are doing at their workplaces after graduation.

Instructional design is both a practical field and a research field. The ADDIE model is typically used to organise the methods, strategies and guidelines that help practitioners in the field of education, such as Inez Delores, to design instruction in its broadest sense, that is, including the analysis of desired outcomes on the one hand and the evaluation whether these goals have been met on the other hand. Yet, empirical research is needed to develop evidence-based methods, strategies and guidelines and to organise these in the instructional design models. The remainder of this chapter will focus on research themes that are pertinent to each of the five phases of the ADDIE model.

## The Analysis phase

In the context of the ADDIE model, the analysis phase refers to the analysis of fixed conditions that cannot be altered by the designer (context, target group, tasks and subject matter to be taught) and the analysis of final attainment levels, that is, the specification of what learners will be able to do after they have finished the educational programme. In this chapter, we focus on two approaches for the specification of final attainment levels: the traditional use of taxonomies of learning for setting learning goals and the use of cognitive task analysis for developing *integrative* learning goals.

### Taxonomies of learning

Traditional models for task and content analysis describe final attainment levels in terms of learning goals. Typically, tasks and contents that must be mastered by the learners after the instruction are first categorised as belonging to a particular domain of learning, such as the cognitive domain, psychomotor domain or affective domain[11], roughly corresponding with the triple knowledge, skills and attitudes. For each of these domains, the desired outcomes are then further analysed in terms of distinct learning goals. For example, in the cognitive domain, Bloom's taxonomy makes a further distinction between (a) knowledge, (b) comprehension, (c) application, (d) analysis, (e) synthesis and (f) evaluation (for an updated version of Bloom's original taxonomy, see[12]).

Gagné[13] introduced another widely used taxonomy in the cognitive domain. His taxonomy makes a distinction between verbal information, intellectual skills, cognitive strategies, attitudes and psychomotor skills. The intellectual skills are at the heart of the taxonomy and include five further subcategories: (a) discriminations, (b) concrete concepts, (c) defined concepts, (d) rules and (e) higher-order rules. This taxonomy reflects the fact that some intellectual skills enable the performance of other, higher-level skills. When you teach an intellectual skill, it is important to identify, in the so-called learning hierarchy, the lower-level skills that enable this higher-level skill. In teaching, one will often start with the skills lower in the hierarchy and successively work towards the skills higher in the hierarchy. For example, when you are teaching how to reattach a finger following a traumatic injury, you might first teach the names of all the relevant bones in the hand and the instruments needed (i.e. concrete concepts) as well as particular complications that may occur (i.e. defined concepts). Then, you might teach the standard procedure for conducting the operation (i.e. rules). And finally, you might teach the decision-making and problem-solving processes needed for dealing with the complications (i.e. higher-order rules).

In addition to those of Bloom and Gagné, there are several other taxonomies of learning goals. With regard to the design of instruction, they all provide the input for condition-based instructional design models[14]. These models are based on the idea of the 'conditions of learning'[13], meaning that there are different instructional methods necessary for reaching different goals. For example, the instructional method for teaching the understanding of one or more principles (e.g. comprehending how the heart–lung system works) is different from the instructional method for teaching the use of a procedure (e.g. conducting a hip replacement). Consequently, when designing instruction, the optimal method is chosen for each goal depending on its classification in the taxonomy, the goals are taught according to their preferred method one-by-one and the overall educational goal is believed to be met after all separate goals have been taught.

This condition-based approach works very well when there are few relationships between the goals. For example, in the field of nursing, the goals of providing stoma care to patients and the goal of scheduling patient admissions/discharges can be taught apart from each other because no integration of these goals is required. However, it may not work well when learning goals are integrated with each other. For example, when a nurse is delivering stoma care to patients, certain goals are involved that relate to correctly using the necessary instruments, dealing with complications, properly communicating with patients and so forth[15]. All related skills must be performed simultaneously and need to be coordinated in order to provide good stoma care. An analysis leading to a list of separate learning goals that are then taught one-by-one is not very helpful in this case: It yields instruction that is experienced by students as fragmented and piecemeal because it does not take the relationships between the goals and their coordination into account. In short, the whole complex skill of providing stoma care is greater than can be expressed in a list of goals because it also includes coordination of the skills related to these goals. For this reason, in the early 1990s, authors in the field of instructional design started to question the value of taxonomies of learning and condition-based models for the teaching of complex skills or professional competencies where 'integrative' goals are at stake (e.g.[1,16]). Amongst other analysis methods, Cognitive Task Analysis (CTA) was put forward as an alternative for using taxonomies of learning, and whole-task instructional design models were put forward as an alternative for condition-based models.

## Cognitive task analysis

Almost 100 different approaches to task analysis have been described in the literature (see[17]). A classification of the different approaches can be made, based on two characteristics of the tasks to be analysed: (a) whether the steps for performing the task show a temporal order or not and (b) whether the steps are observable or not[18]. When the steps necessary for task performance show a fixed temporal order (e.g. performing cardiopulmonary resuscitation), forms of *procedural analysis* are used; when they do not show such a temporal order (e.g. touch typing while using a medical prescribing system), forms of *rule-based analysis* are used. Furthermore, when only observable or overt steps are relevant (e.g. operating a scalpel), forms of *behavioural analysis* are used; when non-observable or covert, mental steps are also relevant (e.g. diagnostic reasoning), forms of *information processing analysis* are used. Forms of analysis that are able to deal with non-temporal steps are also often able to deal with temporal steps, and forms of analysis that are able to deal with covert steps are also often able to deal with overt steps. Thus, some powerful types of CTA can deal with all types, or all different aspects, of complex task performance.

Clark et al.[19] describe such a powerful form of CTA. It distinguishes three phases: (a) decomposition of the complex skill or the competency underlying expert task performance into its different aspects or constituent skills, (b) analysis of the non-routine aspects of the complex skill and (c) analysis of the routine aspects of the complex skill (see Table 17.1). In the first phase, the complex skill that underlies successful task performance is broken down into its constituent skills in a reiterative process and the inter-relationships between constituent skills are identified in a so-called skills hierarchy, where the skills lower in the hierarchy enable the skills higher in the hierarchy (cf. Gagne's learning hierarchy). The distinct constituent skills are classified as 'non-recurrent' when the desired exit performance varies from problem to problem situation and is guided by the use of cognitive strategies and mental models (i.e. non-routine aspects). They are classified as 'recurrent' when the desired exit performance is highly similar from problem to problem situation and is guided by rules or procedures (i.e. routine aspects).

*Table 17.1* Cognitive task analysis

|  | Object of analysis |  | Main question(s) | Analysis results |
|---|---|---|---|---|
| *Phase 1* Skill Decomposition | Constituent skills and their inter-relationships underlying whole-task performance | | –Which constituent skills make up the complex skill? –Which constituent skills enable skills higher in the hierarchy? –What is the temporal relation between constituent skills? | Skills hierarchy |
| *Phase 2* Analysing non-routine aspects of exit performance | Non-recurrent constituent skills | Cognitive strategies | –How do experts systematically approach tasks in the domain? –Which rules-of-thumb might help to complete the task? | Systematic Approaches to Problem Solving (SAP) |
|  |  | Mental models | How is the task domain organised? | Domain models: –conceptual –structural –causal |
| *Phase 3* Analysing routine aspects of exit performance | Recurrent constituent skills | Cognitive rules or procedures | Under which conditions are particular actions performed (IF … THEN …) | Just-in-time information displays |
|  |  | Prerequisite knowledge | What does the task performer need to know in order to apply the rule(s) or perform the procedure correctly? |  |

Documentation analysis, observation and semi-structured interviews with expert task performers provide the information for iteratively building a skills hierarchy, which inter-relates the constituent skills to each other. Figure 17.2 provides a small part of a skills hierarchy that was constructed for performing a nephrostomy (for the full analysis, see[20]). In this hierarchy, recurrent constituent skills can be found in the dark grey boxes. Usually, recurrent constituent skills are at the bottom of the hierarchy because they involve routine behaviours that are basic to many skills higher in the hierarchy; in Figure 17.2, they relate to stabilising the ultrasound (US) probe while introducing the needle and operating the controls of the US machine. The skills hierarchy guides further knowledge elicitation efforts in phases 2 and 3.

In the second phase, non-recurrent aspects of the complex skill are further analysed. Cognitive strategies (how to effectively approach tasks in the domain) can be analysed as Systematic Approaches to Problem-solving or SAPs. They describe a systematic approach to performing particular aspects of the task in terms of subsequent problem-solving phases and rules-of-thumb that may help to successfully complete each phase. For example, a SAP may

be developed for introducing the needle, describing the phases to go through and the rules-of-thumb ('tricks of the trade') that may help to deal with complications and successfully complete each phase. In turn, mental models (how is the domain organised?) can be analysed as domain models. They describe the knowledge necessary for successful task performance as conceptual models (how are things named in the domain? e.g. the names of different parts of the renal system such as the cortex, medulla, calyx, pelvis, etc.), structural models (how are things organised in the domain? e.g. the structure of the kidney) and causal models (how do things work in the domain? e.g. the working of the renal system). Knowledge elicitation methods commonly used with expert task performers to capture data for non-recurrent aspects of a complex skill include think-aloud protocols (for the development of SAPs) and document study and interviews (for the development of domain models).

In the third phase, recurrent aspects of the complex skill are further analysed. Here, analysts first employ techniques to identify the rules and/or procedures that generate highly specific, algorithmic descriptions of routine aspects of task performance. In contrast to SAPs, rules and procedures are

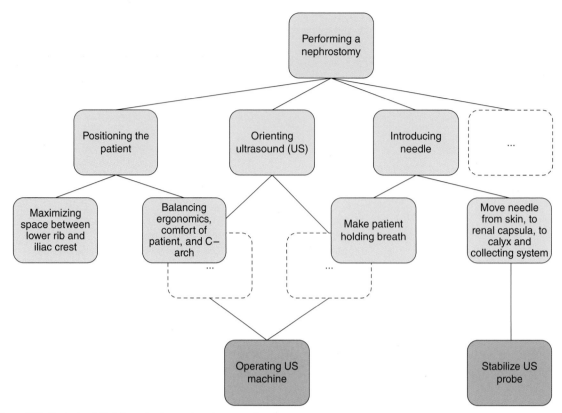

*Figure 17.2* Part of a skills hierarchy for performing a nephrostomy.

algorithmic rather than heuristic: they not only help to effectively perform the task but also, unlike SAPs, *guarantee* success. For example, the analyst may develop rules and procedures for correctly operating the US machine, describing which knobs to turn and which displays to study in order to reach specific objectives. Next, the prerequisite knowledge required to correctly apply the rules or perform the procedures is identified. For example, when a particular rule specifies 'IF you need to switch on the machine, THEN push the power button', prerequisite knowledge might relate to the exact position and appearance of the power button. The analysis results are often expressed in just-in-time information displays with 'how-to instructions' for performing routine aspects of tasks, such as a quick reference guide that is next to the US machine. This type of analysis has much in common with computer programming because it yields algorithmic descriptions of how to perform routine aspects of tasks.

The results of the three phases provide highly detailed information about the constituent skills, cognitive strategies, mental models, rules/ procedures and prerequisite knowledge required for successfully performing the complex task.

Knowledge and skills are fully integrated in the representation of the complex skill and, if necessary, desirable attitudes can be related to the distinct constituent skills. This makes it clear, for example, that for the complex skill of nephrostomy, it is important to be attentive to patient modesty and comfort while positioning the patient (one particular constituent skill), but not when operating the US machine (another constituent skill for which this particular attitude is not important).

Several studies in the health sciences domain have shown that educational programmes based on CTA are particularly effective (for an overview, see[21]). One example is provided by[22]; see also[21]). In a controlled experiment, they studied the expertise of emergency medicine specialists. Participants in the control group were taught an emergency procedure in a traditional modelling and practice strategy by expert emergency physicians and participants in the CTA group were trained with information gathered from a CTA conducted with the same emergency medicine experts who taught the control group. In the following year, the CTA group outperformed the control group on all diagnostic and many performance items by over 50%. Furthermore, the traditionally trained doctors caused four serious medical emergencies in applying the medical protocol to patients, while those from the CTA group made no life-threatening mistakes. Thus, CTA seems to provide a strong basis for the design of educational programmes. The next section discusses the design and development of such programmes.

## The design and development phases

As discussed in the previous section, a distinction can be made between design models that start designing instruction from learning goals (i.e. 'condition-based models'), and design models that start designing instruction from whole, real-life tasks, whose performance can be analysed in a process of CTA. The remainder of this chapter will discuss only whole-task models[23], because in the health sciences, many instructional design projects will deal with the development of professional competencies or complex skills. In whole-task models, all learning tasks provided to students are meaningful, authentic and representative for the tasks that a professional might encounter in the real world. Yet, learning tasks are often not identical to real-life professional tasks because they may contain support and guidance and are carefully designed to optimally support the learning process. The next three subsections discuss relevant research themes pertaining to the design and development phases of the ADDIE model. First, we discuss research on learning tasks. Second, we discuss four-component instructional design as one popular example of a whole-task model. Third, we focus on the development phase, that is, the selection of media and the actual construction of instructional materials.

### Learning tasks

With regard to the design of learning tasks, relevant research themes concern the authenticity of tasks, variation between tasks, different types of tasks, sequencing of tasks and scaffolding of task support and guidance (see Table 17.2). Although the basic idea of whole-task models is that people learn to perform real-life professional tasks by practising on learning tasks that are based on these real-life tasks, the learning tasks need *not* be identical to the real-life tasks. With regard to authenticity of simulation-based learning environments, for example, a distinction can be made between psychological fidelity (the learning environment replicates the psychological factors experienced in the real environment), functional fidelity (the learning environment behaves in the same way as the

*Table 17.2* Research on learning tasks: five themes

| Topic | Example research questions[1] |
| --- | --- |
| Authenticity of tasks | How similar should learning tasks be to real-life tasks? |
| Variation between tasks | How can variation across tasks be best designed to facilitate transfer? |
| Types of tasks | How do different types of learning tasks differentially affect learning? |
| Sequencing of tasks | How can learning tasks be best sequenced to facilitate learning and transfer? |
| Scaffolding of tasks | Which types of scaffolding are most effective to support learning? |

[1]Note that according to the instructional design approach, the answers to these questions will typically be dependent on the characteristics of the target learners, the context and the tasks or subject matter taught.

real environment) and physical fidelity (the learning environment looks, sounds, feels and smells like the real environment). Research indicates that the psychological fidelity should be high for all learners, but a high physical fidelity is especially important for high-expertise learners and can even be detrimental for novice learners[24].

A second theme relates to variation between tasks. Each real-life task is unique: not one patient is identical to another patient, and not one intervention is identical to another intervention. In order to reach transfer, that is, the ability to perform an acquired complex skill in new, unfamiliar situations (e.g. in the workplace rather than in the training setting), it is thus critical that learning tasks differ from each other in all dimensions on which real-life tasks also differ from each other. For example, when practising nephrostomy, it is important that learning tasks use different patients or models (obese or not, septic or not, etc.), different renal problems (kidney stones, scoliosis, cystic kidneys, horseshoe kidneys, etc.), different complications and so forth. This principle is sometimes called 'variability of practice' and there is very strong evidence that preparation for transfer to unknown situations requires variation (see[25]). Although variation is necessary for transfer to occur, it is still an open question how variation across tasks can best be designed to optimise learning and transfer, especially because some types of variation have negative effects on performance during learning but positive effects on transfer (the 'transfer paradox';[26]).

A third research theme concerns the use of different types of learning tasks. Here, the main question is under which conditions particular tasks can be best used. In addition to conventional tasks or problems, where the learner must come up with a solution, learning tasks include modelling examples, case studies, tasks with specific goals, reverse tasks, completion tasks and others (for an overview, see[27]). For learning tasks in nephrostomy, for example, a conventional task would require learners to perform the whole task (with or without guidance from an expert); a modelling example would require learners to closely observe an expert who is performing the task and explaining what s/he is doing and why s/he is doing it, and a completion task would require learners to observe an expert who is performing (difficult) parts of the task but also perform (easier) parts of the task themselves. Research has shown that conventional tasks are not always the best type of task to support learning. One particularly important example can be found in the 'expertise reversal effect', showing that novice learners learn more from studying modelling examples or case studies than from performing the equivalent tasks, while the opposite is true for more experienced learners[28].

A fourth research theme concerns the sequencing of learning tasks. In traditional educational programmes, part-whole sequencing techniques are dominant. In such an approach, learning tasks are organised in such a way that students first practise parts of the whole task and practise only the whole, real-life task at the end of the educational programme. There is, however, accumulating evidence that this approach only works well when there is little coordination between the parts required; for tasks that require much coordination between parts, a whole-task sequencing approach is more effective (for a meta-analysis, see[29]). One may then sequence from simple to increasingly more complex versions of the whole task, an approach that is in line with the concept of the 'spiral curriculum'[30]. For example, when practising nephrostomy, one may work from relatively simple whole tasks (e.g. fixed kidney, small distance between skin and kidney, no scar tissue) to increasingly more complex versions of the whole task (e.g. mobile kidney, large distance between skin and kidney, scar tissue).

A fifth and final research theme concerns scaffolding, that is, the provision of support and guidance to learners who are working on learning tasks – in combination with *fading* this support and guidance as learners acquire more expertise. Thus, the basic idea is that learners who are working on tasks at a particular level of complexity should first receive a sizeable amount of support and guidance but receive increasingly less support and guidance for later tasks at the same level of complexity. Only when they are able to perform the learning tasks at a particular level of complexity independently,

without any support or guidance, they continue to learning tasks at a higher level of complexity. Research has identified many different ways for scaffolding learners, including the use of modelling examples, process worksheets and performance constraints (for an overview, see[27]). Tutor guidance, however, provides the most flexible approach to scaffolding. For example, when learners practise nephrostomy, guidance can be given by a supervisor who closely monitors their task performance and takes appropriate actions when necessary. In case of impasses, the supervisor can point out where the learner should look, take over the task and/or provide useful rules of thumb (cf. modelling examples), lead learners into the next phase (cf. process worksheets) or stop them to ensure that they successfully complete one phase before entering the next (cf. performance constraints).

## Four-component instructional design (4C/ID)

All whole-task models in education emphasise the importance of real-life tasks as the basis for the design of learning tasks and, thus, for fruitful learning. Some models limit themselves to one particular type of learning task, for example, 'problems' in problem-based learning (PBL), 'projects' in project-based learning and 'cases' in the Harvard case method. Other whole-task models that are more strongly rooted in an instructional design tradition prescribe or allow for the use of different types of learning tasks in the same educational programme. Examples are Merrill's first principles of instruction[31]; cognitive apprenticeship learning[32] and van Merrienboer's four-component instructional design model (4C/ID)[18].

4C/ID is a popular whole-task model, claiming that educational programmes that support the acquisition of complex skills or professional competencies can always be constructed from four components:

1 *Learning tasks.* Meaningful whole-task experiences that are based on real-life tasks; they form the 'backbone' of the educational programme.
2 *Supportive information.* Information that is supportive to the learning and performance of non-recurrent aspects of learning tasks (i.e. problem solving, decision making, reasoning).
3 *Procedural information.* Information that is prerequisite to the learning and performance of recurrent aspects of learning tasks (i.e. routine behaviours).
4 *Part-task practice.* Additional exercises for recurrent aspects of learning tasks for which a very

high level of automaticity is required after the instruction.

Vandewaetere et al.[33] describe the development of a large-scale educational programme in general medicine on the basis of 4C/ID. In one of the developed courses, 'Patients with diabetes', learners work on learning tasks both in a simulated task environment (either online or in face-to-face meetings) and in the real task environment, that is, in the doctors' practice. The tasks show a high variability of practice and may be of different types (e.g. from systematically observing an expert performing the task to performing the task yourself). Furthermore, the learning tasks are ordered from a low level of complexity to increasingly higher levels of complexity (i.e. a spiral approach): Higher levels of complexity make an appeal on additional CanMeds roles, such as acting as a collaborator and communicator (e.g. not only diagnosis and treatment of diabetes but also management of patients with diabetes). At each level of complexity, scaffolding ensures that learners receive ample support and guidance in the beginning but less support and guidance as their expertise increases; guidance is given by both the teacher and the peer learners.

Supportive information helps students learn to perform non-recurrent aspects of learning tasks, which involve problem solving, diagnostic reasoning or decision making. For our example, in order to successfully diagnose patients with diabetes, supportive information includes a systematic approach and rules-of-thumb for diagnosing patients with diabetes (i.e. a SAP, which may be based on the analysis of cognitive strategies as part of CTA; see Phase 2 in Table 17.1). It also includes information on different forms of diabetes (i.e. domain models, which may be based on the analysis of mental models as part of CTA; see again Phase 2 in Table 17.1), which may help learners to reason about alternative diagnoses and to make decisions. Supportive information is specified again for each higher level of task complexity because learners need to know *more* about diabetes and how to diagnose and treat it for performing tasks at a higher level of complexity. The supportive information thus provides a bridge between what learners already know about diabetes and what they need to know about it in order to work on the learning tasks. In the field of instructional design, relevant research concerns presentation strategies (e.g. guided discovery, self-explanation and group discussion) that help learners connect new supportive information to what they already know.

Procedural information allows students learn to perform recurrent aspects of learning tasks that are always performed in the same way. For our example, procedural information may include just-in-time information displays that specify how to use the Electronic Health Record (EHR) to propose an adjusted management plan for a patient with diabetes (i.e. how-to instructions, which may be based on the analysis of rules/procedures, and prerequisite knowledge as part of CTA; see Phase 3 in Table 17.1). This can be done by online help, a quick reference guide or a job aid. But for learning tasks that are performed in the doctors' practice, procedural information may also be provided by a supervisor who is 'looking over the learner's shoulder' or by a mobile application. Procedural information is quickly faded as learners gain more expertise. In the field of instructional design, relevant research concerns just-in-time presentation strategies that help learners construct cognitive rules. One example can be found in 'augmented reality', where augmented-reality glasses can be used to project how-to instructions in the learner's visual field precisely when he or she is looking at the scene in which the actions must be performed.

Finally, part-task practice pertains to additional practice of recurrent aspects so that learners can develop routines with a very high level of automaticity for selected task aspects. One of the courses developed on the basis of 4C/ID in general medicine is 'The child with fever'. In this course, part-task practice is used for 'spot diagnoses', where learners practice the quick diagnosis of childhood infectious diseases with prototypical cases. Furthermore, it is often used for constituent skills that play a role in many different whole tasks (e.g. cardiopulmonary resuscitation, auscultation, stitching, liver palpation, venipuncture) and for critical tasks in, for example, emergency medicine. Part-task practice typically provides huge amounts of repetition and only starts after the recurrent aspect has been introduced in the context of whole, meaningful learning tasks. In the field of instructional design, relevant research concerns practice strategies (e.g. overlearning, distributed practice, time compression) aimed at full automation of the recurrent constituent skill.

## Instructional media

In the development phase of the ADDIE model, research typically concerns the use of particular media in relation to learning processes. Some media are better to support, enable or sustain particular learning processes than others. Table 17.3 provides an overview of both traditional and ICT-based media for each of the four components of the 4C/ID model. Suitable media for learning tasks must allow learners to work on those learning tasks and will

*Table 17.3* Some examples of traditional and ICT-based media

|  | Traditional media | ICT-based media |
| --- | --- | --- |
| Learning tasks | Real-task environments, project groups, role play | Computer-simulated task environments, high-fidelity simulation, serious games, virtual reality |
| Supportive information | Textbooks, encyclopaedia, lectures, realia | Video, multimedia, hypermedia (Internet), microworlds, social media |
| Procedural information | Instructor, job aids, quick reference guides, manuals | Mobile technologies, augmented reality, online help systems, pedagogical agents |
| Part-task practice | Skills laboratory, practicals, paper and pencil | Part-task trainers, drill-and-practice computer-based training, computer games for basic skills training |

usually take the form of either a real or simulated task environment. Suitable media for supportive information must allow learners to study and discuss models of a domain and how to approach tasks in that domain. Suitable media for procedural information must allow learners to consult how-to instructions precisely when they need them during task performance. And suitable media for part-task practice must allow learners to repetitively practice selected recurrent task aspects. As can be seen from Table 17.1, educational programmes developed according to a whole-task approach such as 4C/ID will typically make use of a rich mix of different media.

Finally, all instructional materials need to be actually constructed using the selected media. It falls beyond the scope of this chapter to discuss 'instructional message design' and related research. But, highly specific research is done to develop guidelines for the construction of textbooks, manuals, simulators, serious games, multimedia and so forth. For example, van Merriënboer and Kester[34] describe research on 22 principles for the construction of educational multimedia including, for example, the coherence principle (do not include irrelevant seductive details such as music in the presentation), self-pacing principle (let the learner set the pace of the presentation) and segmentation principle (divide longer presentations in meaningful segments).

## The implementation and evaluation phases

The eventual success of instruction depends on how well it is implemented in the educational organisation and whether evaluation results are used for continuous improvement or not. Implementing instruction based on whole-task models is far from easy and will probably fail when teachers, students and the organisation are not well prepared for it[35]. After a whole-task curriculum has been implemented, it should continuously be improved. In order to reach this, it is important to evaluate both the quality of the courses offered within the curriculum and the curriculum as a whole (e.g. connections between courses). But how to evaluate the quality of courses and the curriculum? And, above all, how to ensure that these evaluations result in continuous improvement?

## Preparing staff, students and the organisation

At the staff level, it is important to involve professionals working in the field to design different learning tasks and to train them on how to design a variety of learning tasks, as described above. Staff members furthermore need training to prepare them to fulfil new and different teaching roles. Within whole-task curricula, teachers need to give support and guidance to students and are often involved in small group teaching or coaching of students within a simulated learning environment or at the workplace. Teachers need to be prepared to fulfil these roles by means of a faculty development programme. In these programmes, teachers are encouraged to apply and experience what they have learned, receive feedback, have discussions and build relationships with other teachers and faculty. These programmes are known to enhance positive changes in attitudes towards teaching, lead to increased knowledge about education and skills and above all lead to more involvement in education[36]. These programmes preferably extend over time[37]. Second, it is crucial that staff members collaborate with each other in multidisciplinary teams because whole learning tasks that are based on real-life tasks rarely make an appeal on only one discipline – almost by definition, these tasks are multidisciplinary. Within a whole task curriculum, teachers should thus collaborate with professionals from multiple disciplines when designing professionally relevant learning tasks; good collaborative teaching must reflect the workplace.

Students also need to be prepared. First, students should be well informed about why they are confronted with a variety of whole tasks that are based on professional tasks, and why they should apply what they have learned to a variety of tasks. But it is of course not only a matter of informing students and training students on how to study and prepare themselves for a group meeting, but a simulation training or activities at the workplace are even more important, since students are also often not familiar with their new roles. Second, it is important to involve students in the design and evaluation of the curriculum. Thus, it is important to involve not only professionals working in the field in the design of a curriculum as stated above, but also students actively in designing and redesigning the curriculum. Students can make valuable contributions because of their experiences as a student in the curriculum. Students can play a valuable role within multidisciplinary teams of teachers responsible for designing learning tasks. Ask students to give tips on how to improve the learning tasks; ask students whether these learning tasks build on learning tasks offered earlier in the curriculum.

Finally, it is important to prepare the organisation. One of the biggest challenges is that schools are often characterised by a high level of autonomy of disciplines and that collaboration between disciplines is limited[38]. Many professionals prefer to work autonomously and put their own discipline first, due to which it is not easy to encourage professionals to collaborate with other professions. However, if collaboration between disciplines or professions is lacking, it will be very difficult, if not impossible, to implement an integrated whole-task curriculum, because whole tasks by definition make an appeal on knowledge from different disciplines. When implementing whole-task curricula, it is thus important to reduce the autonomy of individual teachers and disciplines by introducing a central management team responsible for the design, implementation and evaluation of the curriculum – a management team that mandates and delegates responsibilities to multidisciplinary teams of teachers who are responsible for the design of different courses within the curriculum. The management team should also decide which disciplines must collaborate within the specific courses and should appoint teachers as coordinators for the different courses; these coordinators are responsible for designing, implementing and evaluating the courses. In other words, the teams of teachers from different disciplines should to a certain extent limit and reduce the autonomy of the disciplines[38]. A second issue that is important is that educational support is offered to teachers in the area of assessment, evaluation and designing curricular materials.

## Evaluation and quality culture

More too often, curricula are evaluated based on items that are not empirically related to student learning[39]. Often, a list of items is used with no underlying theory about effective teaching and learning[40]. When evaluating courses, it is important to derive evaluation items from whole-task instructional design models, such as Merrill's first principles of instruction[31] or 4C/ID[27], because these models make clear what the key components of effective instruction are. Merrill's first principles of instruction emphasise that learning is promoted when instruction is based on whole tasks, prior knowledge is activated, demonstrations are given, students can apply what they have learned and students are encouraged to integrate what they have learned to a variety of tasks[40]. Evaluations should preferably be based on these principles of effective instruction. Frick et al.[39] developed an evaluation questionnaire that contains scales of items measuring these first principles of instruction, being authentic problems, activation, demonstration, application and integration. The information collected with such an evaluation instrument can help to improve courses within a whole-task curriculum. In other words, when evaluating courses, define the key aspects of effective instruction based on theories or models of current instructional design and evidence about effective instruction.

Another important issue when evaluating whole-task curricula is that different stakeholders should be involved. Not only students but also teachers, alumni and professionals working in the field should be involved. Different stakeholders have different opinions about the extent to which the curriculum prepares well for professional practice. Furthermore, not only one data collection method but various methods should also be used. More too often, only questionnaires are filled out by students. When improving curricula, it is important to collect data from a variety of sources, for instance, from interviews or observations, and from a variety of stakeholders. Various methods and various stakeholders contribute towards rich data providing suggestions for improvement[40].

Yet, only collecting evaluation data is not sufficient to encourage continuous improvements of a curriculum. Nowadays, almost all schools collect evaluation data about the quality of their curriculum, but this does not result in continuous improvement of the curriculum in all schools. Evaluations often lead to a lot of bureaucratic documents or evaluations that look good on paper, but that do not result in actual change[41,42]. Continuously improving curricula is not a matter of evaluating and checking, but it is foremost a frame of mind that should be owned by the people who live it[43]. Ensuring that evaluations result in continuous improvement is not an easy step. It requires the development of an organisational culture based on shared values[41]. But how to develop an organisational culture of quality?

Nowadays, the concept of 'quality culture' is used in higher education. A complex concept that embraces not only instruments but also enabling factors such as commitment, values, communication, participation and both top-down and bottom-up interactions[41]. So far, not much is known about how to enhance continuous improvement and a quality culture, and this area is ripe for research. Kleijnen et al.[44] conducted a study to gain deeper understanding about the question which factors enhance continuous improvement from the teachers' perspective. Interviews with senior staff members demonstrated that active involvement of students and external professionals working in the field, a clear shared vision about the curriculum, a strong commitment and active involvement of staff members in evaluations, clear and shared responsibilities, strong collaborations, short formal and informal communication lines and an external orientation enhance continuous improvement of curricula. Thus, although the level of autonomy of the discipline should be reduced as stated above, it is also important to make sure that teachers feel ownership and are committed to and actively involved in the design, development, implementation and continuous improvement of a whole-task curriculum.

---

**BOX 17.1   Theoretical influences and the ADDIE model**

In the ADDIE model, guidelines and models for the Analysis and Design phases are typically linked to particular research paradigms or perspectives on learning, such as behaviourism, cultural–historical theory, cognitive theory or social-constructivist theory (for an overview of perspectives, see[45]). For example, original taxonomies of learning for the specification of learning goals were based on behaviourist and information-processing approaches. Whole-task approaches such as first principles of instruction,[31] cognitive apprenticeship learning[32] and 4C/ID[27] are typically based on cognitive and/or social-constructivist perspectives. For example, 4C/ID links each of its four components to the construction and automation of cognitive schemas: The construction of cognitive schemas results from inductive learning while performing learning tasks and from elaboration of

new supportive information (i.e. linking it to prior knowledge); the automation of cognitive schemas results from the formation of cognitive rules from procedural information and their subsequent strengthening as a result of part-task practice. In addition, whole-task approaches with a focus on workplace learning often rely on cultural-historical perspectives, for example, activity theory[46] analyses learning as the result of three interacting entities – the individual, the objects and tools used, and the community.

---

## Conclusion

This ends our concise description of research on instructional design in the health sciences. One chapter cannot do justice to such an extensive research field, but nevertheless, we were able to identify some important research themes. For analysis, research aims at the development of analysis methods for integrative goals that often characterise real-life tasks; lists of separate learning goals are replaced by integrated descriptions of desired performance that may result, for example, from CTA. For design, a shift can be found from condition-based models to whole-task models, where learning tasks that are based on real-life tasks provide the backbone of educational programmes. For development, research aims to identify principles for the construction of ICT-based instructional materials, such as multimedia, computer-based simulations, serious games and so forth. For implementation, research highlights the importance of strategies for preparing teachers, students and the organisation for the newly developed instruction. And finally, for evaluation, it stresses the importance of a quality culture so that evaluations do not become a burdensome duty but indeed lead to continuous improvement.

Future research on instructional design in the health sciences will increasingly be aimed at the development of instructional design guidelines and models that allow learners to deal with the fast changes and the ever-increasing complexity of the healthcare professions (new technologies, more inter-professional work, increasing cultural diversity, etc.). Learners must not only be prepared for performing familiar professional tasks at a high level of proficiency, but they must also develop the competencies necessary for performing new, unfamiliar tasks in their professional domain. Such competencies are often called 21st century skills and include adaptive expertise and cognitive readiness[47]. Instructional design research aimed at their development should study how novelty in the form of unfamiliar learning tasks can be introduced after an initial level of proficiency in the domain has been achieved, and how learners should be stimulated to explore these tasks, solve them with limited scaffolding and reflect on errors. Research questions as posed in Table 17.2 should then be answered for novel tasks that re-occur at irregular intervals and '…create occasional impasses which confront the learners with situations where (learned) routines do not work and which train them to switch from an automatic to a problem-solving mode' ([27], p. 265). It is our firm conviction that good research on instructional design might help to develop instructional design models that better prepare learners for their future tasks and that sustain teachers and designers in realising educational innovations. It might bring us one step closer to a situation in which students experience their educational programme no longer as a set of disconnected topics and courses but as a challenging road to their future profession, a profession which will tomorrow be different from today.

## Practice points

- CTA on real-life tasks provides a good basis for the design of whole-task curricula.
- Whole-task curricula can be designed from four inter-related components: (a) learning tasks, (b) supportive information, (c) procedural information and (d) part-task practice.
- Media will be different for each of the four components; thus, whole-task curricula will typically make use of a rich mix of media.
- Successful implementation of whole-task curricula requires a careful preparation of teachers, staff and organisation and a quality culture to ensure that evaluations lead to continuous improvement.
- Good research on instructional design might help to realise future innovations in health sciences education and thus contribute to the quality of care.

## References

1 Gagné, R.M. & Merrill, M.D. (1990) Integrative goals for instructional design. *Educational Technology, Research and Development*, **38**, 23–30.
2 Molenda, M. (2003) In search of the elusive ADDIE model. *Performance Improvement*, **42** (5), 34–37.
3 Tessmer, M. & Richey, R.C. (1997) The role of context in learning and instructional design. *Educational Technology, Research and Development*, **45**, 85–115.
4 Morrison, G.R., Ross, S.M., Kalman, H.K. & Kemp, J.E. (2013) *Designing Effective Instruction*, 7th edn. Wiley, Hoboken, NJ.
5 Norman, G. (2011) CanMEDS and other outcomes. *Advances in Health Sciences Education*, **16**, 547–551.
6 Hartley, J. (1994) *Designing Instructional Text*, 3rd edn. Kogan Page, London.
7 Bartsch, R.A. & Cobern, K.M. (2003) Effectiveness of PowerPoint presentations in lectures. *Computers and Education*, **41**, 77–86.
8 Mayer, R.E. (ed) (2014) *The Cambridge Handbook of Multimedia Learning*, 2nd edn. Cambridge University Press, New York.
9 Jochems, W., van Merriënboer, J.J.G. & Koper, R. (eds) (2004) *Integrated E-Learning*. RoutledgeFalmer, London, UK.
10 Annetta, L.A. (2010) The "I's" have it: A framework for serious educational game design. *Review of General Psychology*, **14**, 105–112.
11 Bloom, B.S. (1956) *Taxonomy of Educational Objectives*. Allyn and Bacon, Boston, MA.
12 Marzano, R.J. & Kendall, J.S. (2007) *The New Taxonomy of Educational Objectives*. Corwin press, Thousand Oaks, CA.
13 Gagné, R.M. (1985) *The Conditions of Learning*, 4th edn. Holt, Rinehart & Winston, New York.
14 Ragan, T.J., Smith, P.L. & Curda, L.K. (2008) Outcome-referenced, conditions-based theories and models. In: Spector, J.M., Merrill, M.D., van Merrienboer, J.J.G. & Driscoll, M.P. (eds), *Handbook of Research on Educational Communications and Technology*, 3rd edn. Erlbaum/Routledge, Mahwah, NJ, pp. 383–400.
15 Fastré, G.M.J., van der Klink, M.R. & van Merrienboer, J.J.G. (2010) The effects of performance-based assessment criteria on student performance and self-assessment skills. *Advances in Health Sciences Education*, **15**, 517–532.
16 Van Merrienboer, J.J.G., Jelsma, O. & Paas, F. (1992) Training for reflective expertise: A four-component instructional design model for complex cognitive skills. *Educational Technology, Research and Development*, **40** (2), 23–43.
17 Jonassen, D.H., Hannum, W.H. & Tessmer, M. (1989) *Handbook of Task Analysis Procedures*. Praeger, New York.
18 Van Merrienboer, J.J.G. (1997) *Training Complex Cognitive Skills*. Educational Technology Publications, Englewood Cliffs, NJ.
19 Clark, R.E., Feldon, D.F., van Merrienboer, J.J.G., Yates, K.A. & Early, S. (2008) Cognitive task analysis. In: Spector, J.M., Merrill, M.D., van Merrienboer, J.J.G. & Driscoll, M.P. (eds), *Handbook of Research on Educational Communications and Technology*, 3rd edn. Erlbaum/Routledge, Mahwah, NJ, pp. 577–594.
20 Tjiam, I., Schout, B., Hendrikx, A., Scherpbier, A., Witjes, J. & van Merrienboer, J.J.G. (2012) Designing

simulator-based training: An approach integrating cognitive task analysis and four-component instructional design. *Medical Teacher*, **34**, e698–e707.

21 Clark, R.E. (2014) Cognitive task analysis for expert-based instruction in healthcare. In: Spector, J.M., Merrill, M.D., Elen, J. & Bishop, M.J. (eds), *Handbook of Research on Educational Communications and Technology*, 4th edn. Springer, New York, pp. 541–551.

22 Velmahos, G.C., Toutouzas, K.G., Sillin, L.F. *et al.* (2004) Cognitive task analysis for teaching technical skills in an inanimate surgical skills laboratory. *American Journal of Surgery*, **187**, 114–119.

23 Van Merrienboer, J.J.G. & Kester, L. (2008) Whole-task models in education. In: Spector, J.M., Merrill, M.D., van Merrienboer, J.J.G. & Driscoll, M.P. (eds), *Handbook of Research on Educational Communications and Technology*, 3rd edn. Erlbaum, Mahwah, NJ, pp. 441–456.

24 Aggarwal, R., Mytton, O.T., Derbrew, M. *et al.* (2010) Training and simulation for patient safety. *Quality and Safety in Healthcare*, **19**, i34–i43.

25 Marton, F. (2006) Sameness and difference in transfer. *Journal of the Learning Sciences*, **15**, 499–535.

26 Van Merrienboer, J.J.G., Kester, L. & Paas, F. (2006) Teaching complex rather than simple tasks: Balancing intrinsic and germane load to enhance transfer of learning. *Applied Cognitive Psychology*, **20**, 343–352.

27 Van Merrienboer, J.J.G. & Kirschner, P.A. (2013) *Ten Steps to Complex Learning*, 2nd rev. edn. Routledge, New York.

28 Kalyuga, S., Ayres, P., Chandler, P. & Sweller, J. (2003) The expertise reversal effect. *Educational Psychologist*, **38 (1)**, 23–31.

29 Wickens, C.D., Hutchins, S., Carolan, T. & Cumming, J. (2013) Effectiveness of part-task training and increasing-difficulty training strategies: A meta-analysis approach. *Human Factors*, **55**, 461–470.

30 Harden, R.M. (1999) What is a spiral curriculum? *Medical Teacher*, **21**, 141–143.

31 Merrill, M.D. (2013) *First Principles of Instruction*. John Wiley and Sons.

32 Collins, A., Brown, J.S. & Newman, S.E. (1989) Cognitive apprenticeship: Teaching the craft of reading, writing and mathematics. In: Resnick, L.B. (ed), *Knowing, Learning, and Instruction: Essays in Honor of Robert Glaser*. Erlbaum, Hillsdale, NJ, pp. 453–493.

33 Vandewaetere, M., Manhaeve, D., Aertgeerts, B., Clarebout, G., van Merrienboer, J.J.G. & Roex, A. (2015) 4C/ID in medical education: How to design an educational program based on whole-task learning: Medical Teacher - AMEE Guide 93. *Medical Teacher*, **37 (1)**, 4–20.

34 Van Merrienboer, J.J.G. & Kester, L. (2014) The four-component instructional design model: Multimedia principles in environments for complex learning. In: Mayer, R.E. (ed), *The Cambridge Handbook of Multimedia Learning*, 2nd edn. Cambridge University Press, New York.

35 Dolmans, D.H.J.M., Wolfhagen, I.H. & van Merrienboer, J.J.G. (2013) Twelve tips for implementing whole-task curricula: How to make it work. *Medical Teacher*, **35**, 801–805.

36 Steinert, Y., Mann, K., Centeno, A. *et al.* (2006) A systematic review of faculty development initiatives designed to improve teaching effectiveness in medical education: BEME guide no 8. *Medical Teacher*, **28**, 497–526.

37 Stes, A., Min-Leliveld, M., Gijbels, D. & van Petegem, P. (2010) The impact of instructional development in higher education: The state-of-the art of the research. *Educational Research Review*, **5**, 25–49.

38 Bland, C.J., Starnaman, S., Wersal, L., Moorhead-Rosenberg, L., Zonia, S. & Henry, R. (2000) Curricular change in medical schools: How to succeed. *Academic Medicine*, **75**, 575–594.

39 Frick, T.W., Chadha, R., Watson, C. & Zlatkovska, E. (2010) Improving course evaluations to improve instruction and complex learning in higher education. *Educational Technology, Research and Development*, **58**, 115–136.

40 Dolmans, D.H.J.M., Stalmeijer, R.E., van Berkel, H.J.M. & Wolfhagen, H.A.P. (2011) Quality assurance of teaching and learning: Enhancing the quality culture. In: Dornan, T., Mann, K., Scherpbier, A. & Spencer, J. (eds), *Medical Education - Theory and Practice*. Elsevier, Edinburgh, UK, pp. 257–264.

41 Ehlers, U.D. (2009) Understanding quality culture. *Quality Assurance in Education*, **17**, 343–363.

42 Spencer-Matthews, S. (2001) Enforced cultural change in academe. A practical case study: implementing quality management systems in higher education. *Assessment and Evaluation in Higher Education*, **26**, 51–59.

43 Harvey, L. & Stensaker, B. (2008) Quality culture: understandings, boundaries and linkages. *European Journal of Education*, **43**, 427–440.

44 Kleijnen, J., Dolmans, D., Willems, J. & van Hout, H. (2014) Effective quality management requires a systematic approach and a flexible organizational culture: A qualitative study among academic staff. *Quality in Higher Education*, **20**, 103–126.

45 Van Merrienboer, J.J.G. & de Bruin, A.B.H. (2014) Research paradigms and perspectives on learning. In: Spector, J.M., Merrill, M.D., Elen, J. & Bishop, M.J. (eds), *Handbook of Research on Educational Communications and Technology*, 4th edn. Springer, New York, pp. 21–29.

46 Engeström, M.Y., Miettinen, R. & Punamaki, R.L. (eds) (1999) *Perspectives on Activity Theory*. Cambridge University Press, Cambridge, UK.

47 Bohle Carbonell, K., Stalmeijer, R.E., Konings, K.D., Segers, M. & van Merrienboer, J.J.G. (2014) How experts deal with novel situations: A review of adaptive expertise. *Educational Research Review*, **12**, 14–29.

# 18 Cognitive load theory: researching and planning teaching to maximise learning

*Jimmie Leppink, Tamara van Gog, Fred Paas and John Sweller*

*A patient reports acute and severe chest pain. Residents have to respond with immediate action, meaning they have to ask the right questions, perform a physical examination, think about the diagnosis – which has implications for further examination and decision making – meanwhile continue monitoring the blood pressure, pulse rate and respiration of the patient, as well as communicate with other people. Doing so requires a considerable mental effort from residents and even more so from students. In fact, by trying to focus on all aspects simultaneously, a student's mind may be easily overloaded, and learning may be hampered. Training that focuses on only one specific aspect (e.g. blood pressure, heart, lungs and CPR) at a time may not be perceived as very complex or difficult, but may not sufficiently facilitate integration and coordination of the composite skills, which are needed for appropriate task performance. The question then is how to manage the excessive working memory load (i.e. the number of information elements that need to be processed simultaneously within a certain amount of time) that is imposed by complex tasks in such a way that students' acquisition of knowledge and skills is improved.*

## Introduction

Cognitive load theory was devised for precisely the conditions under which people must deal with a heavy information-processing load and hence it has implications for both training and practice. In the following, we discuss the cognitive architecture that underlies the theory and some of its consequent general design guidelines before applying it to medical education and practice. By the end of this chapter, you will have acquired knowledge about cognitive load theory; more specifically, about the following four distinct components: (a) A cognitive architecture incorporating those components of human cognition that are relevant to instructional issues and related areas; (b) Categories of cognitive load; (c) Techniques for measuring cognitive load and (d) Cognitive load effects based on randomised controlled trials that compare a new instructional,

learning or problem-solving procedure – which is based on cognitive load theory – against a commonly used procedure. The cognitive load effects lead to the recommended instructional or related procedures. Each of these components is summarised below.

## Cognitive architecture

In recent years, cognitive load theory has placed an increasing emphasis on biological evolution when discussing human cognitive architecture.[1] Firstly, it has used Geary's evolutionary educational psychology to categorise classes of information.[2–4] Geary divides knowledge into two basic categories: biologically primary and biologically secondary. Primary knowledge is knowledge we have evolved to acquire. It tends to be very complex but very easily acquired without conscious effort. It is also modular with different types of knowledge probably acquired at different epochs. Examples are learning to recognise faces, acquire generic skills such as general problem-solving strategies, learning to listen and speak a native language. In contrast, biologically secondary knowledge is knowledge that we are able to acquire but that we have not specifically evolved to acquire, such as writing or algebra. We invented educational establishments in order to provide people with biologically secondary skills that are culturally important but that they otherwise are unlikely to acquire. Every topic taught in a medical course is likely to consist of biologically secondary knowledge.

There are particular structures and functions of biologically secondary knowledge that constitute those aspects of human cognitive architecture relevant to instructional design. They can be described by five principles that describe the information flows that underlie human cognition.

1 *The information store principle.* The human information processing system relies on a vast store of information. The aim of instruction is to change

*Researching Medical Education*, First Edition. Edited by Jennifer Cleland and Steven J. Durning.
© 2015 John Wiley & Sons, Ltd. Published 2015 by John Wiley & Sons, Ltd.

that store of biologically secondary information held in long-term memory, the memory where information elements can be stored for years or decades in the form of cognitive schemata (i.e. knowledge networks) indicating how these elements are related. Working memory, as indicated in point 4 below, can hold a limited amount of new information – obtained through sensory memory – for a limited time but has no known limitations when it comes to retrieving information from long-term memory.

2  *The borrowing and reorganising principle.* The human information processing system obtains its vast store of information by borrowing it from others. Humans imitate other humans, listen to what others say and read what they write to achieve the same aim. Cognitive load theory was designed to assist in these processes. It might be noted that while our tendency to obtain information from others is biologically primary (we are one of the very few species of animals that has evolved to both provide and obtain information from others), what we obtain in an educational context is biologically secondary.

3  *The randomness as genesis principle.* While the human information processing system obtains most of its information by borrowing it from other stores, that information must be created in the first instance. Random generation followed by tests of effectiveness during problem-solving creates the initial source of human knowledge. Humans normally only will use this principle to gain knowledge when knowledge is unavailable using the borrowing and reorganising principle.[5]

4  *The narrow limits of change principle.* The notion of a limited working memory capacity forms the core of cognitive load theory.[6] Working memory load, or cognitive load, is determined by the number of information elements that need to be processed simultaneously within a certain amount of time.[7] When dealing with novel information, the duration and capacity limits are very narrow. No more than two or three elements can be processed at any time and novel information can be held in working memory for no more than about 20 seconds without rehearsal.[8–10] Working memory can determine which novel information affects the system, and ensure that the amount of novel information permitted to be added to the information store is small. Change is incremental. It is of crucial importance that we take the limitations of working memory into account when designing instruction and strive for reducing unnecessary working memory load.

5  *The environmental organising and linking principle.* This principle provides the ultimate justification for the human information processing system. It ensures that appropriate information held in the information store is used to determine action in a particular environment. The capacity and duration limits of working memory are eliminated when it deals with organised information from long-term memory. Once appropriate environmental signals are received, the limits associated with long-term memory disappear.[11]

On the basis of this architecture, cognitive load theory assumes that learning is the gradual development of knowledge stored in long-term memory. Knowledge influences what is considered an information element to be processed by working memory. Take the following series of digits: 0031433885709. On the basis of the narrow limits of change principle, trying to memorise this series as just a random series of digits is very difficult and for most people impossible, because thirteen digits exceeds the capacity of working memory. Using the environmental organising and linking principle, if we add the information that this is a Dutch phone number, the number of digits to be processed is reduced from thirteen to nine for people who hold in long-term memory the knowledge that the 0031 (i.e. '31') is the country code for the Netherlands. If we further add the information that this number is a landline in Maastricht, a city in the south of the country, people who know that (0)43 represents landlines in Maastricht have to process 'only' seven elements. Finally, for those who know that the combination 003143388 indicates that this is a landline number from Maastricht University, the job appears easy; the demand on their working memory capacity is limited to handling the schema of 0031 (Dutch) 43 (Maastricht) 388 (University) stored in long-term memory as one element in working memory and processing the remaining four digits. In this way, via the environmental organising and linking principle, an impossible task can be rendered simple by using appropriate information stored in long-term memory.

Similarly, seeing for the first time an X-ray of someone's lungs, a novice student may perceive an almost unstructured myriad of elements to be processed deliberately. It will require time to process all these elements in an attempt to develop a preliminary schema and make sense of what is presented. For a more experienced student, who has seen similar X-rays before and managed to develop a preliminary schema, the same X-ray is expected to demand less working memory capacity, because the knowledge in long-term memory enables him/her to integrate knowledge of physiology, anatomy, lung disease theory and the projective geometry of an X-ray.[12] In short, compared to a novice, a more experienced student has more working memory resources available for deliberate processing of remaining unknown elements.

## Categories of cognitive load

The number of elements to be processed in a complex material, such as an X-ray, depends not only on the number of elements present in it but also on the extent to which there is interaction between these elements. If there is no interaction between the elements, all elements can be learnt in isolation. For example, learning the names of anatomical structures can be a difficult task because of the large number of structures that must be learnt. Nevertheless, since each name can be learnt independently of every other name, it is not interactions between elements that make the task difficult.

In contrast, some information is difficult to assimilate not because it has a very large number of elements, but rather because the (relatively a small number of) elements interact and so need to be learnt simultaneously. Processing a large number of elements simultaneously (e.g. physiology, anatomy, lung disease theory and the projective geometry of an X-ray) can place a heavy load on working memory. For example, the human body is a complex biological system in which organs interact in a variety of ways. It is therefore difficult to study the functioning of a particular organ in this system in isolation. Given that the hypothalamus links the nervous system to the endocrine system via the pituitary gland, it makes sense to strive for a combined study of the two systems as the neuroendocrine system. In a complex system such as this, element interactivity is typically high and we should take this element interactivity into account when designing instruction and working environments. Cognitive load theory is primarily concerned with difficulty due to high element interactivity. High element interactivity imposes a heavy working memory load, because interacting elements must be processed simultaneously in working memory. In contrast, difficulty due to a large number of isolated elements does not impose a heavy working memory load because each element can be processed individually without reference to the other elements, reducing the impact of cognitive load.

Originally, cognitive load theory distinguished between two sources of cognitive load, namely intrinsic cognitive load and extraneous cognitive load, and later on the concept of germane cognitive load was added.

1 *Intrinsic cognitive load.* Intrinsic cognitive load is a direct function of the number of interacting elements in information on the one hand and the availability of knowledge held in long-term memory on the part of the learner or performer on the other hand.[13] Novice learners, who have little if any knowledge of the type of information presented, have to select, organise and integrate all interacting elements in order to learn or perform. As learning advances, however, information elements gradually become incorporated into knowledge stored in long-term memory that can be handled as a single element in working memory via the environmental organising and linking principle (see earlier). Therefore, the intrinsic cognitive load that is imposed by particular information is much higher for novices than for more advanced learners.

2 *Extraneous cognitive load.* Extraneous cognitive load also is due to element interactivity. However, in this case, the element interactivity is due to instructional procedures or the way in which information is presented. Extraneous cognitive load refers to the learner or performer engaging in cognitive processes that are extraneous to the learning goals.[14,15] One example of such a process is having to mentally integrate spatially or temporally separated but mutually referring information sources. This imposes a very high cognitive load but hampers learning compared to the same information presented in a spatially or temporally integrated form. As another example, information that should be presented visually is presented verbally (e.g. describing anatomical structures such as the vessels of the heart verbally instead of presenting them visually using a diagram) also contributes to extraneous cognitive load; translating the words into a mental diagram requires working memory resources that consequently are not available for learning. Processes that impose an extraneous cognitive load can either hamper learning or performance if intrinsic cognitive load is high or lead to suboptimal learning under conditions in which cognitive load is lower. That is, even though extraneous cognitive load may be managed without hampering learning, a replacement of the extraneous cognitive load by processes that impose a cognitive load that actually contributes to learning should result in better learning.

3 *Germane cognitive load.* This type of cognitive load was added to the cognitive load framework in

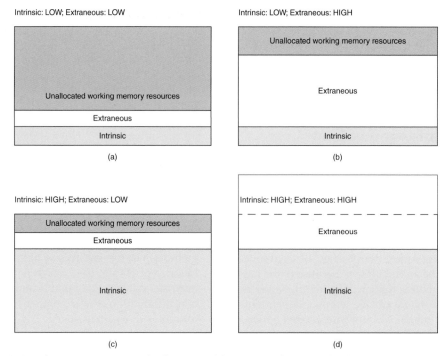

*Figure 18.1* Intrinsic and extraneous cognitive loads as two additive types of cognitive load.

the 1990s[16,17] and referred to cognitive load that contributes to learning. Given that in cognitive load theory, learning is the gradual development of knowledge in long-term memory, this third type of cognitive load is the one that arises from relating relevant information from long-term memory or context to new information elements.[18] In other words, it pertains to the working memory resources allocated to dealing with intrinsic cognitive load.[19] For example, variability in practice with diagnosing complex cases increases cognitive load, but this increase in cognitive load can aid learning. Requiring learners to compare and distinguish between cases rather than dealing with each case individually increases the intrinsic cognitive load of the task requiring more working memory resources (i.e. germane resources) to deal with a new task. Therefore, what was introduced as 'germane cognitive load' in the end of the 1990s is now referred to as 'germane resources' or working memory resources allocated to deal with intrinsic cognitive load and is thus related to intrinsic cognitive load.[20]

In the traditional (i.e. late 1990s) version of the theory, intrinsic cognitive load, extraneous cognitive load and germane cognitive load were assumed to be three additive types of cognitive load. In the recent reconceptualisation, however, only intrinsic

cognitive load and extraneous cognitive load are assumed to be additive: extraneous cognitive load should be minimised so that learners can allocate working memory resources (i.e. germane resources) to dealing with intrinsic cognitive load and engage in learning, and the sum of intrinsic and extraneous cognitive loads should be within the capacities of working memory.

Figure 18.1 provides a graphical representation of (a) low intrinsic and low extraneous cognitive load, (b) low intrinsic and high extraneous cognitive load, (c) high intrinsic and low extraneous cognitive load and (d) high intrinsic and high extraneous cognitive load.

Recall that the amount of intrinsic cognitive load imposed depends on the number of elements and interactions between elements in the information on the one hand and the knowledge available in the learner's long-term memory on the other hand. While intrinsic cognitive load depends on the intrinsic nature of the information the learner is confronted with, the amount of extraneous cognitive load experienced by the learner depends on the way the information is presented to the learner.

In situation (a), the learner is confronted with information that has a low intrinsic cognitive load and the way this information is presented imposes a low extraneous cognitive load. The grey area represents working memory resources that are not used for processing this particular information. A low intrinsic cognitive load can mean two things: either it is very easy information or it is information that would be perceived as complex by a novice learner, but is perceived as easy by the individual learner who has well-developed knowledge for this type of information. The difference between situation (a) and situation (b) is that in the latter the way in which the information is presented requires the learner to engage in processes that are unnecessary and not beneficial for learning. Situation (a) could occur if a cube is presented visually, whereas situation (b) would be more likely if the same cube is described verbally instead of presented visually. The cube itself is not a very complex shape and most people understand what a cube is and have mental representations of how a cube looks like. Providing a verbal instead of visual description of a cube, the learner may or may not realise that the description is about a cube but the processing needed to process a verbal description of a cube is extraneous.

Similarly, for someone who is trained in inspecting X-rays of people's lungs, seeing yet another X-ray may impose a rather low intrinsic cognitive load (much lower than would be the case for a novice learner). When presenting that X-ray as it should be presented, visually, the trained individual may notice an eventual abnormality quite easily, while any verbal description of what can be seen in the X-ray may contribute to extraneous cognitive load. However, for a less-advanced learner, verbal information presented along with the actual X-ray is likely to result in situation (c) if that information is presented appropriately and in situation (d) if not presented appropriately. In the latter case, cognitive overload may occur. In short, the sum of intrinsic and extraneous cognitive loads should be optimised in instructional design by selecting materials that match the learner's prior knowledge, proficiency or expertise, while extraneous cognitive load should be minimised. Doing so, we can challenge learners to engage in cognitive processes that help them to deal with intrinsic cognitive load by relating their knowledge from long-term memory to elements and interactions between elements that are new to them.

Cognitive load theory has led to many guidelines for how to optimise intrinsic cognitive load, how to minimise extraneous cognitive load and how to encourage learners to allocate working memory resources to dealing with intrinsic cognitive load. Details may be found in Van Merriënboer and Sweller[21] and in Van Merriënboer and Kirschner.[22] We will now focus on the measurement of cognitive load as well as on considerations for future research.

## On the measurement of cognitive load

Given that the concept of working memory load lies at the very core of cognitive load theory, measuring working memory load is crucial to test specific hypotheses and provide concrete guidelines for further research and educational practice. In the first two decades of cognitive load theory, cognitive load measurement focused almost exclusively on this core construct of working memory load[6] or mental effort[23] or cognitive load. These three terms have been used interchangeably for referring to cognitive capacity that is actually allocated to deal with the demands imposed by a task, and as such reflects the actual cognitive load.[16,24]

1 *Indirect measures of cognitive load.* In the first years of cognitive load theory, cognitive load was measured mainly indirectly. In the 1980s and early 1990s, it was found that learning strategies that require less problem-solving search (i.e. search needed for problem-solving) tend to result in better learning outcomes and fewer errors during performance than learning strategies that require more problem-solving search.[25–27] Models of cognitive load supported this suggestion.[6] Even though additional demand on working memory resources due to the use of learning strategies that require more problem-solving search imposes a higher cognitive load and may require more learning time, the increase in mental effort is not likely to result in better learning or performance. Two suggestions appear to follow from this finding. Firstly, learning time could provide an indirect measure of cognitive load.[28,29] Secondly, problem-solving search strategies do not change the intrinsic complexity of the information to be learnt. The additional cognitive load as a consequence of more intensive problem-solving search does not contribute to learning or performance and can be expected to be extraneous cognitive load. However, a later study also demonstrated that an increase in intrinsic complexity of information (e.g. many variables in mathematical equations) can also increase error rates.[30] Therefore, it is evident that computational models (e.g. associated with changes in problem-solving search), learning time (or time-on-task) and error rates can serve as indirect measures of cognitive load, although the validity of those measures as indicators of cognitive load may be task dependent.

2 *Subjective rating scales of cognitive load.* Subjective rating scales have been used intensively to estimate cognitive load experienced by learners, ever since the introduction of a nine-point

one-dimensional mental effort rating scale in the early 1990s.[23] Even though it is not entirely clear to what extent workload and cognitive load refer to the same concept across contexts, the multidimensional NASA task load index (TLX) is an example of another instrument that subjectively assesses experienced workload on five (i.e. mental demands, physical demands, temporal demands, own performance and effort and frustration) seven-point rating scales[31] that has been used in cognitive load research.[32–34]

3 *Efficiency measures.* Measuring overall experienced cognitive load by subjective or objective techniques can be very informative, especially in relation to measures of learning outcomes into the so-called efficiency measures.[35–37] Efficiency measures relate performance to the costs (in terms of overall cognitive load) needed to reach that performance. In other words, learning acquired per amount of learning effort expended. Higher efficiency is reached if higher performance is achieved with the same costs or if the same performance is reached with lower costs. However, while extraneous cognitive load is clearly unnecessary, some intrinsic cognitive load is desirable for learning. It is not yet clear to what extent intrinsic cognitive load should be seen as a cost. For example, too little intrinsic cognitive load could make a task appear boring.[38] If we succeed in measuring intrinsic and extraneous cognitive loads separately, we can test specific hypotheses with regard to intrinsic cognitive load (e.g. decreasing element interactivity results in lower intrinsic cognitive load) and extraneous cognitive load (e.g. learning strategies requiring more problem-solving search impose a higher extraneous cognitive load than learning strategies requiring less problem-solving search). This would allow the study of possibilities to express costs in terms of extraneous cognitive load instead of as overall cognitive load which is the sum of intrinsic and extraneous cognitive loads. The distinction between intrinsic and extraneous cognitive loads is important for education and education research. More cognitive load is not necessarily negative for learning. There is a common misunderstanding in the field that cognitive load needs to be as low as possible. Even though extraneous cognitive load needs to be minimised, cognitive load theory-based instruction attempts to use all available working memory resources to deal with intrinsic cognitive load. Intrinsic cognitive load should be optimised in instructional design by selecting materials that align with the learner's prior knowledge or expertise, while extraneous cognitive load should be minimised. In such a context, learners can be challenged to allocate available working memory resources for dealing with intrinsic cognitive load and actually engage in learning.

4 *Measuring categories of cognitive load.* In recent years, several studies have attempted to develop instruments for measuring one or more types of cognitive load.[39–43] A drawback of most of these studies is that one or more types of cognitive load were represented by a single item. The use of multiple indicators of the separate types of cognitive load might yield a more precise measurement and might enable researchers to separate the types of cognitive load more clearly than the use of a single indicator for each scale. Further, when referring to one very specific instructional feature or cognitive process to measure extraneous or germane cognitive load, a conceptual problem may arise, because instructional features that are beneficial for less advanced learners may not be beneficial for more advanced learners (i.e. expertise reversal effects).[44–46] For instance, in some studies, less-experienced medical students outperformed seasoned medical practitioners on recall in specific cases.[47] Recently, a new psychometric instrument was developed that took an alternative approach to the formulation of questions for measuring different types of cognitive load, which may solve the problem of not being able to differentiate between intrinsic and extraneous cognitive loads at least to some extent.[48] There is some support for the assumption that two factors capture intrinsic and extraneous cognitive loads, respectively.[49] Table 18.1 provides the eight items that form these two factors: questions 1–4 focus on intrinsic cognitive load, while questions 5–8 pertain to extraneous cognitive load.

5 *Physiological measures of cognitive load.* Various researchers have suggested the use of physiological measures of cognitive load. A study conducted in the first half of the 1990s suggested that a nine-point mental effort rating scale was more sensitive to differences in task complexity than heart rate variability, in that the former could explain more of the variation in task complexity and performance.[50,51] Some studies have suggested using techniques such as functional magnetic resonance imaging (fMRI) and focus on, for instance, an increase in activity in the dorsolateral prefrontal cortex while the learner is processing information.[52,53] Others have suggested using electroencephalography (EEG).[54]

Using EEG, a study of the use of the so-called hypertext leads (i.e. introductory text linking pieces together) found that the use of such leads resulted in better learning outcomes than using hypertext without leads, and alpha, beta and theta (EEG) measures were significantly lower in the hypertext lead group, suggesting that the use of hypertext leads resulted in a decrease in cognitive load.[55] Further, various researchers have suggested that particular eye-tracking variables could be related to cognitive load.[56–59] For instance, increases in pupil diameter are positively correlated with increases in cognitive load, at least in a non-elderly population.[60,61] It has been suggested that saccade rate and amplitude correlate negatively with cognitive load.[62–64] Finally, average dwell time (i.e. time focusing in the same position or area in a visual stimulus) is also expected to reflect a higher cognitive load.[65] Again, for some of these variables, the relation with cognitive load is highly task dependent. Nevertheless, these and other relations between eye-tracking variables and (categories of) cognitive load need and deserve further study.

6  *Secondary tasks.* An alternative way of measuring cognitive load may be through the study of performance on a secondary task.[66,67] A secondary task requires one to invest additional cognitive effort that is secondary to the primary task of learning or performance. One example of such a task is recognising a tone presented at random during the learning episode.[68] Another example is recalling or remembering letters.[69] The idea is that the less working memory resources the primary task of interest requires the more working memory resources one has available to perform well on the secondary task.

7  *Combining two or more types of measures.* Secondary tasks have not been used as extensively as subjective measures because they require a more complex experimental design and, like physiological measures, more advanced equipment. Moreover, it is not yet clear how the use of secondary tasks or physiological measures can enable us to differentiate between intrinsic and extraneous cognitive loads. In contrast to secondary tasks, subjective measurement tools such as the one presented in Table 18.1 may help us to differentiate between intrinsic and extraneous cognitive loads, but may be more difficult to use in particular contexts than a single-item mental effort rating scale. For example, if individuals have to provide a mental effort rating after each of a series of say eight tasks, it is easier to use

*Table 18.1* A new psychometric instrument for the measurement of intrinsic cognitive load (i.e. questions 1–4) and extraneous cognitive load (i.e. questions 5–8)

All of the following eight questions refer to the activity that just finished. Please take your time to read each of the questions carefully and respond to each of the questions on the presented scale from 0 to 10, in which '0' indicates not at all the case and '10' indicates completely the case:

0 1 2 3 4 5 6 7 8 9 10

[1] The content of this activity was very complex.
[2] The problem/s covered in this activity was/were very complex.
[3] In this activity, very complex terms were mentioned.
[4] I invested a very high mental effort in the complexity of this activity.
[5] The explanations and instructions in this activity were very unclear.
[6] The explanations and instructions in this activity were full of unclear language.
[7] The explanations and instructions in this activity were, in terms of learning, very ineffective.
[8] I invested a very high mental effort in unclear and ineffective explanations and instructions in this activity.

a single-item mental effort scale than having individuals respond to eight items after each of eight tasks. However, it may be possible to use a single-item mental effort rating scale after each of the eight tasks and have individuals respond to the eight-item questionnaire either once at the end of the full procedure or, preferably, after each block of (e.g. four) tasks. This procedure may provide researchers with insight into the extent of mental effort invested in separate tasks as well as in the experienced overall intrinsic and extraneous cognitive loads. Well-designed experiments that combine two or more of the types of measures discussed in this section – indirect measures, subjective response measures, biological measures and secondary task measures – may lead to new insights on convergence and divergence between these different types of measures. If we encounter consistent correlations, for instance, between the two scales presented in Table 18.1 and particular eye-tracking measures and findings on these measures are in line with cognitive load theory, these findings may contribute to the expectation that the measures under consideration indeed capture intrinsic or extraneous cognitive load, eventually leading to further refinement of these measures. If we do not encounter a consistent correlation between measures, this finding may give rise to new research on why and under what circumstances the different types of measures diverge.

## Cognitive load effects

The cognitive load effects are the empirical manifestation of cognitive load theory. The cognitive architecture, categories of cognitive load and techniques for measuring cognitive load are all necessary to generate cognitive load effects. Each consists of a comparison of an instructional procedure generated by cognitive load theory with an alternative, normally but not always, a traditionally used procedure. That comparison always uses randomised, controlled trials at some point.[24,44,49]

A large number of cognitive load theory effects have been generated by the theory with each effect having the potential to change instructional procedures[18] and all of the effects are relevant to medical and healthcare profession education and practice.[20,21]

One of the most widely investigated effects is the worked example effect, which indicates that replacing a number of practice problems with examples in which it is demonstrated how to complete the task (either in writing or by a teacher or more advanced student), makes learning more effective as well as more efficient (i.e. less time or effort investment required) for students who have little or no prior knowledge of a task.[17,70,71] In medical education, example-based learning has proven beneficial with a variety of tasks, such as learning to diagnose certain diseases[72,73], or acquiring bronchoscopy skills through simulation training.[74] Recently, it was also shown that the acquisition of diagnostic knowledge, which had been found to be enhanced by engaging in structured reflection on one's own initial diagnosis[75,76], was made even more effective and efficient by providing students with worked examples of reflection.[77]

Medical decision making requires breadth and depth of knowledge, organisation of knowledge, communication skills and an ability to deal with emotions and stress. As students in the medical domain accumulate experience, their knowledge of diseases and related phenomena becomes more and more elaborate. This influences what is perceived as an element or chunk of information to be processed and may reduce the likelihood of cognitive overload on the part of a student when having to make a decision. The latter may hold particularly in cases where emotion is involved. At first, one might expect that emotion can facilitate the recognition of relevant cues or patterns and as such supports learning or decision making in a particular context. However, if negative emotion (e.g. intense stress) or positive emotion stimulates bias, learning and

decision making may be impaired.[78–80] Further, if negative emotion (e.g. due to learning about a previous misdiagnosis) or positive emotion leads us to think what caused that emotion, that very thought consumes working memory resources and may hamper learning and decision making.[81] As an example, in one study it was found that when teaching medical students using a mannequin, and if the mannequin 'died', the emotional impact of the death increased cognitive load and decreased learning.[82]

In decision making, medical students largely rely on basic science or biomedical knowledge accumulated in various courses, including knowledge of anatomy.[47,83] Anatomy appears a topic that many students find difficult to study. Take, for instance, the anatomy of the human brain. The human brain is a large three-dimensional structure which is very difficult to represent in two-dimensional pictures. Two-dimensional pictures of the brain or of parts of the brain already comprise many interacting elements, and having to mentally build a three-dimensional picture of the brain or of a brain region is something that results in additional intrinsic cognitive load. To avoid excessive intrinsic cognitive load, it is important that students first study two-dimensional pictures of parts of the brain in detail, learn some core functions associated with those parts and learn important jargon. Verbal explanations of how to integrate two-dimensional pictures of parts of the brain to obtain a three-dimensional representation are unlikely to compensate for a lack of time spent on studying two-dimensional pictures of parts of the brain in sufficient detail. Verbal explanations are more likely to impose an extraneous cognitive load, because – like deriving a cube from six squares – deriving a three-dimensional representation of the human brain from two-dimensional pictures is a visual and not a verbal process.

How to train medical students to become experts in this domain is an important challenge. Different approaches to this challenge are encountered in the literature. In a traditional approach, students are expected to memorise large volumes of information and integrate them into structured knowledge. While memorising plays an important role in the medical curriculum, especially in early stages, there is no empirical support for the assumption that having students memorise with a minimum of instructional guidance results in optimal learning. Research in a variety of domains, including medicine, demonstrates that, especially in early stages of knowledge development, students learn much more from the study of well-designed worked examples than from autonomous problem-solving.[84] Autonomous problem-solving can result in very high intrinsic cognitive load due to a lack of prior knowledge and may impose a considerable extraneous cognitive load due to the need for problem-solving search. However, once students have developed sufficient knowledge of a particular phenomenon or situation through instructional guidance, autonomous problem-solving can be expected to yield superior results to the study of worked examples.[44–46] It is for that reason that problem-based learning (PBL)[85,86] could work 'as a supplementary approach with senior students to facilitate their exploration and self-study' (combined with worked examples in the form of clinical presentations) but cannot be expected to yield optimal learning outcomes when used as a single approach in the medical curriculum.[87] In other words, PBL can be a useful approach in the later stage of a medical curriculum, once students (should) have sufficient knowledge of topics under consideration.

A major strength of cognitive load theory is that the guidelines generated by this theory are based on well-designed randomised controlled experiments. Conducting randomised controlled experiments is of great importance in medical education research, because when appropriate – as is the case with measuring and examining the intricacies of cognitive load – and well designed, they allow causal conclusions with regard to effectiveness of instruction or the influence of motivation on learning or performance (see also Cleland, and Stansfield and Gruppen, in this book). Of course, this manifest advantage of using randomised controlled trials to study causality does not negate the use of other techniques based on correlational or qualitative techniques. Such techniques can be important in studying, for example, cognitive processes as well as in the development of measurement tools such as the one presented in Table 18.1. This questionnaire, which was in its original form developed and tested in the context of statistics education[48], resulted from a synthesis of literature review[88,89], qualitative research[90] and subsequently a combination of correlational studies and randomised controlled trials[48,49]. The literature review and qualitative research resulted in a framework of elements that may contribute to either of intrinsic or extraneous cognitive load. This resulted in a questionnaire used in correlational studies (i.e. lectures), and the final scales were used in randomised controlled trials. Although parallel versions for language learning[49]

and medical education (Table 18.1) have been provided, combination of qualitative and correlational studies on the one hand and randomised controlled trials on the other hand may reveal that the questionnaire needs some adjustment or expansion for use in specific settings.

Finally, basing educational practice, when possible, on the results of well-designed randomised controlled trials carried out before the introduction of new teaching procedures, provides an excellent demonstration of the use and application of quantitative research philosophy in healthcare education.

## Conclusion

In this chapter, we have provided an overview of cognitive load theory and its various key components, including how best to measure cognitive load and which research designs are favoured in this field of research. One chapter cannot give justice to this extensive research field but we hope we have illustrated the importance of cognitive load in learning in such a way as to stimulate your interest in research on this topic.

---

**Practice points**

Cognitive load theory has many implications for medical and healthcare professions education research. Through an ongoing interaction between cognitive load theory and carefully designed experiments, medical and healthcare professions education research could make crucial steps forward in its development. Four bullet points summarise the main messages:

- The limitations of human working memory have clear implications for how much and what kind of information students and practitioners can process in a medical context.
- Unnecessary additional demands on working memory resources due to inappropriate ways of presenting information may lead to cognitive overload in a complex environment.
- A combined use of different types of cognitive load measures could lead to new insights with regard to which measures can be used as indicators for which type of cognitive load.
- Educational practice should be based on the results of well-designed randomised controlled trials carried out before the introduction of new teaching procedures rather than afterwards.

# References

1 Paas, F. & Sweller, J. (2012) An evolutionary upgrade of cognitive load theory: Using the human motor system and collaboration to support the learning of complex cognitive tasks. *Educational Psychology Review*, **24**, 27–45.

2 Geary, D. (2007) Educating the evolved mind: Conceptual foundations for an evolutionary educational psychology. In: Carlson, J.S. & Levin, J.R. (eds), *Psychological Perspectives on Contemporary Educational Issues*. Information Age Publishing, Greenwich, CT, pp. 1–99.

3 Geary, D. (2008) An evolutionarily informed education science. *Educational Psychologist*, **43**, 179–195.

4 Geary, D. (2012) Evolutionary educational psychology. In: Harris, K., Graham, S. & Urdan, T. (eds), *APA Educational Psychology Handbook*. Vol. **1**. American Psychological Association, Washington, D.C., pp. 597–621.

5 Sweller, J. (2009) Cognitive bases of human creativity. *Educational Psychology Review*, **21**, 11–19.

6 Sweller, J. (1988) Cognitive load during problem solving: Effects on learning. *Cognitive Science*, **12**, 257–285.

7 Barouillet, P., Bernardin, S., Portrat, S., Vergauwe, E. & Camos, V. (2007) Time and cognitive load in working memory. *Journal of Experimental Psychology: Learning, Memory, and Cognition*, **33**, 570–585.

8 Barouillet, P., Gavens, N., Vergauwe, E., Gaillard, V. & Camos, V. (2009) Working memory span development: A time-based resource-sharing model account. *Developmental Psychology*, **45**, 477–490.

9 Cowan, N. (2001) The magical number 4 in short-term memory: a reconsideration of mental storage capacity. *Behavioral and Brain Science*, **24**, 152–153.

10 Peterson, L. & Peterson, M.J. (1959) Short-term retention of individual verbal items. *Journal of Experimental Psychology*, **58**, 193–198.

11 Ericsson, K.A. & Kintsch, W. (1995) Long-term working memory. *Psychological Review*, **102**, 211–245.

12 Lesgold, A., Rubinson, H., Feltovich, P., Glaser, R., Klopfer, D. & Wang, Y. (1988) Expertise in a complex skill: Diagnosing x-ray pictures. In: Chi, M.T.H., Glaser, R. & Farr, M.J. (eds), *The Nature of Expertise*. Erlbaum, Hillsdale, NJ.

13 Sweller, J. (1994) Cognitive load theory, learning difficulty, and instructional design. *Learning and Instruction*, **4**, 295–312.

14 Sweller, J. & Chandler, P. (1994) Why some material is difficult to learn. *Cognitive and Instruction*, **12**, 185–223.

15 Sweller, J., Chandler, P., Tierney, P. & Cooper, M. (1990) Cognitive load as a factor in the structuring of technical material. *Journal of Experimental Psychology*, **119**, 176–192.

16 Paas, F. & Van Merriënboer, J.J.G. (1994) Instructional control of cognitive load in the training of complex cognitive tasks. *Educational Psychology Review*, **6**, 51–71.

17 Sweller, J., Van Merriënboer, J.J.G. & Paas, F. (1998) Cognitive architecture and instructional design. *Educational Psychology Review*, **10**, 251–296.

18 Sweller, J. (2010) Element interactivity and intrinsic, extraneous, and germane cognitive load. *Educational Psychology Review*, **22**, 122–138.

19 Kalyuga, S. (2011) Cognitive load theory: How many types of load does it really need? *Educational Psychology Review*, **23**, 1–19.

20 Sweller, J., Ayres, P. & Kalyuga, S. (2011) *Cognitive Load Theory*. Springer, New York.

21 Van Merriënboer, J.J.G. & Sweller, J. (2010) Cognitive load theory in health professional education: design principles and strategies. *Medical Education*, **44**, 85–93.

22 Van Merriënboer, J.J.G. & Kirschner, P.A. (2013) *Ten Steps to Complex Learning: A Systematic Approach to Four-Component Instructional Design*, 2nd edn. Routledge, New York.

23 Paas, F. (1992) Training strategies for attaining transfer of problem-solving skills in statistics: A cognitive load approach. *Journal of Educational Psychology*, **84**, 429–434.

24 Paas, F., Tuovinen, J., Tabbers, H. & Van Gerven, P.W.M. (2003) Cognitive load measurement as a means to advance cognitive load theory. *Educational Psychologist*, **38**, 63–71.

25 Ayres, P. & Sweller, J. (1990) Locus of difficulty in multistage mathematics problems. *American Journal of Psychiatry*, **103**, 167–193.

26 Owen, E. & Sweller, J. (1985) What do students learn while solving mathematics problems? *Journal of Educational Psychology*, **77**, 272–284.

27 Sweller, J. & Cooper, M. (1985) The use of worked examples as a substitute for problem solving in learning algebra. *Cognitive and Instruction*, **1**, 59–89.

28 Chandler, P. & Sweller, J. (1991) Cognitive load theory and the format of instruction. *Cognitive and Instruction*, **8**, 293–332.

29 Chandler, P. & Sweller, J. (1992) The split-attention effect as a factor in the design of instruction. *British Journal of Educational Psychology*, **62**, 233–246.

30 Ayres, P. (2001) Systematic mathematical errors and cognitive load. *Contemporary Educational Psychology*, **26**, 227–248.

31 Hart, S.G. & Staveland, L.E. (1988) Development of NASA-TLX (Task Load Index): results of empirical and theoretical research. In: Hancock, P.A. & Meshtaki, N. (eds), *Human Mental Workload*. North-Holland, Amsterdam, pp. 139–183.

32 Gerjets, P., Scheiter, K. & Catrambone, R. (2004) Designing instructional examples to reduce intrinsic cognitive load: Molar versus modular presentation of solution procedures. *Instructional Science*, **32**, 33–58.

33 Gerjets, P., Scheiter, K. & Catrambone, R. (2006) Can learning from molar and modular worked examples be enhanced by providing instructional explanations and prompting self-explanations? *Learning and Instruction*, **16**, 104–121.

34 Kester, L., Lehnen, C., Van Gerven, P.W.M. & Kirschner, P.A. (2006) Just-in-time, schematic supportive information presentation during cognitive skill acquisition. *Computers in Human Behavior*, **22**, 93–112.

35 Hoffman, B. & Schraw, G. (2010) Conceptions of efficiency: Applications in learning and problem solving. *Educational Psychologist*, **45**, 1–14.

36 Paas, F. & Van Merriënboer, J.J.G. (1993) The efficiency of instructional conditions: An approach to combine mental effort and performance measures. *Human Factors*, **35**, 737–743.

37 Van Gog, T. & Paas, F. (2008) Instructional efficiency: Revisiting the original construct in educational research. *Educational Psychologist*, **43**, 16–26.

38 Young, M.S. & Stanton, N.A. (2002) Attention and automation: new perspectives on mental underload and performance. *Theoretical Issues in Ergonomics Science*, **3**, 178–194.

39 Ayres, P. (2006) Using subjective measures to detect variations of intrinsic load within problems. *Learning and Instruction*, **16**, 389–400.

40 Cierniak, G., Scheiter, K. & Gerjets, P. (2009) Explaining the split-attention effect: Is the reduction of extraneous cognitive load accompanied by an increase in germane cognitive load? *Computers in Human Behavior*, **25**, 315–324.

41 De Leeuw, K.E. & Mayer, R.E. (2008) A comparison of three measures of cognitive load: Evidence for separable measures of intrinsic, extraneous, and germane load. *Journal of Educational Psychology*, **100**, 223–234.

42 Eysink, T.H.S., De Jong, T., Berthold, K., Kollöffel, B., Opfermann, M. & Wouters, P. (2009) Learner performance in multimedia learning arrangements: An analysis across instructional approaches. *American Educational Research Journal*, **46**, 1107–1149.

43 Galy, E., Cariou, M. & Mélan, C. (2012) What is the relationship between mental workload factors and cognitive load types? *International Journal of Psychophysiology*, **83**, 269–275.

44 Kalyuga, S., Ayres, P., Chandler, P. & Sweller, J. (2003) The expertise reversal effect. *Educational Psychologist*, **38**, 23–31.

45 Kalyuga, S., Chandler, P., Tuovinen, J. & Sweller, J. (2001) When problem-solving is superior to studying worked examples. *Journal of Educational Psychology*, **93**, 579–588.

46 Leppink, J., Broers, N.J., Imbos, T., Van der Vleuten, C.P.M. & Berger, M.P.F. (2012) Self-explanation in the domain of statistics: An expertise reversal effect. *Higher Education*, **63**, 771–785.

47 Kalyuga, S., Rikers, R.M.J.P. & Paas, F. (2012) Educational implications of expertise reversal effects in learning and performance of complex cognitive and sensorimotor skills. *Educational Psychology Review*, **24**, 313–337.

48 Leppink, J., Paas, F., Van der Vleuten, C.P.M., Van Gog, T. & Van Merriënboer, J.J.G. (2013) Development of an instrument for measuring different types of cognitive load. *Behavior Research Methods*, **45**, 1058–1072.

49 Leppink, J., Paas, F., Van Gog, T., Van der Vleuten, C.P.M. & Van Merriënboer, J.J.G. (2014) Effects of pairs of problems and examples on task performance and different types of cognitive load. *Learning and Instruction*, **30**, 32–42.

50 Paas, F. & Van Merriënboer, J.J.G. (1994) Variability of worked examples and transfer of geometrical problem-solving skills: A cognitive-load approach. *Journal of Educational Psychology*, **86**, 122–133.

51 Paas, F. & Van Merriënboer, J.J.G. (1994) Measurement of cognitive-load in instructional research. *Perceptual and Motor Skills*, **79**, 419–430.

52 Paas, F., Ayres, P. & Pachman, M. (2008) Assessment of cognitive load in multimedia learning: Theory, methods and applications. In: Robinson, D.H. & Schraw, G. (eds), *Recent Innovations in Educational Psychology that Facilitate Student Learning*. Information Age Publishing, Charlotte, pp. 11–35.

53 Whelan, R.R. (2007) Neuroimaging of cognitive load in instructional multimedia. *Educational Research Review*, **2**, 1–12.

54 Antonenko, P., Paas, F., Grabner, R. & Van Gog, T. (2010) Using electroencephalography to measure cognitive load. *Educational Psychology Review*, **22**, 425–438.

55 Antonenko, P. & Niederhauser, D.S. (2010) Using electroencephalography to measure cognitive load. *Computers in Human Behavior*, **26**, 140–150.

56 Holmqvist, K., Nyström, M., Andersson, R., Dewhurst, R., Jarodzka, H. & Van de Weijer, J. (2011) *Eye-Tracking: A Comprehensive Guide to Methods and Measures*. Oxford University Press, Oxford.

57 Underwood, G., Jebbert, L. & Roberts, K. (2004) Inspecting pictures for information to verify a sentence: eye movements in general encoding and in focused search. *Quarterly Journal of Experimental Psychology Section A-human Experimental Psychology*, **57A**, 165–182.

58 Van Gog, T. & Jarodzka, H. (2013) Eye tracking as a tool to study and enhance cognitive and metacognitive processes in computer-based learning environments. In: Azevedo, R. & Aleven, V. (eds), *International Handbook of Metacognition and Learning Technologies*. Springer, New York, pp. 143–156.

59 Van Gog, T. & Scheiter, K. (2010) Eye tracking as a tool to study and enhance multimedia learning. *Learning and Instruction*, **20**, 95–99.

60 Van Gerven, P.W.M., Paas, F., Van Merriënboer, J.J.G. & Schmidt, H.G. (2004) Memory load and the cognitive pupillary response in aging. *Psychophysiology*, **41**, 167–174.

61 Van Orden, K.F., Jung, T.P. & Makeig, S. (2000) Combined eye activity measures accurately estimate changes in sustained visual task performance. *Biological Psychology*, **44**, 85–93.

62 Recarte, M.A. & Nunes, L.M. (2003) Mental workload while driving: Effects on visual search, discrimination, and decision making. *Journal of Experimental Psychology: Applied*, **9**, 119–133.

63 Veltman, J. & Gaillard, A. (1998) Physiological workload reactions to increasing levels of task difficulty. *Ergonomics*, **41**, 656–659.

64  Williams, L.J. (1988) Tunnel vision or general interference? Cognitive load and attentional bias are both important. *American Journal of Psychiatry*, **101**, 171–191.

65  Zwahlen, H.T., Adams, C.C. & DeBald, D.P. (1988) Safety aspects of CRT touch panel controls in automobiles. In: Gale, A.G., Freeman, M.H., Haslegrave, C.M., Smith, P. & Taylor, S.H. (eds), *Vision in Vehicles*. Elsevier, Amsterdam, pp. 335–344.

66  Britton, B.K. & Tesser, A. (1982) Effects of prior knowledge on use of cognitive capacity in three complex cognitive tasks. *Journal of Verbal Learning and Verbal Behavior*, **21**, 421–436.

67  Kerr, B. (1973) Processing demands during mental operations. *Memory and Cognition*, **1**, 401–412.

68  Marcus, N., Cooper, M. & Sweller, J. (1996) Understanding instructions. *Journal of Educational Psychology*, **88**, 49–63.

69  Chandler, P. & Sweller, J. (1996) Cognitive load while learning to use a computer program. *Applied Cognitive Psychology*, **10**, 151–170.

70  Renkl, A. (2014) Towards an instructionally-oriented theory of example-based learning. *Cognitive Science*, **38**, 1–37.

71  Van Gog, T. & Rummel, N. (2010) Example-based learning: Integrating cognitive and social-cognitive research perspectives. *Educational Psychology Review*, **22**, 155–174.

72  Kopp, V., Stark, R. & Fischer, M.R. (2008) Fostering diagnostic competence through computer-supported, case-based worked examples: Effects of erroneous examples and feedback. *Medical Education*, **42**, 823–829.

73  Kopp, V., Stark, R., Kühne-Eversmann, L. & Fischer, M.R. (2009) Do worked examples foster medical students' diagnostic knowledge of hyperthyroidism? *Medical Education*, **43**, 1210–1217.

74  Bjerrum, A.S., Hilberg, O., Van Gog, T., Charles, P. & Eika, B. (2013) Effects of modeling examples in complex procedural skills training: A randomized study. *Medical Education*, **47**, 888–898.

75  Mamede, S., Van Gog, T., Moura, A.S., De Farias, R.M.D. & Peixoto, J.M. (2014) How can students' diagnostic competence benefit most from practice with clinical cases? Effects of structured reflection on future diagnosis of the same and novel diseases. *Academic Medicine*, **89**, 121–127.

76  Mamede, S., Van Gog, T., Moura, A.S. *et al.* (2012) Reflection as a strategy to foster medical students' acquisition of diagnostic competence. *Medical Education*, **46**, 464–472.

77  Ibiapina, C., Mamede, S., Moura, A.S., Eloi-Santos, S. & Van Gog, T. (2014) Effects of free, cued, and modeled reflection on medical students' diagnostic competence. *Medical Education*, **48**, 796–805.

78  Brenner, L., Koehler, D. & Tversky, A. (1996) On the evaluation of one-sided evidence. *Journal of Behavioral Decision Making*, **9**, 59–71.

79  Croskerry, P. (2009) A universal model for diagnostic reasoning. *Academic Medicine*, **84**, 1022.

80  Kahneman, D. (2011) *Thinking, Fast and Slow*. Farrar, Straus and Giroux, New York.

81  Fraser, K., Ma, I., Teteris, E., Baxter, H., Wright, B. & McLaughlin, K. (2012) Emotion, cognitive load and learning outcomes simulation training. *Medical Education*, **46**, 1055–1062.

82  Fraser, K., Huffman, J., Ma, I. *et al.* (2014) The emotional and cognitive impact of unexpected simulated patient death: A randomized controlled study. *Chest*, **145**, 958–963.

83  Patel, V.L., Evans, D.A. & Groen, G.J. (1989) Biomedical knowledge and clinical reasoning. In: Evans, D.A. & Patel, V.L. (eds), *Cognitive Science in Medicine: Biomedical Modeling*. MIT Press, Cambridge, pp. 53–112.

84  Mancin, H., Harasym, P., Eagle, C. & Watanabe, M. (1995) Developing a "clinical presentation" curriculum at the University of Calgary. *Academic Medicine*, **70**, 186–193.

85  Barrows, H.S. (1984) A specific, problem-based self-directed learning method designed to teach medical problem-solving skills, and enhance knowledge retention and recall. In: Schmidt, H.G. & de Volder, M.L. (eds), *Tutorials in Problem-Based Learning*. Van Gorcum, Assen, The Netherlands.

86  Barrows, H.S. (1996) Problem-based learning in medicine and beyond: A brief overview. In: Wilkerson, L. & Gijselaers, W.H. (eds), *New Directions for Teaching and Learning*. Vol. **68**. Jossey-Bass Publishers, San Francisco, pp. 3–11.

87  Qiao, Y.Q., Shen, J., Liang, X. *et al.* (2014) Using cognitive load theory to facilitate medical education. *BMC Medical Education*, **14**, 79–85.

88  Leppink, J. (2010) Adjusting cognitive load to the student's level of expertise for increasing motivation to learn. In: *Proceedings of the Eighth International Conference on Teaching Statistics*. International Association for Statistical Education, Auckland, NZ.

89  Leppink, J. (2012) *Propositional knowledge for conceptual understanding of statistics [PhD Dissertation]*. Boekenplan, Maastricht.

90  Leppink, J., Broers, N.J., Imbos, T., Van der Vleuten, C.P.M. & Berger, M.P.F. (2011) Exploring task- and student-related factors in the method of propositional manipulation (MPM). *Journal of Statistics Education*, **19**, 1–23.

# 19 Deliberate practice and mastery learning: origins of expert medical performance

*William C. McGaghie and Theresa Kristopaitis*

*On 15 January 2009, US Airways Flight 1549 departed LaGuardia Airport in New York City en route to Charlotte/Douglas International Airport in Charlotte, North Carolina. Minutes after takeoff, the aircraft hit a flock of geese, disabling both engines completely. The Airbus A320 lost all power. The aeroplane pilot, Captain Chesley 'Sully' Sullenberger, first officer Jeff Skiles and the cabin crew responded to the crisis without hesitation. Conversation with air traffic control ruled out a ground landing either at LaGuardia or at nearby Teterboro Airport in New Jersey. The only option was ditching the aircraft in the Hudson River. The water landing was successful. All 155 passengers and crew survived the incident, several with minor injuries. Sullenberger and his crew immediately became national heroes for their cool, life-saving response to the crisis under pressure.*

## Introduction

Sullenberger's skill and leadership from the safe water landing of US Airways Flight 1549 are now legendary. Were Sullenberger (and the passengers and crew) simply lucky and fortunate that the Hudson River landing and rescue of all 155 people were flawless? Not at all. In a later magazine interview, Captain Sullenberger reported, '… everything I had done in my career had in some way been a preparation for that moment … everything I'd done in some way contributed to the outcome'.[1] Sullenberger also writes in his memoir, *Highest Duty: My Search for What Really Matters*,[2] that his passion for flying started early in life, 'At sixteen, I was already in the sky alone, practicing and practicing' and is sustained by a key principle, 'never stop learning, either professionally or personally'.

Captain Sullenberger and the flight crew achieved a successful conclusion to a potentially disastrous crisis because they had practiced the situation many times. Commercial airline pilots undergo careful screening and rigorous training before they are awarded a license to fly. Pilots and flight crew also undergo mandatory annual recurrent training throughout their careers to maintain their expertise and licenses. Preflight and recurrent training involve powerful doses of simulation-based practice with feedback, which requires prompt, professional responses to in-flight scenarios, some with life-threatening consequences. In short, airline pilots and crew practice routine flights and flight crisis management throughout their careers. The airline industry's topnotch flight safety record suggests that its history of almost no accidents is no accident.

This chapter uses Captain Sullenberger's flying expertise as an example and for inspiration. It amplifies the US Airways Flight 1549 story by addressing the history of education for clinical skill acquisition in medicine; the definition and expression of expert medical performance; the origins of medical expertise in deliberate practice (DP) of cognitive, motor, social, conative and professional skills towards their acquisition and maintenance and the transfer of skills acquired in classroom, laboratory and clinical settings to patient care practices and patient outcomes.

The chapter uses the critical-realist approach to review, synthesise and report extant literature.[3] The critical-realist approach focuses on the most compelling studies in a research domain and need not be exhaustive. It relies simultaneously on rigorous methodology and professional judgment. Rycroft-Malone and colleagues teach that, 'A realist review focuses on understanding and unpacking the mechanisms by which an intervention works (or fails to work), thereby providing an explanation, as opposed to a judgment, about how it works … the realist approach is particularly suited to the synthesis of evidence about complex implementation interventions'.[4] The evidence we review is therefore selective, focusing on key reports and examples to reinforce our ideas and arguments. The chapter is neither a systematic nor a comprehensive treatment of available literature. Our intent is to achieve three goals: (a) educate the medical and healthcare professions communities about the link

*Researching Medical Education*, First Edition. Edited by Jennifer Cleland and Steven J. Durning.
© 2015 John Wiley & Sons, Ltd. Published 2015 by John Wiley & Sons, Ltd.

between DP and acquisition of medical expertise, (b) report how clinical skills acquired in the medical education laboratory can transfer to patient care practices and patient outcomes and (c) challenge medical education researchers to advance the scholarly agenda. Several practical ideas and suggestions about improved teaching and evaluation practices are also offered.

The chapter has seven sections following these opening, stage-setting remarks. They are: (a) a brief history of clinical medical education and its persistent problems, (b) definition of medical expertise grounded in experience and science, (c) DP – definition, goals, features, role of educators, (d) DP with mastery learning (ML) for clinical skill acquisition and maintenance, (e) translational education outcomes, (f) research agenda and (g) conclusion. There is a coda, a table of five handy hints and practice points for quick application.

## History of clinical medical education

The intellectual foundation of traditional clinical medical education is grounded in 19th century thinking about the acquisition of clinical competence expressed by Sir William Osler in an address to the New York Academy of Medicine in 1903. The address, titled 'The hospital as a college', was published later in a collection of Osler's essays titled *Aequanimitas*.[5] The essay reflects Osler's earlier experience with European medical education, which he judged superior to the extant American model. Osler states, 'The radical reform needed is in the introduction into this country of the system of clinical clerks … ' Osler continues, 'In what may be called the *natural method of teaching* the student begins with the patient, continues with the patient, and ends his studies with the patient (emphasis added). Teach him how to observe, give him plenty of facts to observe, and the lessons will come out of the facts themselves'.

Osler's idea about the *natural method of teaching* was endorsed by his Johns Hopkins surgeon colleague, William Halsted who described 'the training of the surgeon' in 1904.[6] Osler and Halsted argued that the clinical medical curriculum is embodied in patients, that is, that student exposure to patients and experience over time is sufficient to ensure that physicians in training will become competent doctors. This is a passive clinical medical curriculum based solely on longitudinal patient experience. While visionary in their day, Osler and Halsted made no place for structured, graded, educational requirements; skills practice; objective evaluation

with feedback; accountability and guided reflection for novice physicians to master their craft. The Osler clinical curriculum tradition has dominated 20th century medical education and continues with modest variation into the 21st century.[7]

The 19th century model of clinical medical education is expressed in 2014 as undergraduate clinical clerkships, postgraduate residency rotations and fellowship experiences that are structured by time (weeks or months) and location (clinical site). The clinical education experiences operate in a complex healthcare environment where medical education is often subordinate to patient care and financial incentives. Structural and operational expressions of Osler's *natural method of teaching* are seen every day at medical schools, residency and fellowship programs where traditional, 'time-honored' educational practices, such as morning report and professor rounds, are preserved and sustained. Key learning outcomes among medical students or residents (e.g. clinical skill acquisition, medical record documentation and healthcare team communication) are rarely evaluated with rigour, or based on reliable data that permit valid decisions about medical learners and their educational progress.[8,9] However, traditional educational practices have been maintained by accreditation requirements that, until recently, have preserved the status quo and endorsed educational inertia.[10]

Medical education research over the last two decades has produced measured outcomes that question the utility of Osler's *natural method of teaching* based on longitudinal clinical education. Over the past 20 years, rigorous clinical skills evaluations among postgraduate resident physicians produce consistent, concerning results. For example, two large studies published by Mangione and colleagues in 1993 and 1997 were among the first to show that residents in medicine and family medicine and cardiology fellows perform poorly on objective measures of cardiac auscultation.[11,12] Year of resident training had no benefit because senior resident performance did not differ from first year residents. Cardiology fellows performed slightly better (22% correct) than residents (20% correct) on these basic skills. Residents and cardiology fellows in these two studies performed no better than medical students at evaluating heart sounds. Findings from a large and separate study reported in 1999 on resident proficiency at pulmonary auscultation replicated the poor cardiac auscultation results.[13]

Many other studies that objectively measure substandard clinical skill acquisition among physicians in training due to clinical education grounded solely in patient care experience have been published recently. Three examples include (a) a 3-year study of 126 pediatric residents reported in 1996 that showed trainees failed to meet faculty expectations about acquisition of basic skills such as physical examination, history taking, laboratory use and telephone management,[14] (b) two similar but independent studies performed at the University of Michigan in 2004 and Northwestern University in 2013 that revealed deep skill and knowledge deficits including basic proficiency with critical laboratory values, cross-cultural communication, evidence-based medicine, radiographic image interpretation, aseptic technique, invasive procedures (e.g. lumbar puncture (LP)), intensive care unit (ICU) skills and cardiac auscultation among new PGY-1 residents,[15,16] and (c) research involving 81 PGY-1 residents in internal medicine, emergency medicine, anaesthesiology and general surgery beginning postgraduate training at Northwestern University in 2013 that shows the residents, 'could not reliably identify 10 basic [ECG] findings. This is despite graduating almost exclusively from US medical schools and performing at high levels on standardised tests'.[17]

The educational ineffectiveness of reliance on clinical experience alone as a proxy measure of medical skill acquisition is evident in a recent study by Richard Bell and colleagues.[18] In this research, surgery residency program directors graded 300 operative procedures A, B or C using these criteria:

A – graduating general surgery residents should be competent to perform the procedure independently, B – graduating residents should be familiar with the procedure, but not necessarily be competent to perform it and C – graduating residents neither need to be familiar with nor competent to perform the procedure.

The actual operative experience of all US residents ($n = 1022$) completing general surgery training in June 2005 was reviewed and compared with the three procedural criteria.

The study results are sobering and address Osler's *natural method of teaching* directly. Bell and colleagues[18] state:

One-hundred twenty-one of the 300 operations were considered A level procedures by a majority of the program directors (PDs). Graduating 2005 US residents ($n = 1022$) performed only 18 of the 121 A procedures an average of more than 10 times during residency; 83 of 121 procedures were performed on average less than five times and 31 procedures

less than once. For 63 of the 121 procedures, the mode (most commonly reported) experience level was 0. In addition, there was significant variation between residents in operative experience for specific procedures.

Bell and colleagues conclude:[18]

Methods will have to be developed to allow surgeons to reach a basic level of competence in procedures which they are likely to experience only rarely during residency. Even for commonly performed procedures, the numbers of repetitions are not very robust, stressing the need to determine objectively whether residents are actually achieving basic competency in these operations.

The message from these and other studies on clinical medical education is clear and consistent. Clinical experience alone is insufficient to guarantee the acquisition of clinical competence among medical trainees.[19,20] Osler's *natural method of teaching* based only on longitudinal clinical experience without curriculum objectives and management, performance expectations, learner practice and supervision, rigorous assessment with feedback, high achievement standards and clear educational milestones is insufficient and must be restructured and improved.

## Medical expertise

In this chapter, we acknowledge that expertise in clinical medicine is defined in two different ways: (a) professional consensus and (b) scientific study captured by the expert performance approach.

### Professional consensus

Reliance on professional consensus has been used for decades as a source of authority to define medical curriculum goals and objectives, the content and structure of general and specialty medical board examinations and accreditation requirements for undergraduate medical schools and postgraduate medical training programs.[7,10] Consensus among medical professional experts, weighted heavily by physicians located in academic health science centres, is the current 'gold standard' for defining medical expertise embodied in educational curricula, test and examination criteria and standards and accreditation requirements for schools and programs.[21]

A recent expression of professional consensus as an approach to define medical expertise operationally is a 2014 report published by the

Association of American Medical Colleges (AAMC) titled *Core Entrustable Professional Activities for Entering Residency* (CEPAER).[22] The CEPAER report identifies 13 core entrustable professional activities (EPAs), which are units of professional work rather than attributes of medical people (competencies), that new graduates of US medical schools should be able to perform without direct supervision on the first day of postgraduate education. This is a call to account for US undergraduate medical schools, none of which can now certify their graduates' readiness to fulfil the EPA expectations. The EPAs range from history taking and performing a physical examination to entering and discussing orders and prescriptions, giving or receiving a patient handover, and performing general procedures of a physician. The EPAs are foundational units of medical professional work that are reasonable expectations for all new medical school graduates, expressed by an expert and representative panel of clinical physicians, endorsed and published by the AAMC.[22]

## Expert performance approach

A new method to define medical expertise empirically is embodied in the *expert performance approach*. This is a systematic framework to study expertise and to structure and operationalise the definition of expertise in medicine.[23–25] The expert performance approach relies on neither clinical experience nor peer nomination to ascribe expertise to medical doctors. Many studies, summarised by Choudhry *et al.*,[26] show that even decades of clinical experience are not a proxy for medical expertise measured objectively. Research dating from the 1970s[27] to the present[28] also finds consistently that physicians named by their peers to be 'superior' or 'expert' clinicians, or psychotherapists who have advanced degrees or specialty credentials, perform no better than other professionals [or some laypersons] when clinical skills are evaluated under controlled conditions. The expert performance approach eschews a doctor's clinical experience and status among peers as valid expertise metrics.

By contrast, the expert performance approach to study and ascribe medical expertise is grounded in scientific principles and methods. It focuses on objectively measured superior performance on clinical tasks or problems that account for expertise in a professional domain.[29] This strategy of measuring and designating medical expertise avoids using questionable criteria based on professional experience or peer reputation to identify reproducibly superior performance. As noted by Causer and Williams,[29] 'The intention in the

expert-performance approach is to recreate an environment that enables researchers to empirically quantify performance and to compare individuals under the same performance conditions'.

The expert performance approach has three connected phases to (a) isolate features of expertise, (b) identify mechanisms that produce or are responsible for expert performance and (c) create educational environments that facilitate acquisition of expertise by individuals and teams via practice, assessment, feedback and coaching.[29]

The first phase involves identifying and studying physician responses to clinical medical problems in representative situations that require prompt action. Superior performance observed in real-world settings is later replicated as standardised, simulated medical challenges under controlled laboratory conditions. Physicians with varied levels of age and experience respond to the clinical challenges, their behaviour is measured objectively and metrics are developed and refined to capture successful performance. Examples of studies to identify and isolate features of medical expertise include research in radiology (radiograph image interpretation),[30] surgery (laparoscopic and robotic procedures)[31,32] and investigations of clinical cognition (amount and organisation of knowledge, such as renal physiology).[33]

The second phase is put in place after investigators have successfully reproduced the superior performance of medical experts on representative clinical tasks. It seeks to identify mechanisms that are responsible for superior performance. This is done using process tracing methods such as 'think aloud' protocols, verbal reports, eye movements, haptic sensors and video recordings of doctors at work.[20,34] Data obtained using such procedures are used to derive theories and models to understand and explain doctors' acquisition and expression of clinical competence. For example, cognitive rehearsal, a form of mental practice, can exert a positive impact on skill acquisition and subsequent performance.[35]

The third phase of the expert performance approach involves the design, implementation and management of training environments that allow individual physicians and medical teams to acquire clinical expertise. The phase's intent is to create and manage an educational program, a curriculum, that produces doctors with knowledge, clinical skills and professionalism attributes that are measured against a high standard, generalisable across clinical situations and robust to decay. A key feature of such a clinical medical curriculum is to provide opportunities for physicians in training to

*Table 19.1* Expert performance approach phases for undergraduate (UME), graduate (GME) and continuing (CME) medical education

| Phases | UME | GME | CME |
| --- | --- | --- | --- |
| 1. Isolate features of expertise | Cardiac auscultation, that is, discriminate heart sounds[86] | Basic clinical skills for internal medicine residents: physical examination findings, procedural skills, management of critically ill patients, communication with patients[16] | Diagnostic imaging of the bronchial tree and image interpretation using ultrasonography[87] |
| 2. Identify mechanisms that produce or are responsible for expertise | Auditory acuity, prior knowledge of cardiac physiology, achievement motivation | M.D. degree, prior knowledge measured by USMLE Step 1 and Step 2 scores, brief clinical experience, achievement motivation | Licensed healthcare professionals, extensive clinical experience, achievement motivation, opportunity for institutional recognition |
| 3. Create an educational environment that promotes acquisition of expertise | High-fidelity cardiology simulator, deliberate practice with coaching, measurement, feedback and minimum performance standards[86] | Three-day clinical 'boot camp' with small group teaching, deliberate practice, evaluation, feedback and minimum performance standards[16] | Prerequisite readings, simulated critical care scenarios, pre-post evaluations, deliberate practice, feedback, self-assessment, self-directed online portfolio[87] |

work hard under controlled conditions to acquire clinical skills identified and elaborated from the first and second expert performance approach phases.[21]

Table 19.1 gives examples of the three phases of the expert performance approach for undergraduate, graduate and continuing medical education.

The expert performance approach is establishing roots as a new strategy to define medical expertise criteria and shape expectations, structures and outcome measures for medical education curricula at all levels. Whether they originate from experience or empirical study, achievement of medical learning objectives can now be advanced by a new concept from learning science – DP – which provides a clear, evidence-based technology for skill and knowledge acquisition.

## Deliberate practice

DP is a term conceived and advanced by psychologist K. Anders Ericsson[36–38] and his colleagues. Ericsson sought to study and explain the acquisition of expertise in a variety of skill domains including sports, music, writing, science and the learned professions including medicine and surgery.[39] The research goal was to isolate and explain the variables responsible for the acquisition and maintenance of superior reproducible (expert) performance. Ericsson and his colleagues found consistently that the origins of expert performance across skill domains do not reside in measured intelligence, scholastic aptitude or longitudinal experience. Instead, the

acquisition of expertise stems from approximately 10,000 hours of DP in a focused skill domain.[40]

Ericsson writes that his research group '

> … identified a set of conditions where practice had been uniformly associated with improved performance. Significant improvements in performance were realized when individuals were (a) given a task with a well-defined goal, (b) motivated to improve, (c) provided with feedback, and (d) provided with ample opportunities for repetition and gradual refinements of their performance. Deliberate efforts to improve one's performance beyond its current level demands full concentration and often requires problem-solving and better methods of performing the tasks'.[38]

DP in medical education settings means that learners are engaged in difficult, goal-oriented work, supervised by teachers, who provide feedback and correction, under conditions of high achievement expectations, with revision and improvement. Maintenance of the clinical status quo is insufficient. To illustrate, the world famous cardiac surgeon Denton A. Cooley[41] writes in his memoir *100,000 Hearts* about the countless hours of practice in animal and cadaver laboratories, biomedical engineering laboratories, carpentry shops and focused surgical practice with feedback from different sources he experienced to master and advance his craft. This far exceeds the 10,000-hour rule that Ericsson has set as a minimum requirement for the acquisition of expertise in a variety of domains. Another example from the sports world is the DP of basketball star Michael Jordan. Despite his physical gifts and commitment to teamwork, Michael Jordan shot 500 free-throws (practice baskets) every day of his professional career.[42] Similarly, Captain Sullenberger, Denton Cooley and Michael Jordan never stopped practicing and always tried to improve.

A more practical, and granular, definition of DP is presented here for medical educators who intend to embed the approach in learner educational experiences. This list of *10 essential features of DP* is a distillate drawn from several sources.[38,43,44]

## Ten essential features of deliberate practice

1 Highly motivated learners with good concentration and active coaching;

2 Engagement with a well-defined learning objective or task; at an

3 Appropriate level of difficulty [emphasis on difficult aspects]; with

4 Focused, repetitive practice [stop and start]; that leads to

5 Rigorous, precise educational measurements; that yields

6 Immediate, informative feedback from educational sources (e.g. simulators and teachers) focused on areas of weakness; and where

7 Trainees also monitor their learning experiences and current strategies, errors and levels of understanding; and

8 Consciously engage in more DP with gradual refinements in performance; and continue with

9 Evaluation to reach a mastery standard and then

10 Advance to another task or unit.

The comparative effectiveness evidence about medical education grounded in DP versus traditional clinical education leaves no doubt that DP yields better results. A recent head-to-head meta-analytic investigation reported in *Academic Medicine* in 2011 compared outcomes derived from 14 studies of traditional clinical education versus simulation-based clinical education with DP.[45] The quantitative results are unequivocal and without exception. Traditional, Oslerian clinical education fell short in every individual comparison and across all 14 studies. The overall effect size ($r = 0.71$) translates to a Cohen's *d* coefficient $= 2.00$, which is very large.[46] These and other empirical data that demonstrate a dose–response relationship between DP and medical skill acquisition[47] strongly suggest that the traditional Oslerian approach to medical education featuring clinical experience alone is obsolete.

Medical educators are responsible for creating the conditions where learners can undergo the DP needed to acquire and maintain essential clinical skills, judgment and professionalism – the core objectives of medical education. This is a behavioural engineering problem. The question is, given learning objectives for individual medical learners or clinical care teams, how can educational experiences be designed, implemented and calibrated to help learners acquire the competencies? The answer stems from thoughtful curriculum planning, DP management, reliable measurement, feedback, learner achievement to a mastery standard and advancement to next objectives.

Medical educators work hard to fulfil DP responsibilities on behalf of learners. Passive experience has no place either for learners or teachers in a DP environment. Educators are active mentors and coaches.[48] Recent examples that illustrate the power of DP to increase knowledge and skill acquisition among clinical medical learners include studies on patient handoff communication,[49] pediatric resuscitation[50] and technical performance in surgery.[51] In these and other studies featuring DP, learners are engaged trainees, not passive observers.

A second sports analogy about the importance of coaching in DP is instructive for medical education researchers. This example is taken from the book *Basketball: Multiple Offense and Defense,*[52] written by legendary University of North Carolina basketball coach Dean Smith (Michael Jordan's mentor). Smith writes, 'The organization, the preparation, the execution, plus a coach's entire philosophy is implemented in the all-important practice session'. He continues, 'Each player's motivation should be to walk off the practice floor a better player than he was when he arrived for the session. The coach has the responsibility of helping every player meet this goal'. Smith continues to describe the daily, 2-hour practice sessions that are goal-directed, planned to the minute, involving praise and peer pressure, having no idle time, with two 90-second water breaks. Coach Smith asserts, 'Coaches must push players to a point beyond which the players would like to stop'. 'This kind of effort builds *mental toughness* … the harder a team works to achieve its goals, the stronger will be its determination to accomplish them'.

DP experiences reported in medical education approximate, but do not duplicate, the intensity found in competitive sports programs. An example is the work of internist Diane B. Wayne[53] and her education team, which used the DP model to educate internal medicine residents to perform thoracentesis to high and uniform ML standards. The dose of deliberate thoracentesis skills practice in the medical simulation laboratory was at least 4 hours for each trainee. Several of the residents (3/40 = 8%) 'needed extra time ranging from 20 to 90 minutes to reach mastery'. The end result is that at the conclusion of training, all of the residents met or exceeded the clinical skill acquisition goals, without exception. The research report concludes, '... residents strongly agreed that practice with the medical simulator boosts clinical skills and self-confidence, that they received useful feedback from the training sessions, and that DP using the simulator is a valuable educational experience'.[53]

## Deliberate practice and mastery learning

ML in medical education is an especially stringent form of competency-based education.[54] ML requires 'excellence for all', knowledge and skill acquisition to high achievement standards without regard to learning time. As stated elsewhere,[55,56] the ML model has at least eight properties, which include DP, to promote high achievement among medical learners.

### Eight properties of mastery learning

1 Baseline, that is, diagnostic testing
2 Clear learning objectives, expressed as units ordered by difficulty
3 Educational activities (e.g. deliberate skills practice) focused on the objectives
4 Minimum passing *mastery* standard (MPS) for each unit
5 Formative testing with feedback to assess progress towards the MPS for each unit
6 Advancement if performance ≥MPS or
7 Continued practice or study until the MPS is reached
8 Learning time can vary among trainees, but outcomes are uniform.

The goal of ML is to certify that all medical learners achieve all educational objectives with little or no variation in outcome. This is a practical, operational definition of acquiring expert medical performance from a curriculum. The amount of time needed to reach the mastery standard for a unit's educational objectives varies among the learners.[55,56]

In medical education, ML has been used primarily for acquisition and maintenance of clinical procedural skills, such as advanced cardiac life support (ACLS),[57] paracentesis[58] and central venous catheter (CVC) insertion.[59] However, ML with DP has also been used to help learners acquire and refine cognitive and affective education outcomes. Research shows, for example, that competence to engage a family in a difficult conversation about end-of-life issues is a clinical skill that improves with DP with standardised patients, just like performance of an invasive procedure.[60]

A recent study by Barsuk and colleagues illustrates the power of DP with ML to help PGY-1 internal medicine (IM) residents acquire skills with a basic clinical procedure – LP.[61] The study also contrasts the IM residents' LP competence with the LP skills of PGY-2, -3 and -4 neurology residents who learnt the procedure using traditional clinical education. As expected, the IM residents expressed much variation at baseline pretesting using an LP simulator. However, after a minimum 3-hour education session featuring DP with feedback, all IM residents met or surpassed an LP mastery standard at post-test. By contrast, only 2 of 36 (6%) traditionally trained PGY-2, -3 and -4 neurology residents met the passing standard although they had much more LP clinical experience. The investigators also report that 42% of the traditionally trained neurology residents did not even specify routine laboratory tests for cerebrospinal fluid after the specimen was obtained. The article concludes, 'Few [traditionally trained] neurology residents were competent to perform a simulated LP despite clinical experience with the procedure'.[61]

An editorial titled, 'Does experience doing LPs result in expertise? A medical maxim bites the dust', accompanied publication of the LP ML research report.[62] The editorial states, 'The Barsuk *et al.*[62] study is clearly a wake-up call for all of us who were trained in the era of 'see one, do one, teach one' – the so-called 'apprenticeship' model of clinical training. The old training methods are no longer enough to ensure the best education, and thus the best care for patients'.

A growing body of research evidence now shows that medical education featuring ML with DP can lead to better health for individuals and populations.[63] This line of investigation casts medical education research as translational science because the outcomes of powerful educational interventions are linked directly with better and safer patient care practices and patient outcomes.[64]

## Translational education outcomes

Translational outcomes are educational effects measured at progressively distal levels beginning in a classroom or simulation laboratory (T1) and moving downstream to improved and safer patient care practices (T2), better patient outcomes (T3)[64] and collateral effects (T4), such as cost savings,[65] skill retention[66,67] and systemic educational and patient care improvements.[68,69]

At least five recent review articles, which address translational outcomes, that derive from powerful medical education interventions have been published recently.[70–74] Most of the reports of original research that are synthesised in the reviews employ simulation-based medical education, frequently with DP, many grounded in the ML model. The common message from this growing body of medical education science is that rigorous medical education including reliable measures can have a direct effect on patient and public health outcomes that really matter, for example, reduced ICU infection rates,[75] lower childbirth complications,[76] faster surgical recovery,[77] reduced hospital length of stay[78] and fewer blood transfusions and ICU admissions.[78] We anticipate that the list of translational outcomes resulting from medical education interventions featuring DP and ML will expand as the training model spreads and the science advances.

Translational education outcomes are difficult to reach and cannot be achieved from isolated, one-shot studies. Instead, translational results in medical education research come from integrated education and health services research programs that are thematic, sustained and cumulative. Such research programs usually involve interdisciplinary teams, composed of a diverse group of scientists and scholars, and must be carefully designed and managed to yield strong results.[79]

## Research agenda

The research agenda needed to fully address the DP and ML origins of expert medical performance is both broad and deep. Other publications have started the agenda-setting discussion.[43,74] The following short list covers only those topics where we believe the need for solid research evidence is most acute. We choose to highlight seven key issues that warrant research attention.

1 More studies are needed that use the expert performance approach to better identify reproducibly superior medical performance (expertise) in laboratory settings. The volume of such work today is very modest. We need to place greater reliance on evidence-based approaches to ascribe expertise given the known flaws and sources of

bias that affect peer nominations and socially ascribed expertise designations.

2 Development of measures that yield reliable data which permit valid decisions to be made about the effects of educational interventions is a chronic problem. Most of the studies covered in this chapter used observational checklists as principal outcome measures. There is an acute need to create measures that capture expert performance with complex clinical cases (e.g. management of a diabetic patient with multiple interacting problems) that cannot be reduced to dichotomous (done/not done) responses.

3 DP is not a uniform construct. DP has many possible variations depending, for example, on the knowledge or skill set being acquired and studied. Research is needed to isolate the conditions, intensity, duration, feedback features and other moderator variables that make DP effective.

4 Healthcare is now a team-based enterprise rather than being delivered by solo practitioners. Thus there is a need for rigorous research to determine if the ML model works for team-based competencies. We also need to learn more about the translational potential of team-based competencies in healthcare, although early research is promising.[76,80]

5 Research is needed to identify and measure the skill set and DP experiences that make simulation instructors effective. This is expert performance approach research focused on expertise among medical simulation teachers versus medical experts in clinical practice. Evidence is needed to better understand the expertise of individual instructors and educational teams.

6 Institutional research framed by principles of implementation science is needed to better comprehend how innovative educational programs featuring DP and ML are created, implemented, sustained and evaluated.[81] Quantitative and qualitative research programs are needed not only to demonstrate that innovations such as simulation-based ML with DP produce intended results, but also to show how and why the results are transferred and achieved in different settings.[82,83]

7 The expert performance approach to capturing and measuring expertise in the laboratory has limits because it emphasises focused skill domains and standardised tasks. This approach works well for healthcare professionals who work in focused skill domains (e.g. radiology) but less well for those who are active in less-controlled professional environments (e.g. family medicine and emergency medicine). Professional performance

in uncontrolled or unfamiliar domains is very complex and must be *adaptive*.[84,85] Medical education research is needed to better understand and measure adaptive expertise among clinicians. Educational models are also needed to promote the acquisition of adaptive expertise among healthcare professionals from DP.

## Conclusion

This chapter began with a heroic anecdote about expertise in aviation and how Captain Sullenberger attributed his flying expertise to many years of practice beginning in adolescence. The discussion continued with a short history of clinical medical education to reveal Osler's legacy of passive clinical learning that persists today in many forms. We then addressed how the definition of medical expertise is usually based on professional consensus while a new research paradigm, the expert performance approach, is beginning to define medical expertise empirically. DP, grounded in learning science, is defined in detail including its marriage with ML to reach learning goals of clinical skill acquisition and maintenance. The chapter concludes with brief discussions about translational education outcomes and a proposed research agenda.

A large body of research evidence now shows clearly that DP coupled with ML can produce strong, sometimes translational outcomes when designed, implemented and evaluated with thought and care. We encourage other educational scientists to join the research collaboration on this innovation in clinical medical education.

### Practice Points

1 DP and ML can produce powerful and lasting results among medical learners in classrooms and medical simulation laboratories (T1 outcomes).

2 Carefully designed and executed medical education and health services research programs can produce downstream results measured as improved patient care practices, better patient outcomes and collateral effects (T2, T3 and T4 outcomes). Such research programs need to be thematic, sustained and cumulative.

3 Medical education and research featuring DP and ML can be accomplished using modest resources. Careful research planning and nimble colleagues are more important for success than a big budget.

4 The medical educator role is critical in environments that feature DP and ML. Setting goals, active coaching, measuring progress, giving feedback and acknowledging success by learners are all key educational activities that must be fulfilled.

5 The research agenda needed to fully address DP and ML in medical education is broad and deep with many opportunities for significant scholarship.

## References

1 Shiner L. (2009) *Sully's Tale: Chesley Sullenberger talks about that day, his advice for young pilots, and hitting the ditch button (or not)*. URL http://airspacemag.com/as-interview/aamps-interview-sullys-tale-53584029/?no-ist [accessed on 15 April 2014]

2 Sullenberger, C. (2009) *Highest Duty: My Search for What Really Matters*. Harper, New York.

3 McGaghie, W.C. (2015) Varieties of integrative scholarship. *Academic Medicine*, **90**, 294–302.

4 Roycroft-Malone, J., McCormack, B., Hutchinson, A.M. *et al.* (2012) Realist synthesis: illustrating the method for implementation research. *Implementation Science*, **7**, 33.

5 Osler, W. (1932) The hospital as a college. In: Osler, W. (ed), *Aequanimitas*. P. Blakiston's Son & Co., Philadelphia.

6 Halsted, W.S. (1904) The training of the surgeon. *Bulletin of the Johns Hopkins Hospital*, **15**, 267–275.

7 Ludmerer, K.M. (1996) *Learning to Heal: The Development of American Medical Education*. Johns Hopkins University Press, Baltimore.

8 Downing, S.M. (2004) Reliability: on the reproducibility of assessment data. *Medical Education*, **38**, 1006–1012.

9 Downing, S.M. (2003) Validity: on the meaningful interpretation of assessment data. *Medical Education*, **37**, 830–837.

10 Nasca, T.J., Philibert, I., Brigham, Y. & Flynn, T.C. (2012) The next GME accreditation system—rationale and benefits. *New England Journal of Medicine*, **366**, 1051–1056.

11 Mangione, S., Nieman, L.Z., Graceley, E. *et al.* (1993) The teaching and practice of cardiac auscultation during internal medicine and cardiology training. *Annals of Internal Medicine*, **119**, 47–54.

12 Mangione, S. & Nieman, L.Z. (1997) Cardiac auscultatory skills of internal medicine and family practice trainees: a comparison of diagnostic proficiency. *JAMA*, **278**, 717–722.

13 Mangione, S. & Nieman, L.Z. (1999) Pulmonary auscultatory skills during training in internal medicine and family practice. *American Journal of Respiratory and Critical Care Medicine*, **159**, 1119–1124.

14 Joorabchi, B. & Devries, J.M. (1996) Evaluation of clinical competence: the gap between expectations and performance. *Pediatrics*, **97**, 179–184.

15 Lypson, M.L., Frohna, J.G., Gruppen, L.D. *et al.* (2004) Assessing residents' competencies at baseline: identifying the gaps. *Academic Medicine*, **79**, 564–570.

16 Cohen, E.R., Barsuk, J.H., Moazed, F. *et al.* (2013) Making July safer: mastery learning of clinical skills during intern bootcamp. *Academic Medicine*, **88**, 233–239.

17 Wilcox, J.E., Raval, Z., Patel, A.B. *et al.* (2014) Imperfect beginnings: incoming residents vary in their ability to interpret basic electrocardiogram findings. *Journal of Hospital Medicine*, **9**, 197–198.

18 Bell, R.H. Jr., Biester, T.W., Tabuenca, A. *et al.* (2009) Operative experience of residents in U.S. general surgery programs: a gap between expectation and experience. *Annals of Surgery*, **249**, 719–724.

19 Kyser, K.L., Lu, X., Santillan, D. *et al.* (2014) Forceps delivery volumes in teaching and nonteaching hospitals: are volumes sufficient for physicians to acquire and maintain competence? *Academic Medicine*, **89**, 71–76.

20 Ericsson, K.A. (2014) Necessity is the mother of invention: video recording firsthand perspectives of critical medical procedures to make simulated training more effective. *Academic Medicine*, **89**, 17–20.

21 Kern, D.E., Thomas, P.A. & Hughes, M.T. (eds) (2009) *Curriculum Development for Medical Education: A Six-Step Approach.* The Johns Hopkins University Press, Baltimore.

22 Flynn, T., Chair, Drafting Panel. (2014) *Core Entrustable Professional Activities for Entering Residency* (CEPAER). Washington, DC, Association of American Medical Colleges.

23 Ericsson, K.A. & Smith, J. (1991) Prospects and limits of the empirical study of expertise: an introduction. In: Ericsson, K.A. & Smith, J. (eds), *Toward a General Theory of Expertise: Prospects and Limits.* Cambridge University Press, New York, pp. 1–38.

24 Ericsson, K.A. & Ward, P. (2007) Capturing the naturally occurring superior performance of experts in the laboratory. *Current Directions in Psychological Science*, **16**, 346–350.

25 Ericsson, K.A. & Williams, A.M. (2007) Capturing naturally occurring superior performance in the laboratory: translational research on expert performance. *Journal of Experimental Psychology Applied*, **13**, 115–123.

26 Choudhry, N.K., Fletcher, R.H. & Soumerai, S.B. (2005) Systematic review: the relationship between clinical experience and quality of health care. *Annals of Internal Medicine*, **142**, 260–273.

27 Elstein, A.S., Shulman, L.S. & Sprafka, S.A. (1978) *Medical Problem Solving: An Analysis of Clinical Reasoning.* Harvard University Press, Cambridge, MA.

28 Dawes, R.M. (1994) *House of Cards: Psychology and Psychotherapy Built on Myth.* Free Press, New York.

29 Causer, J. & Williams, A.M. (2013) Professional expertise in medicine. In: Lanzer, P. (ed), *Catheter-Based Cardiovascular Interventions.* Springer-Verlag, Berlin, pp. 97–112.

30 Lesgold, A., Glaser, R., Rubinson, H. *et al.* (1988) Expertise in a complex skill: diagnosing X-ray pictures. In: Chi, M., Glaser, R. & Farr, M.J. (eds), *The Nature of Expertise.* Erlbaum, Hillsdale, NJ, pp. 311–342.

31 Schijven, M. & Jakimowicz, J. (2003) Construct validity: experts and novices performing on the Xitact LS500 laparoscopy simulator. *Surgical Endoscopy*, **17**, 803–810.

32 Verner, L., Oleynikov, D., Holtman, S. *et al.* (2003) Measurements of the level of surgical expertise using flight path analysis from *da Vinci*™ robotic surgical system. In: Westwood, J.D., *et al.* (eds), *Medicine Meets Virtual Reality 11.* IOS Press, Amsterdam, pp. 373–378.

33 Norman, G.R., Eva, K., Brooks, L. & Hamstra, S. (2006) Expertise in medicine and surgery. In: Ericsson, K.A., Charness, N., Feltovich, P.J. & Hoffman, R.R. (eds), *The Cambridge Handbook of Expertise and Expert Performance.* Cambridge University Press, New York, pp. 339–353.

34 Ericsson, K.A. (2006) Protocol analysis and expert thought: concurrent verbalizations of thinking during experts' performance on representative tasks. In: Ericsson, K.A., Charness, N., Feltovich, P.J. & Hoffman, R.R. (eds), *The Cambridge Handbook of Expertise and Expert Performance.* Cambridge University Press, New York, pp. 223–241.

35 Driskell, J.E., Cooper, C. & Moran, A. (1994) Does mental practice enhance performance? *Journal of Applied Psychology*, **79**, 481–492.

36 Ericsson, K.A., Krampe, R.T. & Tesch-Römer, C. (1993) The role of deliberate practice in the acquisition of expert performance. *Psychological Review*, **100**, 363–406.

37 Ericsson, K.A. (2004) Deliberate practice and the acquisition and maintenance of expert performance in medicine and related domains. *Academic Medicine*, **79**, S70–S81.

38 Ericsson, K.A. (2008) Deliberate practice and acquisition of expert performance: a general overview. *Academic Emergency Medicine*, **15**, 988–994.

39 Ericsson, K.A., Charness, N., Feltovich, P.J. & Hoffman, R.R. (eds) (2006) *The Cambridge Handbook of Expertise and Expert Performance.* Cambridge University Press, New York.

40 Ericsson, K.A., Prietula, M.J. & Cokely, E.T. (2007) The making of an expert. *Harvard Business Review*, **85**, 115–121.

41 Cooley, D.A. (2012) *100,000 Hearts: A Surgeon's Memoir.* Dolph Briscoe Center for American History, University of Texas at Austin, Austin, TX.

42 Jordan, M. (1998) *For the Love of the Game.* Crown Publishers, New York.

43 McGaghie, W.C. (2008) Research opportunities in simulation-based medical education using deliberate practice. *Academic Emergency Medicine*, **15**, 995–1001.

44 Shadrick, S.B. & Lussier, J.W. (2009) Training complex cognitive skills: a theme-based approach to the development of battlefield skills. In: Ericsson, K.A. (ed), *Development of Professional Expertise: Toward Measurement of Expert Performance and Design of Optimal*

*Learning Environments.* Cambridge University Press, New York, pp. 286–311.

45 McGaghie, W.C., Issenberg, S.B., Cohen, E.R. *et al.* (2011) Does simulation-based medical education with deliberate practice yield better results than traditional clinical education? A meta-analytic comparative review of the evidence. *Academic Medicine,* **86**, 706–711.

46 Borenstein, M. (2009) Effect sizes for continuous data. In: Cooper, H., Hedges, L.V. & Valentine, J.C. (eds), *The Handbook of Research Synthesis and Meta-Analysis,* 2nd edn. Russell Sage Foundation, New York, pp. 221–236.

47 McGaghie, W.C., Issenberg, S.B., Petrusa, E.R. & Scalese, R.J. (2006) Effect of practice on standardized learning outcomes in simulation-based medical education. *Medical Education,* **40**, 792–797.

48 Gifford, K.A. & Fall, L.H. (2014) Doctor coach: a deliberate practice approach to teaching and learning clinical skills. *Academic Medicine,* **89**, 272–276.

49 Sawatsky, A.P., Mikhael, J.R., Punatar, A.D. *et al.* (2013) The effects of deliberate practice and feedback to teach standardized handoff communication on the knowledge, attitudes, and practices of first-year residents. *Teaching and Learning in Medicine,* **25**, 279–284.

50 Hunt, E.A., Duval-Arnould, J.M., Nelson-McMillan, K.L. *et al.* (2014) Pediatric resident resuscitation skills improve after "rapid cycle deliberate practice" training. *Resuscitation,* **85**, 945–951.

51 Palter, V.N. & Grantcharov, T.P. (2014) Individualized deliberate practice on a virtual reality simulator improves technical performance of surgical novices in the operating room: a randomized controlled trial. *Annals of Surgery,* **259**, 443–448.

52 Smith, D. (1999) *Basketball: Multiple Offense and Defense.* Allyn and Bacon, Boston.

53 Wayne, D.B., Barsuk, J.H., O'Leary, K.J. *et al.* (2008) Mastery learning of thoracentesis skills by internal medicine residents using simulation technology and deliberate practice. *Journal of Hospital Medicine,* **3**, 48–54.

54 McGaghie, W.C., Miller, G.E., Sajid, A. & Telder, T.V. (1978) *Competency-Based Curriculum Development in Medical Education.* Public Health Paper No. 68. World Health Organization, Geneva.

55 McGaghie, W.C., Siddall, V.S., Mazmanian, P.E. & Myers, J. (2009) Lessons for continuing medical education from simulation research in undergraduate and graduate medical education: Effectiveness of continuing medical education: American College of Chest Physicians evidence-based educational guidelines. *CHEST,* **135**, 62S–68S.

56 Wong, B.S. & Kang, L. (2012) Mastery learning in the context of university education. *Journal of NUS Teaching Academy,* **2**, 206–222.

57 Wayne, D.B., Butter, J., Siddall, V.J. *et al.* (2006) Mastery learning of advanced cardiac life support skills by internal medicine residents using simulation technology and deliberate practice. *Journal of General Internal Medicine,* **21**, 251–256.

58 Barsuk, J.H., Cohen, E.R., Vozenilek, J.A. *et al.* (2012) Simulation-based education with mastery learning improves paracentesis skills. *Journal of Graduate Medical Education,* **4**, 23–27.

59 Barsuk, J.H., McGaghie, W.C., Cohen, E.R. *et al.* (2009) Use of simulation-based mastery learning to improve the quality of central venous catheter placement in a medical intensive care unit. *Journal of Hospital Medicine,* **4**, 397–403.

60 Szmuilowicz, E., Neeley, K.J., Sharma, R.K. *et al.* (2012) Improving residents' code status discussion skills: a randomized trial. *Journal of Palliative Medicine,* **15**, 768–774.

61 Barsuk, J.H., Cohen, E.R., Caprio, T. *et al.* (2012) Simulation-based education with mastery learning improves residents' lumbar puncture skills. *Neurology,* **79**, 132–137.

62 Nathan, B.R. & Kincaid, O. (2012) Does experience doing lumbar punctures result in expertise? A medical maxim bites the dust. *Neurology,* **79**, 115–116.

63 McGaghie, W.C., Issenberg, S.B., Cohen, E.R. *et al.* (2011) Medical education featuring mastery learning with deliberate practice can lead to better health for individuals and populations. *Academic Medicine,* **86**, e8–e9.

64 McGaghie, W.C. (2010) Medical education research as translational science. *Science Translational Medicine,* **2**, 19–8.

65 Cohen, E.R., Feinglass, J., Barsuk, J.H. *et al.* (2010) Cost savings from reduced catheter-related bloodstream infection after simulation-based education for residents in a medical intensive care unit. *Simulation in Healthcare,* **5**, 98–102.

66 Ahya, S.N., Barsuk, J.H., Cohen, E.R. *et al.* (2012) Clinical performance and skill retention after simulation-based education for nephrology fellows. *Seminars in Dialysis,* **25**, 470–473.

67 Moazed, F., Cohen, E.R., Furiasse, N. *et al.* (2013) Retention of critical care skills after simulation-based mastery learning. *Journal of Graduate Medical Education,* **5**, 458–463.

68 Barsuk, J.H., Cohen, E.R., Feinglass, J. *et al.* (2011) Unexpected collateral effects of simulation-based medical education. *Academic Medicine,* **86**, 1513–1517.

69 Cohen, E.R., Barsuk, J.H., McGaghie, W.C. & Wayne, D.B. (2013) Raising the bar: reassessing standards for procedural competence. *Teaching and Learning in Medicine,* **25**, 6–9.

70 McGaghie, W.C., Draycott, T.J., Dunn, W.F. *et al.* (2011) Evaluating the impact of simulation on translational patient outcomes. *Simulations in Healthcare,* **6**, 42–47.

71 McGaghie, W.C., Issenberg, S.B., Cohen, E.R. *et al.* (2012) Translational educational research: a necessity for effective healthcare improvement. *CHEST,* **142**, 1097–1103.

72 Zendejas, B., Brydges, R., Wang, A.T. & Cook, D.A. (2012) Patient outcomes in simulation-based medical education: a systematic review. *Journal of General Internal Medicine,* **28**, 1078–1089.

73  Griswold, S., Ponnuru, S., Nishisaki, A. *et al.* (2012) The emerging role of simulation education to achieve patient safety: translating deliberate practice and debriefing to save lives. *Pediatric Clinics of North America*, **59**, 1329–1340.

74  McGaghie, W.C., Issenberg, S.B., Barsuk, J.H. & Wayne, D.B. (2014) A critical review of simulation-based mastery learning with translational outcomes. *Medical Education*, **48**, 375–385.

75  Barsuk, J.H., Cohen, E.R., Feinglass, J. *et al.* (2009) Use of simulation-based education to reduce catheter-related bloodstream infections. *Archives of Internal Medicine*, **169**, 1420–1423.

76  Draycott, T.J., Sibanda, T., Owen, L. *et al.* (2006) Does training in obstetric emergencies improve neonatal outcome? *British Journal of Obstetrics and Gynaecology*, **113**, 177–182.

77  Zendejas, B., Cook, D.A., Bingener, J. *et al.* (2011) Simulation-based mastery learning improves patient outcomes in laparoscopic inguinal hernia repair: a randomized controlled trial. *Annals of Surgery*, **254**, 502–511.

78  Barsuk, J.H., Cohen, E.R., Feinglass, J. *et al.* (2013) Clinical outcomes after bedside and interventional radiology paracentesis procedures. *American Journal of Medicine*, **126**, 349–356.

79  Page, S.E. (2007) *The Difference: How the Power of Diversity Creates Better Groups, Firms, Schools, and Society.* Princeton University Press, Princeton, NJ.

80  Siassakos, D., Fox, R., Bristowe, K. *et al.* (2013) What makes maternity teams effective and safe? Lessons from a series of research on teamwork, leadership and team training. *Acta Obstetricia et Gynecologica Scandinavica*, **92**, 1239–1243.

81  Bonham, A.C. & Solomon, M.Z. (2010) Moving comparative effectiveness research into practice: implementation science and the role of academic medicine. *Health Affairs*, **29**, 1901–1905.

82  Dixon-Woods, M., Bosk, C.L., Aveling, E.L. *et al.* (2011) Explaining Michigan: developing an ex post theory of a quality improvement programme. *Milbank Quarterly*, **89**, 167–205.

83  Barsuk, J.H., Cohen, E.R., Potts, S. *et al.* (2014) Dissemination of a simulation-based mastery learning intervention reduces central line-associated bloodstream infections. *BMJ Quality and Safety*, **23**, 749–756.

84  Ericsson, K.A. (2014) Adaptive expertise and cognitive readiness: a perspective from the expert performance approach. In: O'Neil, H.F., Perez, R.S. & Baker, E.L. (eds), *Teaching and Measuring Cognitive Readiness.* Springer, New York, pp. 179–197.

85  Carbonell, K.B., Stalmeijer, R.E., Könings, K.D. *et al.* (2014) How experts deal with novel situations: a review of adaptive expertise. *Education Research and Reviews*, **12**, 14–29.

86  Butter, J., McGaghie, W.C., Cohen, E.R. *et al.* (2010) Simulation-based mastery learning improves cardiac auscultation skills in medical students. *Journal of General Internal Medicine*, **25**, 780–785.

87  American College of Chest Physicians (2014). *Critical care ultrasonography live learning course materials, update 2014.* URL http://www.chestnet.org/Education/ [accessed 16 July 2014]

# 20 Reframing research on widening participation in medical education: using theory to inform practice

*Sandra Nicholson and Jennifer Cleland*

*At the interview for medical school that I went to, most of the other students were middle class … Well, I don't know if they were middle class. They came across to me as middle class. But sometimes it feels like they have links that you don't. They've been to all these different things; they've met all these different people. Sometimes it feels like medicine is like this game, where if you have links to enough people, you have an advantage. Because you can get work experience with this person or you can get an advantage in that way. I know it sounds as though I'm playing the smallest violin but it does make a difference who you know* (Focus group participant, inner city London school, p. 12 interview 3.)[1]

## Introduction

The concerns of this UK applicant to medicine are typical of those who come from 'non-traditional' lower socio-economic (see later for definition) backgrounds. Their perceptions of the disadvantages they face, or may face, in the medical admission process are also expressed by medical admission faculty.[2,3] Moreover, this issue is not unique to the United Kingdom: across the world, young people with the academic and personal attributes to successfully study medicine and be doctors face disadvantages associated with demographic factors such as ethnicity, minority group membership and/or low income.[4]

These 'disadvantages' often have a common key factor: inequalities in pre-university education. It is argued that this factor underlies the under-representation of medical school applicants from diverse ethnicities, low income or other demographic disadvantaged groups.[5,6] It is, therefore, important to understand, and address, the educational disadvantages and the inequalities experienced by certain medical school applicants in order to bring about change in terms of increasing medical student diversity globally. Expanding upon the inequalities in pre-university education

experienced by many under-represented groups is beyond the scope of this chapter but includes under-resourced schools[7] and schooling that occurs within a culture of low aspiration.[8]

The goal of this chapter is to introduce how the currently under-theorised field of widening access (WA) to medicine could progress by the use of theoretical and conceptual frameworks. Because of the relative lack of robust research on this topic, this chapter differs from others in this book as we present the issues first, and then outline how research could move beyond the existing evidence by the use of theory and conceptual frameworks to inform practice and future research. This is primarily achieved by illustrating how three theoretical lenses are used separately to examine one dataset. While cognisant that the focus of this book is healthcare education research, the issue of WA is mostly relevant to medicine and hence our focus in this chapter is medical education. However, first, some definitions are presented to aid clarity.

> ### BOX 20.1   Key definitions
>
> Widening participation (WP) refers to the policy that people such as those coming from disadvantaged backgrounds, mature students, students from ethnic and cultural groups and disabled students should be encouraged to take part, and be represented proportionately, within higher education (HE). This is based on ensuring equality of opportunity, and relates to improving social mobility that can be defined as breaking the transmission of disadvantage from one generation to the next.[9] When a society is mobile, individuals have more opportunities of progressing in terms of income or occupation. Summer Schools and activities designed to increase educational aspiration in under-represented groups are examples of initiatives derived from WP policies.

*Researching Medical Education*, First Edition. Edited by Jennifer Cleland and Steven J. Durning.
© 2015 John Wiley & Sons, Ltd. Published 2015 by John Wiley & Sons, Ltd.

WA, on the other hand, emphasises more the equality or fairness of the selection processes that act as a gateway to HE. This may refer to specific selection policies that increase the matriculation of certain unrepresented groups. Affirmative action policies that existed in the United States before the US Supreme Court ruled them as illegal[10] proved successful in increasing the numbers of Black and Minority Ethnicities (BME) enrolled at medical schools.[11] Some Australian medical schools have specific number of places reserved for applicants from rural backgrounds who because of educational disadvantage may not successfully compete due to collective lower GPA scores.[12]

The term non-traditional when used in the context of medical students refers to those students whose gender, race, ethnicity, culture, socio-economic status or disability sets them apart from the main cohort of medical students, highlighting their under-representation within those that apply, and consequently, within the medical profession.

Bearing this in mind, by the end of the chapter, the reader will be able to:

- Appreciate how the issues associated with WP and WA may vary internationally, but the approaches to tackling these issues often share commonalities across contexts.
- Appreciate the contribution of current research while recognising the need to increase the sophistication of empirical work in this field.
- Consider the utility of different theoretical lenses in progressing understanding and affording fresh insight into how social change may be successfully implemented, using UK data as case study material.

## Why is widening participation to medicine important?

The call for increased student diversity in medical school has been made internationally.[13–16] Medical student diversity is a multifaceted, hugely complex issue that is driven by both the sociological concepts of social justice, mobility and equality (see below for definitions), and improving healthcare internationally.

### Social justice

Evidence from the wider literature suggests that aspiring to medicine and attaining the necessary academic and non-academic entry requirements are hugely complex, intersecting issues that are tied up with wider societal issues of social justice and social equality,[17] sociological issues of cultural and social capital and 'insider knowledge'.[3,18]

The capital a student possesses is a key concept within WP, and usually is classified as either cultural or social, so we take a moment to define these here. Puttman[19] defines social capital as features of social organisation such as network norms and trust that facilitate coordination and cooperation for mutual benefit. Bourdieu's[20] concept of cultural capital refers to the collection of symbolic elements such as skills, tastes, posture, clothing, mannerisms, material belongings or credentials that one acquires through being part of a particular social class or group in society. Sharing similar forms of cultural capital with others creates a sense of collective identity and group position ('people like us'). Put simply, social capital is about relationships, whereas cultural capital can be just about anything, from accent to address to relationships. Importantly for this discussion, both social and cultural capital are unevenly distributed among different societal groups, and as having capital can help one's social mobility, not having capital can hinder progress in society. In terms of applicants to medical school, those from 'traditional' backgrounds (e.g. a medical family, a relatively privileged education) have capital in terms of being able to, for example, 'phone a friend' (of Dad or Mum) to organise work experience or advice on how best to write their application essay. They have networks of peers who are also applying to medicine, and teachers who can give knowledgeable advice on the processes. They are encouraged to aspire to a medical career by family, home and school.[8] They know how to talk to doctors.[21] Applicants from 'non-traditional' backgrounds have no such social or cultural advantages. Indeed, the decision to aim for medical school may be counter-cultural if progressing to university education is not a tradition in the school or family.[18] University may be viewed as an unfamiliar environment with an alien ethos and medical school may be seen as 'not for the likes of me'.[22] Unfortunately, evidence indicates that this is not an unreasonable assumption: medicine and medical school culture are still unwelcoming to under-represented students.[23–25]

The concepts of social and cultural capital highlight that there are social and emotional risks to going to medical school, as well as financial risks. This indicates that the approaches to widen access that focus solely on providing financial support for applicants from certain groups,[26] while clearly addressing one major barrier to medical school, only address part of the problem.

## Improving healthcare

Educating and training, with their implied differences, a diverse, culturally competent healthcare workforce, which is well equipped to understand and address social determinants of health, is essential to improving healthcare quality.[27] Improving healthcare provision is considered possible by ensuring 'doctors should be as representative as possible of the society they serve in order to provide the best possible care'.[28–31] This assumes that increasing the diversity of the medical workforce will improve healthcare, based on the assumption that 'like would treat like',[32] and providing culturally and linguistically appropriate care increases patient satisfaction.[33,34] While, currently, this may appear to be rather an unachievable goal given all the different dimensions of similarity and difference between doctor and patient (e.g. gender, race, class, first language, cultural upbringing), students who train in more diverse medical schools appear to gain a greater understanding of other people from different socio-cultural backgrounds, and this increases their ability to provide healthcare to people with backgrounds different from their own.[11,29,20,35] Although increasing minority representation in medicine has been identified as an opportunity to both improve clinical care and reduce healthcare disparities, these outcomes are dependent on such students, once qualified, choosing to practise in areas of diversity and deprivation.[36–38]

However, although addressing issues of social justice/equality and improving healthcare are laudable, there is clear evidence that significant under-representation of some social, cultural and ethnic groups in medical schools and medicine worldwide persists despite a variety of national initiatives (e.g. quota systems, legislation, centralised funding for pipeline or WA activities, political imperatives) and local activities (e.g. pipeline/WA programmes, mentoring) to ameliorate such under-representation. For example, a recent survey conducted by the UK General Medical Council confirmed that there remains a significant under-representation of people from lower socio-economic groups within UK medicine.[39] Similarly, the Association of American Medical Colleges (AAMC) found that under-represented minorities (URM), who make up more than a quarter of the US population, continue to account for less than 13% of the students enrolled in US MD degree granting medical schools, and less than 9% of the practising physicians in the United States.[40,41]

How can so much investment and activity in WP and WA to medicine over the last decades have made so little impact? There are, no doubt, a number of reasons for this, one of which is, in our opinion, the nature of the approaches adopted to do so. Hopefully, it is clear from the above section that the issues associated with the persistent inequalities in participating in medical education reflect significant sociological complexity. Conversely, many of the approaches used to address the issues of WP and WA to medicine have been relatively simplistic and/or weakly conceived in terms of the quality of the related research. We support this statement with data from a review of the literature.

## Evaluating the quality of WP and WA to medicine research: a UK case study

We carried out a qualitative synthesis[42] of published studies reporting UK medical school WA initiatives.[43] The focus of the review was local rather than national-level change initiatives such as the establishment of public bodies to safeguard and monitor fair access to HE generally[44]; affirmative action legislation[10] or the use of compensatory approaches at the point of application to medicine.[45] Qualitative synthesis was considered an appropriate approach given the heterogeneous study designs and methods reported in the 10 studies identified within the parameters of our search.[3,25,46–53]

Of the 10 studies, two were observational, quantitative studies, analysing existing datasets to examine if structural changes (the introduction of graduate entry and Foundation programmes (where the length of the programme is extended to allow for preparatory and support activities [52]) or the use of a particular aptitude test as part of the admissions process [51] had had any impact on the demographic profile of UK medical students.

The other studies focused on reaching out and helping potential applicants from underrepresented groups using various approaches, summarised in Table 20.1. Typically in-reach activities are where pre-applicants are invited to activities based at the medical school/university campus whereas outreach activities are where medical school staff/students go out to the educational institutions of the pre-applicants. For interested readers, the varieties of initiatives are discussed further by Cleland *et al.*[43]

The studies identified had clear design and theoretical limitations (e.g. all but one of the studies

*Table 20.1* An overview of different types of WA interventions identified

| Type of intervention | Intensity | Examples | Aims |
|---|---|---|---|
| In-reach | High | Residential courses | To provide students with information, advice and guidance (IAG), and samples of university experiences to raise aspirations and develop appropriate expectations of university life |
|  | Low | Open days, talks, conferences held at the medical school |  |
| Outreach | High | Extended programmes Mentoring schemes | To support students who meet specified WA criteria to develop the necessary knowledge, skills and requirements to enter the medical course |
|  | Low | Talks, conferences held at schools and other external locations |  |

used an observational design [see Chapter 1 for an explanation of the limitations of this approach]; no study had a theoretical underpinning), linked to this and probably more importantly, in that the whole is bigger than the parts, they looked only at the proximal challenge to be addressed (e.g. increasing the number of WA applicants to the author's medical school). The studies were not cumulative, but rather local evaluations of local initiatives: we did not identify any study within UK medical education that looked at the issues of WP and WA to medicine in a way that would expand the understanding or provide generalisable messages. Moreover, they predominantly examined the psychosocial aspects of the participant experience, neglecting to acknowledge any institutional relational aspects of the medical school environment or culture that may affect the practising agenda and hence participant experiences and learning.[54–57] None of the studies were sufficiently strong 'to warrant change of opinion or practice or theory'[58] (p. 753). If 'determining whether or not progress is being made in an area of study requires judging whether or not empirically unsupported ideas are being discarded, whether or not the conversations stimulated by the research efforts have changed and whether or not the focus of our research efforts continue to evolve'[59] (p. 295), we can comment that our understanding of WA to medicine remains relatively unsophisticated compared with that of other topics in medical and healthcare education, illustrated elsewhere in this book.

Our intention in the remainder of this chapter is to illustrate how taking a more sophisticated approach to WA research can provide a deeper understanding of the area and make the hidden visible and the implicit explicit. In this way, WA research can illuminate the reasons why initiatives in this area have largely failed to achieve their admirable aims and stimulate better-informed efforts in the future.

It is also timely to state here that, although each country may have its own particular issues – race in the United States and South Africa, socio-economic class (SEC) in the UK, the need to recruit to remote and rural practice in Australia, indigenous populations in many countries, for example – the overarching goals of WP are largely shared. One of the few advantages of this common issue is that at least some of the evidence and lessons from different countries may be transferable or generalisable across different contexts – if the studies that provide this evidence and these lessons are appropriately conceptualised.

## The importance of theory

*Theories give researchers different 'lenses' through which to look at complicated problems and social issues, focusing their attention on different aspects of the data and providing a framework within which to conduct their analysis*[60] (p. 631).

Illumination of current practice, providing us with a more nuanced and clearer understanding of how and why we do things the way we do them, is an important step in any research programme, which ultimately wishes to encourage change. To this end, a variety of theories can be used to help design a research question, guide the selection of relevant data, interpret the data and propose explanations of the underlying causes or influences of the observed phenomena. Moreover, 'the use of theory makes it possible for researchers to understand, and to translate for policy makers and healthcare providers, the processes that occur beneath the visible surface and so to develop knowledge of underlying (generating) principles.'[60] (p. 634). This is particularly relevant to WP research where outcomes can in fact inform policy.[61] Consequently, from this point onwards, this chapter aims to illustrate how original and rigorous research in this field could be significant in influencing WP policies and bringing about successful change.

We do so by providing three examples from our own research, purposely selected because they illustrate the use of different theoretical frameworks to interpret the data.[62] Different frameworks will obviously emphasise different things and a programme of research into WA (or indeed any topic) might draw on a number of theories as each will cast light on certain elements of the problem.[63]

In these examples, the data are the same: qualitative data from 26 telephone interviews with admission deans and/or admission staff from UK medical schools, which we carried out in 2012.[43] We begin with a critical pedagogical analysis,[64,65] continue by examining how different philosophies of inclusion can have different implications for understanding and addressing WP[66,67] and finally draw on the heuristic of policy enactment of Braun *et al.* to explain the differing approaches to WA.[68,69] Each example includes a brief introduction to the theory, a description of how it was used and what it added to the research process and outcomes.

## Example 1: Critical pedagogy

If education is fundamentally linked to societal advantage, then it is crucial to look beyond the individual student(s), to groups and group processes and organisational structures and systems that maintain social and educational context/structures.[70] Friere's conceptual framework of critical pedagogy[64,65] is ideal for this as it allows issues of power relations, social justice, deeper meanings, root causes as well as over-arching organisational and policy matters, to be explored.

Critical pedagogy has been likened to a 'prism that reflects the complexities between teaching and learning which sheds light on the hidden subtleties that might have escaped our view previously. The prism has a tendency to focus on shades of social, cultural, political, and even economic conditions, and it does all of this under the broad view of history'[71] (p. 26).

In short, critical pedagogy is a process of appraising the relevant context, including the socio-political and organisational context in which education occurs, highlighting what is required to create a more equal society.

For Freire, and other critical pedagogues, pedagogy, the structures and processes concerned with teaching, should focus on providing the student the appropriate knowledge and skills to become a 'critical citizen', a process that also promotes democracy, rather than preparing students to principally take tests.[66] This goes to the very heart of what education is and what the purposes of education are. Is education providing an economic workforce, maintaining society's structure or providing a means for self-determinism (the process by which a person controls his/her own life)? In this way, critical pedagogy provides the means to explore why some members of society are consistently marginalised in medical admissions processes by focusing on power.

Focusing on power relations across the organisational structures associated with medical education provides opportunities to explore not only the views of stakeholders but also why certain decisions and policies are implemented and, importantly, why some are not. This involves the exploration of possible areas of tension which, when elucidated and better understood, may then be used as potential effective drivers for change.[66]

Using critical pedagogy as a conceptual framework will increase the understanding of the organisational structural issues affecting WP, which, in turn, can inform where to focus efforts to address the WP gulf within medical education.

We now provide an illustration of how critical pedagogy can provide a theoretical lens by which to examine the relations, or tensions, between the individual (micro: in this case, applicants and their teachers), group (meso: medical schools, medical admissions and selection policies) and institutional or national (macro: political agendas, national policies and influences) organisational levels within WP, with the intention of highlighting areas of disagreement and differences that reflect the inherent power struggles within and between these structures.[72]

### Micro-meso-level tensions

Admission deans commented on the challenges of encountering established cultural norms of both the school children and their educational milieu that did not entertain expectations of university education in general, and medical school in particular. For example:

> I spoke recently to a final year medical student, who told me that, when she said that she wanted to do medicine, she was told by her school, oh, children from this school don't do medicine. Why don't you become a nurse? That is very much the attitude and this is reinforced by the experience of the schools (Interview 17)

Another interviewee explained how she tried to engage schools and those schools in particular that have limited experience of preparing students for university.

> I did actually issue an open invitation at the summer school for any teachers who wanted to come along, and nobody did. Which didn't surprise me. I think, there's a lot of work to do … There is, I think a certain amount of, I wouldn't say suspicion but maybe alienation that secondary school teachers have for universities, I think, for higher education in general. (Interview 18)

### Meso-level tensions

One of the most commonly discussed issues was the difficulty of gaining medically-related work experience. Work experience was noted as a tension at both the micro-meso and meso-macro levels. Applicants from non-traditional socio-economic groups have often described obtaining appropriate work experience as difficult due to the lack of medical social connections (or social capital, see earlier). In addition, many interviewees also described how access to relevant medical work experience was made more difficult by their NHS partners who sometimes tried to restrict provision and/or numbers due to the lack of general resources. This interviewee confirmed this but also described how she was trying to overcome these issues.

> If the Trust (hospital) isn't prepared to speak to us, then they're not going to speak to kids. That's very sad. So that's why I'm trying to sort of sidestep it, and see if I can now go the alumni route first … because as I say, I think it's frustrating for doctors too, because they want to help people, you know, they want to help kids get in there, but if they're coming up against the barriers, it's how to try and move round those barriers (Interview 25)

Further difference and disagreements were highlighted between the interviewees at the meso-level where tensions between a genuine desire to widen participation and that of 'paying lip service' to appease authorities were identified. Some of this ambivalence seemed to be driven by a perceived lack of evidence and consequently a genuine hesitancy about how best to WP.

> I hope the kind of research manages to help us move forward, because … because it's also hearts and minds, you know, and … and yes, we need a good evidence base, but we also need the engagement of people actually responsible for admissions, who

are kind of prepared to kind of step forward and maybe converge a bit, in at least some of these areas (Interview 2).

### Meso-macro tensions

If, at the meso level, there is ambivalence because medical schools are either waiting for or questioning evidence concerning the underlying premises and goals of WP, then the implementation of WP initiatives may be neglected. This is illustrated by what interviewees called 'political rhetoric' where interviewees perceived that WP practices were being used as a vehicle to deliver political agendas that were lacking in evidence and not seen as central to the main medical selection process. For example, the assumption that medical students coming from disadvantaged areas are more likely to want to work as doctors in those areas was questioned.

> We need to ask ourselves whether that actually happens. If somebody comes from an inner city somewhere, has grown up in a council house, poor family, not the best education and so on, and has yet succeeded, do they go back, and want to work there? Do they actually carry with them that background and that understanding? I would expect that some would indeed do so, but I don't actually know whether the majority do or don't. (Interview 2)

The final illustration provides an example of tension between developing effective medical school selection strategies, desire to widen participation and how these aims may not always be compatible with overarching national policies. It also by way of highlighting the critical issues paves the way for policy developers to consider how to introduce effective change.

> You're put in a position to recruit the people that are most likely to succeed rather than having 20% of your students where you expect that there's a higher dropout rate. And you … do you see what I mean? … The sort of perverse incentives. Yes, that's what's going on; on the one hand you want to improve widening access but you're almost going to be penalised by government policy because of how it works (Interview 7)

### Example 2: Exploring conflicting widening participation philosophies

WP aims to encourage an inclusive HE system compared with a previously-perceived tradition of elitism, where a much narrower segment of the population was educated by a smaller number of more selective institutions.[61,73,74] However, philosophies of inclusion differ and these different philosophies have different implications for understanding and addressing WP. We draw here upon the conceptualisations of Friere again, including those of Giroux[66] and Habermas,[67] who make the link between transformative learning and the transformation of society.

Transformative learning is concerned with the individual's personal growth and is hence not necessarily dependent on the acquisition of instrumental knowledge required to gain a qualification or do a job. This is associated with professional development – medical students learn many things that do not solely reflect the technicalities of their everyday job. Within this context, transformative learning highlights how disadvantaged students can engage with education in a way that both enhances their own social mobility and influences the nature of the medical profession. We return to this later.

Sheeran[61] identifies two categories of inclusive educators: 'meritocrats' and 'democrats'. The meritocratic model is more about 'fair access' (WA) than WP per se (see Box 20.1). The concern is to ensure that able candidates are facilitated in gaining places to study rather than devoting much, if any, support following their matriculation or reflection on the purposes for such action. This is well illustrated by top universities and medical schools who seek what Sheeran[61] has called the 'rough diamonds' by trying to attract the brightest students from disadvantaged groups, giving them taster experiences and preparation to equalise their chances of entry. This promotes the notions that students from non-traditional backgrounds are in some way deficient and, therefore, need educationally 'topping up' before being considered satisfactory or that these students face 'barriers' because institutions are still not trying hard enough in implementing effective WA.[75] Meritocrats also subscribe to the concerns that WP threatens to lower standards by admitting students with lower or non-traditional qualifications and ultimately has the potential to undermine a system of medical education with a proven track record. 'Why mend something that isn't broken?' could be the plaintive cry of the meritocrat.

The position of the democrats is very different. Democrats see education as an essentially emancipatory or transformative experience, as per Habermas and Giroux.[66,67] From their perspective, WP in HE is not simply about increasing the representation of students from lower socio-economic groups but rather 'a form of pedagogy that is concerned to democratise knowledge and learning, in ways that redefine the very parameters of what counts as higher education'[76] (p. 10). Under this philosophy, non-traditional students have knowledge, experiences and perspectives that may help align themselves with more patients from diverse backgrounds and also contribute to the education of their peers by presenting views and acting as a resource that challenges the persistent medical culture. Transformative educators resist 'pathologising' non-traditional students as lacking in essential prerequisite skills or characteristics and challenge established perceptions of what constitutes a good medical student, and indeed what constitutes legitimate medical knowledge.[77]

We argue that making a difference in terms of WA to medicine requires first an exploration of what established members of the medical culture understand by inclusion, how this understanding may or may not be consistent with current practice and how any desired change in practice may be successfully implemented. Sheeran[61] points out that the 'philosophies of inclusion', including the assumptions and political commitments to which contributors subscribe, are frequently not explicit and this risks leaving the implicit uncontested. If we do not really understand what stakeholders think about WA, what opinions and values they hold, then we also cannot ensure that any proposed change or initiative stands the best possible chance of successful implementation.

To illustrate this, we drew out the implicit meanings of many of the uncontested selection practices and WP initiatives from the interview data.

> I think we need to stop ourselves and say so what's the objective here? What's the goal? And what's the evidence or the rationale for the goal, per se, and so on? Because a goal which says, Widening Access it about making sure that we're not missing people who would really be excellent doctors, I don't think anybody would have any trouble just signing up to that.(interview 2)

This reflection from the participant indicates her understanding and agreement with one of the goals of WA being about ensuring that any candidate irrespective of his/her background who will make an excellent doctor is considered. This corresponds to a meritocratic approach, which the participant goes on to indicate would be readily accepted by society. However, this participant also further elaborates on what she calls the 'political goal', which is seen as something that is distinct, and perhaps separate, to the aims of medical school selection and WP policies:

> But what is often perceived as the political goal is something different, and it's ... it's more people with, who come from sort of, you know, socio ... uh, poorer, more deprived socioeconomic groups, in terms of their families, or their communities, or their own origin, and that ... and that somehow, success will be defined when you have greater numbers from those backgrounds. But actually, success shouldn't be defined quite that way. There is a ... perceived, at least, to be a political agenda, in that it's just about numbers against demography, and so on, but I don't think anybody ... I suspect there'd be very few people anyway, uh, in medical schools are responsible for admissions, or possibly, even, you know, more, uh, in the profession, more generally, who would say, that is a defensible goal in itself (Interview 2).

Her opinions highlight the existence of conflicting philosophies of WP within medical education. This is reinforced by another participant, who takes a different view where the ethos of transformative education and social justice appear.

> The system has to recognise the outcome of the inequalities within our system and our educational systems in particular. So it doesn't bother me that there appears to be a bit of re-engineering going on. I think there should be a, a debate about the point at which that should be set. There has to be a discussion about, well, how far should we try and balance it? (Interview 14).

Another participant confirms the existence of conflicting philosophies briefly identifying both a meritocratic and democratic position with the additional description of the roles that individuals, medical schools and government may have within policy making.

> There are certain decisions that are either political decisions or judgments about the role of selection. Are we selecting the best people who would cope with medical education and are we hoping to select people who would make the best doctor. Or are we really trying to select on the basis that we want to make the, the composition of medical schools as close to the cross-section of society as possible; is that a reasonable aim? Is that a political decision; if it is then is that university's role to go along with that? Um, so, so, um, I, I don't know.

> It would be nice to debate all of these things and I have my personal view but, but that, that doesn't matter at all (Interview 20)

The participant ends with the comment that her view 'doesn't matter at all', which helps us understand how some faculty and senior staff responsible for medical selection may feel excluded from decisions concerning policy, or possibly may engage in practices that subvert change where there is disagreement.

## Example 3: Policy enactment

Our final example shows how the interview data indicated that individual medical schools interpret and put WP policy into practice very differently. For example, as illustrated earlier, some schools run extended medical programmes for students from certain backgrounds[3,25]; others accredit preparatory programmes[52]; others explicitly use contextual factors in decision making; some run mentoring programmes.[50]

Viewed through the lens of policy enactment, this diversity of approaches is unsurprising: '*Policies do not normally tell you what to do, they create circumstances in which the range of options available in deciding what to do are narrowed or changed, or particular goals or outcomes are set*'[78] (p. 19). Putting macro-level policy decisions into micro-level practice is a complex process to address an issue as required by legislation or other national drivers but usually without explicit guidance as to how to do so. Putting policies into practice is not only a creative, sophisticated and complex but also a constrained process, which is enacted (rather than implemented) in original and creative ways within institutions. In terms of WA, medical schools must interpret policy, drawing on their own culture, within the limitations and possibilities of their context, such as available resource.[68] In other words, context is core to how government-dictated WA policy is implemented 'on the ground'.

Braun *et al.*[69] suggest a four-dimensional heuristic framework where situation (e.g. setting), professional (e.g. commitment), material (e.g. resources) and external (e.g. performance pressures) interact to influence policy enactment. We used this framework to illustrate how context is important in asking questions about the circumstances of WP policy enactment in medical education.[79]

Our data suggested that the locality of the medical school was very relevant to WP policy enactment in terms of general institutional ethos and which societal groups were specifically targeted in WP activities.

> Interviewee 'I do think we have got a background in it (WP) and I think it's probably because of the location, unfortunately [laughs]. Er, you know, there's quite a lot of disadvantage in the area'.

The ultimate goal of WP activities was the same – to attract medical students who would go on to be doctors 'as representative as possible of the society they serve in order to provide the best possible care to the UK population'[25,26] – but who this was differs, to some extent, by the location of the medical school.

The professional concept refers to the individual interviewee's outlook and attitudes and how these might influence how WP policy is enacted. The majority of our interviewees were committed to the principle of WP, taking this serious as a core part of their role. However, they discussed the limits of what medical schools could do to address societal inequalities and were realistic about what their WP activities could do to address issues beyond the control of the medical school.

> Interview 22 'we can only select from those who apply ...'

Materiality refers to practicalities such as budget, staffing and infrastructure, that can have a considerable impact on policy enactment on the ground (compare this to the concept of materiality presented by Nimmo and Fenwick elsewhere in this book, what are the similarities and differences?). Views and experiences of funding for WP varied across our participants. Some were quite positive: for example, our participants talked about the availability of university-wide resources, whereas others spoke about national WP initiatives, which came with funding. It seemed to be the case that some medical schools had more resource for WP than others. However, this clearly intersected with the situation of the school, in terms of locality, and that of historical and external context. It was clear from the data that, generally, medical schools tended to focus their available WP resources on developing and rolling out WP activities, but not evaluating the impact of these activities (see earlier). Thus, our participants talked about the WA activities of their school, but were unable to tell us if these actually had had any impact on their student population.

The last dimension is that of external context. Medical schools do not exist in a vacuum. There are pressures and expectations from a range of key stakeholders (e.g. applicants, students, the government; the wider university). Some, but not all, schools were worried that students from WP backgrounds would struggle academically, and hence the reputation of the medical school in the league tables would be tarnished.

> Interview 7 'You're put in a position to recruit the people that are most likely to succeed ...'

Use of the policy enactment framework allowed us to provide a better understanding as to why WP policy processes are played out differently across medical schools. This better understanding may inform decision making as to what might be open to change, and how best to direct change.

## Summary and research implications

This chapter has broadly outlined some of the issues associated with WP and WA worldwide and indicated how medical education research currently inadequately examines these issues. To this end, we have briefly illustrated how using three different theoretical lenses can give a more in-depth understanding of such a complex topics.

The critical pedagogic approach highlighted some of the tensions within UK medicine's attempts to increase the representation of students from disadvantaged backgrounds and furthermore shed light on possible reasons why such WP initiatives have largely failed. Significant ambivalence within some admission staff concerning some national and governmental policies was uncovered and tensions were highlighted between meso- and macro-organisational levels. Such a structural analysis had been previously neglected within medical education. We have also shown how medical education's obsession with meritocracy can be explored by examining admission staff's views on 'inclusion' and highlighted the value of a more 'transformative' educational perspective if WP is truly to be instigated. Our third example, policy enactment, provided a further framework to explore both how medical schools interpret WA policy within their own individual context and the factors associated with implementation.

By using theoretical lenses to examine problems associated with WP and WA to medicine, we have moved research on this topic forward by identifying some of the attitudes and beliefs, and structural issues, which may be acting as barriers to change. By making these barriers explicit, we can consider how best to address them in future research studies that seek to better understand how medical culture and the practice of medicine affect WP[80]

These lenses have been used to explicitly examine issues associated with WP and WA but they could equally well be used to illuminate and magnify[63] other aspects of healthcare profession education. Using a critical pedagogic approach to explore tensions between organisational levels may be helpful in examining how change occurs (e.g. implementing new assessment systems, introducing a new curriculum) or looking at how structural issues affect processes within institutional structures (e.g. how does the hierarchy of the medical school influence curriculum development and delivery). Critical pedagogy could also be used to compare power dynamics across medical schools (e.g. how some schools position themselves as elite compared with others). Using a policy enactment framework within medical education research would readily lend itself to more robust research that intends to explore the neglected areas of policy and organisational structures (e.g. how guidance on assessment in the workplace is enacted in different contexts).

One word of caution: selecting a conceptual framework to illuminate a particular problem or situation can be daunting.[63] We did not select our three lenses lightly but rather systematically and critically surveyed the pertinent literature to identify potential frameworks. Through examining the evidence, and much discussion, we identified the frameworks that best illuminated our problem.

## Conclusion

WP and access to medicine is an example of an area of healthcare research and practice where we need to be concerned with not only if something works (although we need more research on this question), but also to dig deeper, to see how something works, for whom and under what circumstances. Advancing knowledge in this way requires rigorous research and more sophisticated theoretical approaches, which draw on knowledge and resources from different fields and disciplines.

### Practice points

- WA to medicine is a global issue but one that has been poorly researched to date: we still do not know what works, for whom.
- The reasons for under-representation of certain groups in medicine are complex but the research

and approaches to address the issue have, generally, been inappropriately simplistic.
- This chapter illustrates how a number of theoretical perspectives drawn from the education literature can provide a deeper understanding of the topic under study: critical pedagogy, transformative learning and policy enactment.
- We urge researchers to increase the sophistication of both qualitative and quantitative research on this topic by considering and integrating an appropriate theoretical perspective in their research philosophy, design and process.

## References

1 Cleland J.A. and Nicholson S. (2013) *A report of current practice to support Widening Participation in medicine to the UK Medical Schools Council (MSC)*. URL http://www.medschools.ac.uk/Publications/Documents/MSC-Selecting-for-Excellence-End-of-year-report.pdf

2 Reay, D. (1998) 'Always knowing' and 'never being sure': familial and institutional habituses and higher education choice. *Journal of Educational Policy*, **13**, 519–529.

3 Garlick, P.B. & Brown, G. (2008) Widening participation in medicine. *BMJ*, **336**, 1111–1113.

4 Scott, I., Yeld, N., McMillan, J. & Hall, M. (2005) Equity and excellence in higher education: the case of the University of Cape Town. In: Bowen, W., Kurzweil, M. & Tobin, E. (eds), *Equity and Excellence in American Higher Education*. University of Virginia Press, Charlottesville, VA, pp. 261–284.

5 Chowdry, H. & Goodman, A. (2013) Widening participation in higher education: analysis. *Journal of Royal Statistical Society*, **176**, 1–26.

6 Sacker, A., Schoon, I. & Bartley, M. (2002) Social inequality in educational achievement and psychosocial adjustment throughout childhood: magnitude and mechanisms. *Social Science and Medicine*, **55**, 863–880.

7 Howard, T. (2002) "A tug of war for our minds": African American high school students' perceptions of their academic identities and college aspirations. *High School Journal*, **87**, 4–17.

8 Hill, N.E., Castellino, D.R., Lansford, J.E. *et al.* (2004) Parent academic involvement as related to school behaviour, achievement, and aspirations: demographic variations across adolescence. *Child Development*, **75**, 1491–1509.

9 Millburn, A. (2012) *Fair access to professional careers. A progress report by the independent reviewer on social mobility and child poverty*.

10 Rosenbaum, S.D., Teitelbaum, J.J.D. & Scott, J. (2013) Raising the bar on achieving racial diversity in higher

education: The United States Supreme Court's decision in Fisher v University of Texas. *Academic Medicine*, **88**, 1792–1794.

11  Cohen, J.J. & Steinecke, A. (2006) Building a diverse physician workforce. *JAMA*, **296**, 1135–1136.

12  Laven, G. & Wilkinson, D. (2003) Rural doctors and rural backgrounds: how strong is the evidence? A systematic review. *Australian Journal of Rural Health*, **11**, 277–284.

13  Carrasquillo, O. & Lee-Rey, E.T. (2008) Diversifying the medical classroom: is more evidence needed? *JAMA*, **300**, 1203–1204.

14  Cohen, J.J. (2003) The consequences of premature abandonment of affirmative action in medical school admissions. *JAMA*, **289**, 1143–1149.

15  Burrow, G.N. (1998) Medical student diversity – elective or required? *Academic Medicine*, **73**, 1052–1053.

16  Sikakana, C.N.T. (2010) Supporting student-doctors from under-resourced educational backgrounds: an academic development programme. *Medical Education*, **44**, 917–925.

17  Archer, L. & Leathwood, C. (2003) Identities, inequalities and higher education. In: Archer, L., Hutchings, M. & Ross, A. (eds), *Higher Education and Social Class: Issues of Exclusion and Inclusions*. Routledge Falmer, London, pp. 175–191.

18  Reay, D., David, M. & Ball, S. (2001) Making a difference?: institutional habituses and higher education choice. *Sociological Research Online*, **5**. URL http://www.socresonline.org.uk/5/4/reay.html

19  Putman, R.D. (1995) Bowling alone: America's declining social capital. *Journal of Democracy*, **6**, 65–78.

20  Bourdieu, P. (1986) The forms of capital. In: Richardson, J. (ed), *Handbook of Theory and Research for the Sociology of Education*. Greenwood Press, New York, pp. 241–258.

21  Hafferty, F.W. (1988) Cadaver stories and the emotional socialization of medical students. *Journal of Health and Social Behaviour*, **29**, 344–356.

22  Greenhalgh, T., Russell, J., Boynton, P., Lefford, F., Chopra, N. & Dunkley, L. (2006) "We were treated like adults"-development of a pre-medicine summer school for 16 year olds from deprived socioeconomic backgrounds: action research study. *BMJ*, **332**, 762–767.

23  Orom, H., Semalulu, T. & Underwood, W. III, (2013) The social and learning environments experienced by underrepresented minority medical students: a narrative review. *Academic Medicine*, **88**, 1765–1777.

24  Greenhalgh, T., Seyan, K. & Boynton, P. (2004) "Not a university type": focus group study of social class, ethnic and sex differences in school pupils' perceptions about medical school. *BMJ*, **328**, 1541–1544.

25  Brown, G. & Garlick, P.B. (2007) Changing geographies of access to medical education in London. *Health and Place*, **13**, 520–531.

26  Long, B. (2008) *The effectiveness of financial aid in improving college enrolment. Lessons for policy [Internet]*. Harvard Graduate School of Education. URL http://gseacademic.harvard.edu/~longbr/ Long_._Effectiveness_of_Aid_Lessons_for_policy_ (I-08) [accessed 14 October 2014]

27  Mahon, K.A., Henderson, M.K. & Kirch, D.G. (2013) Selecting tomorrow's physicians: the key to the future health care workforce. *Academic Medicine*, **88**, 1806–1811.

28  British Medical Association. *Equality and diversity in UK medical schools*. 2009.

29  Whitla, D.K., Orfield, G., Silen, W., Teperow, C., Howard, C. & Reede, J. (2003) Educational benefits of diversity in medical school: a survey of students. *Academic Medicine*, **78**, 460–466.

30  Saha, S., Guiton, G., Wimmers, P.F. & Wilkerson, L. (2008) Student body racial and ethnic composition and diversityrelated outcomes in US medical schools. *JAMA*, **300**, 1135–1145.

31  Xu, G., Fields, S.K., Laine, C., Veloski, J.J., Barzansky, B. & Martini, C.J.M. (1997) The relationship between the race/ethnicity of generalist doctors and their care for underserved populations. *American Journal of Public Health*, **87**, 817–822.

32  James, D., Ferguson, E., Powis, D., Symonds, I. & Yates, J. (2008) Graduate entry to medicine: widening academic and socio-demographic access. *Medical Education*, **42**, 294–300.

33  Laveist, T.A. & Nuru-Jeter, A. (2002) Is doctor–patient race concordance associated with greater satisfaction with care? *Journal of Health and Social Behavior*, **43**, 296–306.

34  Cooper, L.A., Roter, D.L., Johnson, R.L., Ford, D.E., Steinwachs, D.M. & Powe, N.R. (2003) Patient-centered communication, ratings of care, and concordance of patient and physician race. *Annals of Internal Medicine*, **139**, 907–915.

35  Niu, N.N., Syed, Z.A., Krupat, E., Crutcher, B.N., Pelletier, S.T. & Shields, H.M. (2012) The impact of cross-cultural interactions on medical students' preparedness to care for diverse patients. *Academic Medicine*, **87**, 1530–1534.

36  McGrail, M.R., Humphreys, J.S. & Joyce, C.M. (2011) Nature of association between rural background and practice location: A comparison of general practitioners and specialists. *BMC Health Services Research*, **11**, 63.

37  De Vries, E. & Reid, S. (2003) Do South African medical students of rural origin return to rural practice? *South African Medical Journal*, **93**, 789–793.

38  Wade, M.E., Brokaw, J.J., Zollinger, T.W. *et al.* (2007) Influence of hometown on family physicians' choice to practice in rural settings. *Family Medicine*, **39**, 248–254.

39  GMC report National Training Survey (2013) *Socio-economic status questions* URL http://www .gmc-uk.org/publications/23538.asp

40  Association of American Medical Colleges (2011) *Table 31: Total enrollment by U.S. medical school and race and ethnicity*. URL https://www.aamc.org/download/160146/data/ table31-enrll-race-sch-2011.pdf [accessed 23 July 2013].

41  American Medical Association (2008) *Total physicians by race/ethnicity 2008*. URL http://www.ama-assn .org/ama/pub/aboutama/our-people/member-

groups-sections/minority-affairs-consortium/ physicianstatistics/total-physicians-raceethnicity.page [accessed 23 July 2013]

42 Baumeister, R.F. & Leary, M.R. (1997) Writing narrative literature reviews. *Review of General Psychology*, **1**, 311–320.

43 Cleland J. A., Dowell J., McLachlan J., Nicholson S. and Patterson F. (2012) Identifying best practice in the selection of medical students (literature review and interview survey). http://www. gmc-uk.org/about/research/14400.asp

44 Office for Fair Access (2008) *Access agreement monitoring: outcomes for 2006-7*. Bristol, UK.

45 Gale T. and Parker S. (xxxx) *Widening participation in Australian Higher Education*. Report to the Higher Education Funding Council for England (HEFCE) and the Office of Fair Access (OFFA), England. CFE (Research and Consulting) Ltd, Leicester UK and Edge Hill University, Lancashire, UK. URL http://www.deakin.edu.au/arts-ed/efi/pubs/wp-in-australian-he.pdf

46 Beedham, C., Diston, A. & Services, C. (2006) Widening participation in medicine: the Bradford Leeds. *The Clinical Teacher*, **3**, 158–162.

47 Holmes, D. (2002) Eight years' experience of widening access to medical education. *Medical Education*, **36**, 979–984.

48 Day, E., Hunt, L., Islam, S. & Vasanth, N.C. (2005) Widening participation in medicine. *Medical Education*, **39**, 505–533.

49 Dunkley, L., Dacre, J., Russell, J. & Greenhalgh, T. (2006) Widening access to medical school: Dick Whittington Summer School. *The Clinical Teacher*, **3**, 80–87.

50 Kamali, A.W., Nicholson, S. & Wood, D.F. (2005) A model for widening access into medicine and dentistry: the SAMDA-BL project. *Medical Education*, **39**, 918–925.

51 Tiffin, P.A., Dowell, J.S. & McLachlan, J.C. (2012) Widening access to UK medical education for under-represented socioeconomic groups: modelling the impact of the UKCAT in the 2009 cohort. *BMJ*, **344**, e1805.

52 Mathers, J., Sitch, A., Marsh, J.L. & Parry, J. (2011) Widening access to medical education for under-represented socioeconomic groups: population based cross sectional analysis of UK data, 2002-6. *BMJ*, **342**, 918–918.

53 Wright, S.R. & Bradley, P.M. (2010) Has the UK Clinical Aptitude Test improved medical student selection? *Medical Education*, **44**, 1069–1076.

54 Maudsley, G. & Strivens, J. (2000) Promoting professional knowledge, experiential learning and critical thinking for medical students. *Medical Education*, **34**, 535–544.

55 Howe, A. (2002) Professional development in undergraduate medical curricula – the key to the door of a new culture? *Medical Education*, **36**, 353–359.

56 Bleakley, A. (2006) broadening conceptions of learning in medical education: the message from teamworking. *Medical Education*, **40**, 150–157.

57 Brosnan, C. & Turner, B.S. (eds) (2009) *Handbook of the Sociology of Medical Education*. Routledge, Oxon and New York.

58 Eva, K.W. & Lingard, L. (2008) What's next? A guiding question for educators engaged in educational research. *Medical Education*, **42**, 752–754.

59 Eva, K.W. (2009) Broadening the debate about quality in medical education research. *Medical Education*, **43**, 294–296.

60 Reeves, S., Albert, M., Kuper, A. & Hodges, B.D. (2008) Why use theories in qualitative research. *BMJ*, **377**, a949.

61 Sheeran, Y., Brown, B.J. & Baker, S. (2007) Conflicting philosophies of inclusion: the contestation of knowledge in widening participation. *London Review of Education*, **5**, 249–263.

62 Lingard, L. (2007) Qualitative research in the RIME community: critical reflections and future directions. *Academic Medicine*, **82**, 128–130.

63 Bordage, G. (2009) Conceptual frameworks to illuminate and magnify. *Medical Education*, **43**, 312–319.

64 Freire, P. (1985) *The Politics of Education: Culture, Power, and Liberation*. Bergin & Garvey, South Hadley, MA.

65 Freire, P. (1986) *Pedagogy of the Oppressed*. Continuum, New York.

66 Giroux, H. A. (2010) *Rethinking education as the practice of freedom: Paulo Freire and the promise of critical pedagogy*. URL http://truth-out.org/archive/ component/k2/item/87456:rethinking-education-as-the-practice-of-freedom-paulo-freire-and-the-promise-of-critical-pedagogy [accessed 19 August 2014]

67 Habermas, J. (1990) *Moral Consciousness and Communicative Action (C. Lenhardt & S. Weber Nicholsen, Trans)*. Cambridge, Polity Press.

68 Braun, A., Maguire, M. & Ball, S.J. (2010) Policy enactments in the UK secondary school: examining policy, practice and school positioning. *Journal of Education Policy*, **25**, 547–560.

69 Braun, A., Ball, S.J., Maguire, M. & Hoskins, K. (2011) Taking context seriously: towards explaining policy enactments in the secondary school. *Discourse: Studies in the Cultural Politics of Education*, **32**, 585–596.

70 Goho, J. & Blackman, A. (2006) The effectiveness of academic admission interviews: an exploratory meta-analysis. *Medical Teacher*, **28**, 335–340.

71 Wink, J. (2005) *Critical pedagogy: Notes from the real world*, 3rd edn. Allyn and Bacon, Boston, MA.

72 Trowler, P. (2008) *Cultures and change in higher education*. Palgrave Macmillan, Basingstoke and New York.

73 Newby H. (2004) *Doing widening participation: social inequality and access to higher education*. Colin Bell memorial lecture, given at the University of Bradford, 30 March. URL www.hefce.ac.uk/news/events/ 2004/bell.doc [accessed 29 April 2006]

74 Thomas, L. (2005) *Higher education widening participation policy in England: transforming higher education or reinforcing elitism?*, Ad-Lib, 29, Article 1. URL www. cont-ed.cam.ac.uk/BOCE/ adlib29/article1 [accessed 30 April 2006]

75  Baker, S., Brown, B.J. & Fazey, J.A. (2006) Individualisation in the widening participation debate. *London Review of Education*, **4**, 169–182.

76  Thompson, J. (2000) *Stretching the Academy: The Politics and Practice of Widening Participation in Higher Education*. National Institute for Adult Continuing Education, Leicester.

77  Brosnan, C.J. (2009) Pierre Bourdieu and the theory of medical education: Thinking "relationally" about medical students and medical curricula. In: Brosnan, C.J. & Truner, B.S. (eds), *Handbook of the Sociology of Medical Education*. Routledge, Abingdon, United Kingdom, pp. 51–68.

78  Ball, S.J. (1994) *Education Reform. A Critical and Post-Structural Approach*. Open University Press, Buckingham, UK.

79  Cleland, J.A., Nicholson, S., Kelly, N. & Moffat, M. (2015) Taking context seriously: explaining widening access policy enactments. *Medical Education*, **49**, 25–35.

80  Krupat, E. (2010) A call for more RCTs (research that is conceptual and thoughtful). *Medical Education*, **44**, 852–855.

# 21 Qualitative research methodologies: embracing methodological borrowing, shifting and importing

*Lara Varpio, Maria Athina (Tina) Martimianakis and Maria Mylopoulos*

*You are familiar with qualitative methods and methodologies. You have read several introductory texts and have carried out some qualitative research projects. While you continue to learn about the intricacies of qualitative research, you no longer consider yourself a novice. Recently, your interest in how trainees deal with uncertainty has led you to question if there is more to understand about this particular learner experience. You want to explore this further and decide that a qualitative study will be required. However, in looking at your setting and reflecting on the body of research already published, you are not sure which qualitative methodology would be best suited to investigating your interests. None of the methodologies commonly used in health professions education (HPE) seem to perfectly fit your research question and context. You aren't sure what to do. You question to what extent you should bring existing theories to bear on your data collection and analysis. You wonder about the impact of the broader training context on individual experiences. You question whether the results should be used to generate a description of experience, a new model, or a revision of an existing theory. In the end, to develop a strong research design, you realise you will have to develop a qualitative study that flexibly employs qualitative methodologies, while also maintaining appropriate markers of qualitative rigour. But how to do this?*

## Introduction

Over the past decade, scholars working in healthcare profession education (HPE) have witnessed the qualitative–quantitative debate slowly moving towards resolution.[1] Scholars have agreed that each approach can be usefully applied to different research questions, each offering informative insights to the field.[1,2] The field has acknowledged that these different approaches are just that – simply different.

This truce has been supported by a proliferation of texts articulating the differences between qualitative and quantitative paradigms, epistemologies, ontologies and methodologies[3–5] (see the chapter by McMillan in this book, and additional reading suggestions at the end of this chapter). Qualitative method guides[6–9] are increasingly available in HPE-based publications, helping scholars to effectively participate in and evaluate qualitative scholarship (see Recommended Reading for some resources we find particularly useful).

But as qualitative methodologies and methods are employed with more frequency, the HPE community must continually 'critique our cultural expectations about how it [qualitative research] should be done'[10] (p. S130). Qualitative methodologies and methods are complex structures in-and-of themselves. Each qualitative methodology has its own history of development, involving disputes that influence the methodology's structures and operational techniques. HPE scholars using qualitative methodologies ought not to gloss over these differences-that-make-a-difference because these variations enable carefully directed research.

In this chapter, we explore some of the qualitative methodological differences-that-make-a-difference. We do not describe the many qualitative methodologies and methods available to HPE scholars. There are other texts that do so skilfully, and in considerable detail (see Recommended Reading for some suggested readings). Instead, we examine how methodological flexibility can be employed in qualitative studies. We identify and describe three ways in which this flexibility is realised in HPE research: (a) methodological *borrowing*, (b) methodological *shifting* and (c) methodological *importing*. We explore each of these flexibility techniques by analysing its application to a specific qualitative methodology. We examine methodological borrowing in relation to qualitative description. We look at methodological shifting as it relates to Grounded Theory (GT). We study methodological importing as it has influenced

*Researching Medical Education*, First Edition. Edited by Jennifer Cleland and Steven J. Durning.
© 2015 John Wiley & Sons, Ltd. Published 2015 by John Wiley & Sons, Ltd.

the use of discourse analysis. We illustrate these flexibility approaches using comparative sets of published HPE research articles to demonstrate the differences-that-make-a-difference. We conduct this analysis neither to praise nor to critique the selected publications; instead, we aim to illustrate the methodological variability that is possible.

## Methodological borrowing

In keeping with the established tradition,[11,12] we conceive of the boundaries that divide qualitative methodologies as permeable. As Denzin and Lincoln propose, qualitative research involves engaging with

'a wide range of interconnected interpretive practices, hoping always to get a better understanding of the subject matter at hand. It is understood, however, that each practice makes the world visible in a different way. Hence there is frequently a commitment to using more than one interpretive practice in any study'[12] (pp. 3–4).

Given this premise, we propose that it is appropriate to borrow elements of one methodology to inform research conducted using another methodology. For example, a study can engage in qualitative description (a methodology that does not seek to develop theory) and borrow techniques associated with GT (a methodology that seeks to develop theory) such as the constant comparison approach for analysis. This mixing of methodologies is not a marker of poor study design. Quite the opposite – it means that the researcher is drawing intentionally on specific methodologies to construct a study that will answer a specific research question.

For successful methodological borrowing to be achieved, *the borrowing should be done explicitly and intentionally.* Methodological borrowing requires that scholars be skilled with both methodologies – both the primary methodology being used, and the methodology being borrowed from. Such expertise is required so that the scholar can articulate the purpose(s) and extent of the borrowing.

To illustrate the practices of methodological borrowing, we examine how it has been applied to qualitative description. We describe qualitative description as a methodology, and then illustrate how scholars have borrowed from other methodologies to enhance their qualitative description studies (this comparison is provided in Box 21.1). Although these publications illustrate how methodological

borrowing can generate different kinds of qualitative description studies, they do not explicitly acknowledge nor describe the purposes of the borrowing. We suggest that researchers must identify, describe and justify the methodological borrowing used in their research in order for this methodological flexibility to be appropriately employed.

---

### BOX 21.1  Methodological borrowing in qualitative description studies

#### Example 1

Colbert *et al.* (2009) The patient panel conference experience: What patients can teach our residents about competency issues. *Academic Medicine* **84(12)**, 1833–1839.

The purpose of this study was to describe (a) the patient panel experience that had been locally developed for resident education and (b) the results of the mixed methods pilot study that involved the examination of residents' experiences with the patient panel innovation. The authors label the study's methodology as a qualitative description. Although the authors do not explicitly describe borrowing from experimental methodology, their descriptions of the methods clearly indicate its influence.

This study's methodological borrowing is evident in its data collection and data analysis approaches. First, all study data were collected via a questionnaire that incorporated both Likert scale questions (generating quantitative data) and open-ended free-text entry questions (generating qualitative data). Questionnaires are commonly used by quantitative research methodologies with post-positivist roots. As Creswell confirms, in post-positivist experiments, 'the researcher collects information on instruments based on measures completed by the participants.'[1] (p. 7) Second, the borrowing from experimental methodology is evident in the structures employed in the qualitative coding process to ensure objectivity and validity. To 'enhance validity'(p. 1834), the authors describe using specific techniques to 'reduce investigator bias' (p. 1834) including collecting data from a 'relatively large number of participants' (p. 1834) thus 'enhancing sample representation,' (p. 1834) and involving multiple investigators with diverse backgrounds in the content analysis process (p. 1834) 'thus reducing investigator bias' (p. 1834). This description echoes the post-positivist tradition of critical multiplism,[2] which involves the use of multiple triangulation techniques (including data, investigator, theory and method triangulation) to generate undistorted, more objective data interpretations.

## Example 2

Killam L.A. & Heerschap C. (2013) Challenges to student learning in the clinical setting: a qualitative descriptive study. *Nurse Education Today*, 684–691.

The purpose of this study was to describe the perceptions of senior nursing students' learning challenges within the clinical setting. It used focus group discussions to generate this description. It labels the work as a qualitative description study.

Although not explicitly stated, the study unmistakably borrows from phenomenology. The authors borrow from this methodology the focus on the lived experiences of a phenomenon (in this case, challenges to learning in the clinical setting) as experienced by a small group of individuals. Phenomenologists aim to '[describe] what all participants have in common as they experience a phenomenon.'[3] (p. 76) The authors summarise the participants' reports into a 'universal essence'[4] (p. 76) of the challenges that nursing students experience, but the descriptions remain at the level of reporting, not interpreting.

The borrowing from phenomenology is also evident when the authors present participants' experiences through multiple data citations. This borrowing is furthered in the presentation of a composite 'universal essence' description that voices both *what* the participants experienced and *how* they experienced it, in its complexity.[5] They visualise the relationships between themes, but avoid oversimplifying the thematic inter-connections that the participants described.

## Qualitative description

With paradigmatic roots in naturalistic inquiry,[13,14] qualitative description rests on the premises that all inquiry reflects specific values, that all knowledge is inextricably linked to the contexts in which it was generated and that all phenomena need to be examined holistically in their natural settings (see Chapters by Cleland, McMillan, Mann and MacLeod earlier in this book). Although it has a long history, interest in qualitative description was most recently renewed by Sandelowski.[11,15]

The purpose of qualitative description is to describe a phenomenon in the common language of the participants, with sufficient detail and nuance to accurately describe the complexity of the phenomenon, but without the interpretive influence of a theoretical framework.[11,15] It generates a description that is 'a comprehensive summary of an event in the everyday terms of those events'[11] (p. 336) and without the shaping power of theoretical interpretations. As Sandelowski summarises, qualitative description emphasises 'readings *of* [data] lines as opposed to *into*, *between*, *over*, or *beyond* [data] lines'[11] (p. 78). The markers of good qualitative description are the precise reporting of events and the un-interpreted reporting of the meanings that participants attributed to those events.[11]

This 'straight' reporting of data does not mean that qualitative description is an atheoretical methodology.[15] Choosing a research question is the start of the interpretive process (see Chapter 3). Similarly, deciding on data collection methods is an interpretive act. Thus, qualitative description involves interpretation just as every research effort does; however, the aim of qualitative description is to describe events in their own terms. These descriptions should not involve the addition of 'spin'[11] that can come from applying an external theory to data analysis.

The dimensions and practices of qualitative description are less regimented than those of many other research methodologies (such as GT). Sandelowski describes qualitative description as resisting simple categorisation and neat delineation of methods-related techniques:

> Given its various guises and the eclectic combinations of sampling, data collection, and data analysis techniques characterizing it, qualitative description could never be described as any one method that any one person invented[15] (p. 78).

Qualitative description does not dictate specific processes for data collection and analysis. It is open to any and all qualitative sampling, data collection and data analysis techniques that will generate the most appropriate means for developing a near-data[11] description of the phenomena being studied. This is where methodological borrowing is often realised in qualitative description. A scholar can borrow elements or techniques from another methodology to inform their qualitative description data collection and analysis processes. In Sandelowski's terms, borrowing would be 'the hues, tones, and textures'[11] (p. 337) from other research methodologies that become 'overtones' to the qualitative description.

Borrowing from different methodologies results in qualitative description studies that look very different from each other. Both the publications described in Box 21.1 generate 'straight,' 'near-data' qualitative descriptions, but do so in very different ways.

## Methodological shifting

We conceive of each methodology as existing on a *shifting* continuum. As paradigms, ontologies and epistemologies (see Chapter 2 by McMillan) change over time, and as methodologies are adopted by different disciplines, methodological traditions shift in accordance with those developments. For instance, Edmund Husserl developed transcendental phenomenology in the early 1900s. Transcendental phenomenology focuses on examining an individual's conscious experiences to uncover the essential meaning of a phenomenon. To accomplish this, the researcher brackets off of prior personal knowledge and attitudes. Soon after Husserl, Martin Heidegger proposed a new variation of phenomenology – hermeneutic phenomenology. This tradition posits that it is impossible to separate the individual from the external world. Therefore, the hermeneutic phenomenologist examines personal knowledge and attitudes in relation to a phenomenon instead of bracketing them off. Today, when a scholar engages in phenomenology, he/she must choose which tradition will enable them to best answer his/her research question – transcendental or hermeneutic. Choosing to engage in transcendental phenomenology does *not* mean that a scholar is using an outdated form of phenomenology. Instead, the scholar is choosing an approach from the methodology's shifting continuum. What is required is that the scholar understands how the methodology has shifted so as to choose the appropriate tradition to employ in his/her study.

We use GT to illustrate methodological shifting. First, we describe the continuum of the GT methodology. We then use two publications (see Box 21.2) to showcase the paradigmatic shifts that have occurred within the methodology and the resulting types of work that each tradition of GT affords.

---

### BOX 21.2   Methodological shifting in grounded theory studies

#### Example 1

Mahant, S., Jovcevska, V., & Wadhwa, A. (2012) The nature of excellent clinicians at an academic health science center: a qualitative study. *Academic Medicine* **87(12)**, 1715–1721.

The purpose of this study was to 'understand the nature of excellent clinicians at an academic health science center by exploring how and why peer nominated 'excellent' clinicians achieve high performance (p. 1715).' This study exemplifies the post-positivist tradition of GT, marked most prominently by the *tabula rasa* approach of the researchers in exploring their phenomenon of interest, and their positioning of the results as representation of a reality.

From the introduction, the rationale for the study is the belief that 'exploring the personal experiences and the ethos of excellent clinicians may reveal important insights into what elements make and contribute to their expert performance (p. 1715).' Accordingly, the data were collected and analysed inductively, with the aim of developing theory grounded in the experiences and perceptions of the participants. The discussion describes overlaps between the model developed from the data and the existing theoretical frameworks of expertise, leadership and motivation. However, and importantly, the authors do not seek to build on those frameworks but rather draw on them to make meaning of the theory developed in the current study. Finally, the 'holistic model' of excellent clinicians is presented as a situated reality (i.e. within a paediatric Academic Health Sciences Centre).

#### Example 2

Mylopoulos M. *et al.* (2012) Renowned physicians' perceptions of expert diagnostic practice. *Academic Medicine* **87(10)**, 1413–1417.

This study sought to 'further the development of a substantive theory of expert diagnostic practice' (p. 1413) by exploring how physicians nominated as exceptional by their peers conceptualised their own diagnostic practice and diagnostic excellence more broadly. While the research question was similar to that of Mahant *et al.* (2012) present in Example 1 of

Box 21.2, this was a constructivist GT study; therefore, the question was explored in a markedly different way. Most notably, the inquiry was framed in theories of adaptive expertise and the results were positioned within current discourses of medical education.

In the introduction, the authors used theories of adaptive expertise to frame the rationale for their research question and data collection approach. Data analysis involved a combination of deductive and inductive analyses to generate themes that were meaningful within the theoretical framework of adaptive expertise. Moreover, the particular perspectives of the researchers involved in the data analysis were described to make transparent the lenses that the research team brought to bear on the data. The discussion foregrounds features of the developed model of diagnostic excellence that are most salient to current discourses within medical education: informing understanding of the intersection between adaptive expertise and competency-based education and articulating how the results support and build on the existing theories of adaptive expertise.

## Grounded theory

GT is an inductive methodology aimed at generating substantive theory using qualitative or quantitative data generated from some combination of interviews, observations and text.[16] It is perhaps the best known and the most commonly used qualitative methodology in HPE research. This popularity is likely due to GT's clearly defined data collection and analysis techniques that were originally laid out by Glaser and Strauss.[16] These techniques, which include some borrowed from other qualitative methodologies, were assembled and clearly defined in a step-by-step text that demystified qualitative research.[17] They include an iterative, constant comparative approach to data collection and analysis, theoretical sampling, theoretical saturation and a four-step, inductive coding process culminating in the generation of theory to understand social phenomena. Generally, when assessing the quality of a GT study, researchers determine if these techniques have been employed effectively.

However, rigour is not solely about fulfilling checklists in the 'doing' of qualitative research.[18] Furthermore, multiple traditions of GT methodology have emerged, reflecting shifts in the underlying epistemologies and ontologies guiding the research process.[19] These shifts have resulted in the modification of GT techniques to reflect the paradigms within which they are being enacted. Thus, it is crucial to understand the underlying paradigms of each tradition within the methodology, how the application of techniques reflects that paradigm and what knowledge is being generated as a result. As researchers, we must situate ourselves paradigmatically (i.e. know our own epistemological and ontological position) in order to select the GT tradition that best allows us to explore our phenomena of interest.

GT's origins in the theory of Symbolic Interactionism[20] significantly shaped the methodology's initial epistemological underpinnings and the development of the techniques that guide its use. Symbolic Interactionism posits that people act towards things based on the meaning that those things have for them; and that these meanings are derived from social interaction and are modified through interpretation.[20] To understand social phenomena, we must explore the meanings that people impose on objects, events and behaviours. Accordingly, the first tradition of GT is underpinned by the question 'what is the *basic social process* that underlies the phenomenon of interest?'[16] As such, GT is a post-positivist methodology, aimed at inductive theory generation that is 'grounded and rigorous,' reflective of an emergent reality. This orientation is manifested in GT's dictates that the researcher is a *tabula rasa*, and that theory generation is an entirely inductive process of discovery generated through systematic analysis of the data being collected from participants. While there has been debate about the particulars of the systematic analysis (most famously, a schism between Glaser and Strauss centred on the issue of verification and abduction in GT[21]), GT remained relatively entrenched within the post-positivist mode of discovering reality until the more recent development of constructivist GT.[22]

As the name suggests, the constructivist GT tradition, developed most notably by Kathy Charmaz, shifts the methodology from post-positivism to constructivism. Constructivist GT retains many of the techniques of the original GT methodology; however, Charmaz's modifications aim for interpretive understanding and situated knowledge (rather than explicit generalities or sparse explanations – criticisms often levelled at the original GT). Constructivist GT positions inquiry in its historical, cultural, social, situational and interactional location. And, perhaps most importantly, rather than demanding the researcher begin as a *tabula rasa*, constructivist GT acknowledges the perspectives and positions of the researcher as well as the researched. In these ways, constructivist GT focuses on 'recognizing prior knowledge and theoretical preconceptions and subjecting them to rigorous scrutiny.'[23] (p. 402) Constructivist GT has gained immense popularity as researchers seek to use the methodology to advance (i.e. refine and elaborate) the existing theory, rather than generate new theories to account for social phenomena.[24]

Some researchers, most notably Clarke,[25] have questioned 'how grounded theory is grounded?', suggesting that grounded theorists must move beyond basic social processes and include 'the *situation* broadly conceived.' In doing so, Clarke has shifted the latest GT tradition into post-modernism. This shift that has yet to find a significant foothold in HPE research, but weak footings are common when methodologies are first imported into a field (see description of methodological importing below).

The publications described in Box 21.2 illustrate how HPE scholars have navigated the methodological shifting that has evolved within the GT methodology. The first publication engages in the post-positivist GT tradition, while the second uses the constructivist GT approach.

## Methodological importing

In interdisciplinary fields such as HPE, scholars often import methodologies from other disciplines and fields. Methodological importing involves the large-scale transfer of a methodology's concepts and tools from a field where it was developed or frequently used, to a field where the methodology is largely unknown. Such importing is valuable because it provides opportunities for raising new questions, for addressing old problems in new ways, and for generating epistemic debates that may lead to conceptual renewal or innovation. However, methodological importing is *not* a simple process. When uprooting a methodology and importing it to a new field, the foundational conditions that underpinned the approach can be left behind. The ontological and epistemological orientation of the importing field is often different from the one imported from. This means that the rationale for using the methodology and its associated markers of rigour may not be accepted in the new field. The importing field may be unfamiliar with both the content and the type of knowledge generated by the imported methodology in its original field. Therefore, using an imported methodology entails re-negotiating the ontological and epistemological basis for its use in the new discipline. It also entails finding ways to link it to a relevant pre-existing knowledge to construct its utility in the new field.

When a methodology is imported into a field, it often seems incomplete in its methodological articulation. Over time, as the methodology attracts followers and is used more frequently in the new context, a tradition around its use is formed and more context-specific ontological and epistemological roots take shape. For example, in HPE, such a tradition has arguably been generated around GT but has not been developed around qualitative description. When methodological importing is in its earliest phases, scholars need to engage in considerable descriptive and justification work. For instance, when importing a methodology, the researcher should explicitly explain what markers of rigour should be used to judge the research generated and should be prepared to modify these markers to accommodate the expectations of the importing field.

To illustrate both the challenges and the possibilities of methodological importing, we examine Foucauldian discourse analysis (FDA). We discuss FDA in the context of other forms of discourse analysis and provide an overview of how it has been imported into the HPE field. We discuss some ways in which the FDA methodology has been used in our field, signposting the negotiations that scholars have had to make in order to legitimate FDA as a rigorous approach for understanding and addressing HPE concerns.

## Discourse analysis

Discourse analysis is a broad term that encompasses a variety of approaches to the study of language. One way to differentiate between different discourse analysis approaches is to identify what the researcher is hoping to accomplish through the study of language. For example, Hodges *et al.*[26] organise discourse analysis approaches in three categories:

1 Formal linguistic discourse analysis (such as sociolinguistics), which focuses on language use and meanings of text at the level of enunciation (what is being said and how it is being said)

2 Empirical discourse analysis (such as conversation analysis and genre analysis), which focuses on ways in which language and texts construct social practices

3 Critical discourse analysis (CDA) (such as Foucauldian analysis), which focuses on ways in which systems of meaning emerge and operate in various contexts, including constructing the limits of what can be said or done by individuals or organisations

In this chapter, we discuss the third form of discourse analysis, the CDA, specifically the Foucauldian analysis.

In CDA, the term *discourse* denotes an inter-related set of texts and practices that have constitutive powers – in other words, the texts and practices of a particular discourse bring people (i.e. subjects) and things (i.e. objects) into being in specific kinds of ways. Broadly speaking, discourses are systems of meaning that have the appearance of truth. Take, for example, the discourse of accountability. This discourse organises people's activities and interactions around processes that hold individuals and institutions accountable to society for their actions (e.g. for the way they conduct their work, the way they operate their business or the way they handle decision making). People take on different roles in enacting or resisting accountability. These roles (or identity constructions) are immediately recognisable and are linked to accountability processes. For instance, when an individual takes on the role of an oncologist, he/she engages with the texts and practices of their professional bodies, of hospitals where they practice, of healthcare teams and of patients. The discourse of accountability is part of these texts and practices. That discourse influences the oncologist's thinking and actions, requiring that he/she recognise and accept being accountable for providing *what the discourse defines* as high quality, ethical patient care. The discourse of accountability requires the oncologist to act (and even just to *be*) in certain kinds of ways in order to be labelled as a 'good and responsible' oncologist.

Consistent with a constructivist paradigm (see the chapter by Mann and MacLeod), CDA methodologies examine texts to understand how versions of reality, society and identity are produced and reproduced. CDA methodologies seek to understand how these versions of reality, society and identity support the power of specific institutions, practices and conceptions of knowledge. To continue our

example, in an accountability culture, individuals who study and create evidence for robust accounting processes gain visibility and are valued for their expertise. The evidence they produce reinforces the dominance of the discourse of accountability. In the process, they may also become implicated in potential unintended effects linked to a culture of accountability, such as overinvestment in surveillance of workers and their work productivity. To illustrate, the oncologist who creates a checklist for safer and more effective chemotherapy treatments will be accorded respect and social capital by his/her professional bodies, hospitals, colleagues and patients. The checklist bolsters the accountability culture of the hospital since there is now a 'standard' to uphold. However, this oncologist might inadvertently also contribute to increased inter-professional tensions because using the checklist requires a new division of labour and care responsibilities in the team. In summary, in a CDA study, *knowledge making* is understood to be implicated in (a) broader socio-political relationships and (b) developing boundaries about what counts as natural, acceptable and desirable behaviour.

FDA refers to textual analytic methodologies inspired by the work of Michel Foucault. As a starting point, FDA acknowledges that reality is ambiguous, diverse and culturally specific. While FDA focuses its analysis on language, the purpose of this methodology is to make visible the way power flows and operates in various contexts, constructing objects and subject positions. FDA problematises truisms and totalising explanations of phenomena. The goal of FDA is to make visible the processes by which worldviews become uncontested truths. Taking up the accountability discourse example yet again, it would be difficult in today's North American healthcare context to argue that a physician is not accountable for his/her actions. A study using FDA methodology might ask: How did this 'truth' discursively come into being? What is created as a result of this 'truth'? How does the discourse continue to uphold this 'truth'?

Foucault challenged linear notions of history that assume the natural progression or evolution of ideas. Indeed, a central organising principle of FDA is to treat the emergence of ideas as relational and contingent. This poses a challenge to scholars, particularly those who have aligned with positivist/post-positivist paradigms (see Chapter 1). To revisit our example, discourse analysts do not evaluate the merits of accountability per se, but instead examine how valuing accountability is generative. For example, FDA can illustrate how reproducing the importance of accountability can open up conceptual space for the construction of new concepts (e.g. accountability reporting requirements) and new objects (e.g. performance checklists) or validate certain subject/identity positions (e.g. good documenter). In the process, scholars using FDA methodologies will endeavour to also show ways in which a commitment to accountability may hide other ways of ensuring high quality, ethical patient care.

Methodologically, FDA researchers attend to language, but not to extract the individual meanings that people ascribe to their words. Instead, this methodology focuses on language to distil and describe how drawing on specific narratives about the world affects individuals, their interactions and the spaces within which they function. In other words, analytical focus is placed on making visible the circulation of power through individuals, organisations and objects. Foucauldian-inspired researchers working in HPE have used discourse analysis to make visible the unintended effects of dominant discourses (e.g. competence, and evidence-based medicine) and to challenge the field's taken-for-granted assumptions.[27–32]

FDA does not have a distinct set of methodological techniques associated with it. This has implications for how researchers demonstrate rigour in their work, particularly when they are importing the FDA methodology into an interdisciplinary field that has had little previous experience with the approach. As the papers mentioned in Box 21.3 demonstrate, HPE scholars devote considerable space in their publications to establishing FDA's methodological credibility. They do so by describing in detail what steps were taken and by rationalising their selections. Such is the price of methodological importing.

---

**BOX 21.3  Methodological importing in Foucauldian discourse analysis studies**

**Example 1**

Rowland, P. & Kitto, S. (2014) Patient safety and professional discourses: implications for interprofessionalism. *Journal of Interprofessional Care.* Early online: 1–8.

This study, relying on Foucault's concepts of discourse and governmentality, sought to explore three inter-related research questions: ' (a) how is patient safety made visible and constituted as part of the delivery of healthcare practices? (b) how does

patient safety make it possible to think in particular ways about professional practice, and the provision of health care? and (c) how do the strategies and knowledges that have become associated with patient safety create truths about professional practice (p. 2)?' The authors begin by problematising the mainstream conceptions of patient safety. They do not set out to understand what elements of the healthcare system pose challenges to patient safety processes. Instead, the authors seek to study 'what constitutes patient safety in the first place (p. 2).' The authors make visible the profession-specific interests in specific visions for patient safety, how these visions may be in tension with one another, their function and role in safeguarding the interests of different professions and the effects (intended and unintended) of making one vision of patient safety more visible than others.

The authors dedicate an entire section of the paper to educating the reader on the key tenets of FDA. They define the concept of discourse, how it relates to the concept of governmentality and explain why discourse analysis can offer a useful perspective on patient safety issues. The authors align their research with that of other social scientists exploring ways 'patient safety policy and programmes are located within wider systems of practice (p. 2).' They detail how they constructed the archive of texts from pre-existing published texts and empirically generated texts. They supplement this description with two tables, one showing an abbreviated list of the documents analysed, and the other providing demographic details of the empirically generated texts. They provide information on their location as authors (conceptually, geographically and professionally) and describe ways in which they encouraged reflexivity in their process. Describing their orientation to the work and their methodological process in such detail is indicative of the effort it takes to import a methodology (in this case, FDA) into a field that will not automatically recognise its legitimacy.

**Example 2**

Haddara, W. & Lingard, L. (2013) Are we all on the same page? A discourse analysis of interprofessional collaboration. *Academic Medicine* **88**, 1509–1515.

The purpose of this study was 'to explore whether a shared interprofessional collaboration [IPC] discourse' (p. 1509) underpinned the efforts to incorporate IPC in competency-based educational frameworks and hospital accreditation models. The authors did not set out to chart the emergence of inter-professional collaboration, but rather to make visible its multiplicity. In the process, they implicitly problematise the unconditional acceptance of inter-professionalism as taking a single form and draw out the implications for healthcare delivery and inter-professional education. These authors only incorporate published peer-reviewed literature in their archive of texts. They provide a rationale for this delimitation by stating that 'the published literature represents a domain within which individuals' ideas, and methods interact, and it is, therefore, a defensible research starting point' (p. 1510). They also delimited their archive to nurse–physician IPC because it was 'arguably the dominant interprofessional axis in modern health care' (p. 1510) and because 'the nurse-physician relationships ... historically predates the emergence of some other professions now participating in the health care workplace (p. 1510).' They make a case for including articles that speak to both the United States and the Canadian healthcare contexts and for reviewing papers published in the period of 1960–2011. Indeed, the description of the delimitation of the archive, the compilation of the archive and the analytical steps used to make sense of the archive takes the authors several paragraphs to articulate. They explain to the reader that it is important to go to these lengths because their methodology resists 'formulaic rules for analysis (p. 1510).' The authors describe that the pivotal point of departure for judging the rigour and trustworthiness of research conducted using CDA is the alignment between the research question, the conceptual framing of the work and the methodological choices. To help the reader visualise the analytical process, and similar to many scholars who employ FDA in HPE, they include a table to contrast the features of the two dominant discourses of IPC on which their discussion is focused.

## Conclusion

In this chapter, we have defined, described and illustrated three ways for flexibly employing qualitative methodologies in HPE scholarship: methodological borrowing, shifting and importing. Our identification and reporting of these approaches was possible in great part because of our experiences of engaging in reflexive practices as qualitative scholars working in HPE. In our efforts to report qualitative research to the community, we have had to attend to and negotiate with the larger HPE context. Ours is a field with deep post-positivist roots. And while the qualitative-quantitative debate might be ending, the influence of HPE's post-positivist paradigm runs deep. This influence is seen even in this chapter when, for instance, we use the term 'rigour' and not 'trustworthiness.' The influence is similarly felt when journal reviewers asks authors to define and describe 'ethnography,' or 'a theme,' but do not ask for the same description of 'an experiment' or 'a p value.' We understand the need for linguistic compromises and for explanatory descriptions in our methods sections. Qualitative research methodologies and methods are still relatively new to the HPE field. Qualitative researchers working in HPE must explain our methodologies and methods in order to make our ways of contributing to the development of knowledge accessible to the larger community.

But it is equally important that HPE's qualitative scholars critique their own practices and traditions. We hope that methodological borrowing, shifting and importing provide scholars with ways of thinking about the differences-that-make-a-difference between and within qualitative methodologies. Just as there is room in the HPE domain for mixed methods research – combining both qualitative and quantitative epistemologies, ontologies and methodologies – there is room for qualitative studies that draw from multiple qualitative traditions (be it by borrowing from across multiple methodologies, by selecting from a methodology's shifting traditions or by importing different methodologies into the field). Furthermore, just as mixed methods researchers must find ways of demonstrating both rigour and trustworthiness, qualitative research that draws on multiple traditions has to demonstrate the markers of trustworthiness that are foundational to each methodology.

---

### Practice points

- Methodological flexibility can be employed in qualitative studies to take advantage of the differences-that-make-a-difference between qualitative methodologies.

- It is appropriate to *explicitly and intentionally* borrow elements of one methodology to inform research conducted using another methodology.

- Scholars must make an *informed* choice, from along a methodology's shifting continuum, of the tradition that will best answer a specific research question.

- When importing a methodology into a new field, researchers must *explicitly explain* what markers of rigour should be used to judge the research generated and should be prepared to modify these markers to accommodate the expectations of the importing field.

## Recommended reading

### Paradigms, ontologies, and epistemologies

Bunniss, S. & Kelly, D.R. (2010) Research paradigms in medical education research. *Medical Education*, **44**, 358–366.

For introductory overviews or summaries:

Bergman, E., de Feijter, J., Framback, J. *et al.* (2012) AM last page: a guide to research paradigms relevant to medical education. *Academic Medicine*, **87**, 545.

For more in depth explanations:

Howell, K.E. (2013) *An Introduction to the Philosophy of Methodology*. SAGE Publications, Thousand Oaks, CA.

### Qualitative methods and methodologies

Ng, S., Lingard, L. & Kennedy, T.J. (2014) Qualitative research in medical education: Methodologies and methods. In: Swanwick, T. (ed), *Understanding Medical Education: Evidence, Theory and Practice*, 2nd edn. The Association for the Study of Medical Education, Wiley Blackwell, pp. 371–384.

For introductory overviews or summaries:

Pope, C. & Mays, N. (eds) (2006) *Qualitative Research in Health Care*, 3rd edn. Blackwell Publishing, Malden, MA.

For more in depth explanations:

Creswell, J. (2013) *Qualitative Inquiry & Research Design: Choosing Among Five Approaches*, 3rd edn. SAGE Publications, Thousand Oaks, CA.

Denzin, N.K. & Lincoln, Y.S. (eds) (2000) *Handbook of Qualitative Research*, 2nd edn. SAGE Publications, Thousand Oaks, CA.

## References

1 Bordage, G. (2006) Moving the field forward: going beyond quantitative-qualitative. *Academic Medicine*, **8**, S126–S128.

2 Norman, G. (2010) Interpretation and inference: towards an understanding of methods. *Advances in Health Sciences Education*, **15**, 465–468.

3 Illing, J. (2014) Thinking about research: theoretical perspectives, ethics and scholarship. In: Swanwick, T. (ed), *Understanding Medical Education: Evidence, Theory and Practice*, 2nd edn. The Association for the Study of Medical Education, Wiley Blackwell, pp. 331–347.

4 Bunniss, S. & Kelly, D.R. (2010) Research paradigms in medical education research. *Medical Education*, **44**, 358–366.

5 Bergman, E., de Feijter, J., Framback, J. *et al.* (2012) AM last page: a guide to research paradigms relevant to medical education. *Academic Medicine*, **87**, 545.

6 Ng, S., Lingard, L. & Kennedy, T.J. (2014) Qualitative research in medical education: methodologies and methods. In: Swanwick, T. (ed), *Understanding Medical Education: Evidence, Theory and Practice*, 2nd edn. The Association for the Study of Medical Education, Wiley Blackwell, pp. 371–384.

7 Barbour, R.S. (2005) Making sense of focus groups. *Medical Education*, **39**, 742–750.

8 Harris, I. (2003) What does "The Discovery of Grounded Theory" have to say to medical education? *Advances in Health Sciences Education*, **8**, 49–61.

9 DiCicco-Bloom, B. & Crabtree, B.F. (2006) The qualitative research interview. *Medical Education*, **40**, 314–321.

10 Lingard, L. (2006) Qualitative research in the RIME community: critical reflections and future directions. *Academic Medicine*, **8**, S129–S130.

11 Sandelowski, M. (2000) Whatever happened to qualitative description? *Research in Nursing & Health*, **23**, 334–340.

12 Denzin, N.K. & Lincoln, Y.S. (2000) The discipline and practice of qualitative research. In: Denzin, N.K. & Lincoln, Y.S. (eds), *Handbook of Qualitative Research*, 2nd edn. SAGE publications, Thousand Oaks, CA.

13 Guba, E.G. & Lincoln, Y.S. (1982) Epistemological and methodological bases of naturalistic inquiry. *Educational Technology Research and Development*, **30**, 233–252.

14 Lincoln, Y.S. & Guba, E.G. (1985) *Naturalistic Inquiry*. SAGE, Beverly Hills, CA.

15 Sandelowski, M. (2010) What's in a name? Qualitative description revisited. *Research in Nursing & Health*, **33**, 77–84.

16 Glaser, B.G. & Strauss, A.L. (1967) *The Discovery of Grounded Theory: Strategies for Qualitative Research*. Aldine de Gruyter, Hawthorne, NY.

17 Merriam, S. (2009) *Qualitative Research: A Guide to Design and Implementation*. Jossey-Bass, San Francisco, CA.

18 Barbour, R. (2001) Checklists for improving rigour in qualitative research: a case of the tail wagging the dog. *British Medical Journal*, **322**, 1115–1117.

19 Birks, M. & Mills, J. (2011) *Grounded Theory: A Practical Guide*. SAGE, Los Angeles, CA.

20 Blumer, H. (1969) *Symbolic Interactionism; Perspective and Method*. Prentice-Hall, Englewood Cliffs, NJ.

21 Strauss, A. & Corbin, J. (1998) *Basics of Qualitative Research: Techniques and Procedures for Developing Grounded Theory*. SAGE Publications, Thousand Oaks, CA.

22 Charmaz, K. (2006) *Constructing Grounded Theory*. SAGE Publications, London.

23 Charmaz, K. (2008) Constructionism and the grounded theory method. In: Holstein, J.A. & Gubrium, J.F. (eds),

*Handbook of Constructionist Research.* Guildford Press, New York.

24 Thornberg, R. (2012) Informed grounded theory. *Scandinavian Journal of Educational Research*, **56**, 243–259.

25 Clarke, A.E. (2005) *Situational Analyses: Grounded Theory after the Postmodern Turn.* Sage Publications, Thousand Oaks, CA.

26 Hodges, B., Kuper, A. & Reeves, S. (2008) Qualitative Research: Discourse Analysis. *BMJ*, **337**, a879. doi:10.1136/bmj.a879

27 Haddara, W. & Lingard, L. (2013) Are we all on the same page? A discourse analysis of interprofessional collaboration. *Academic Medicine*, **88**, 1509–1515.

28 Hodges, B.D., Martimianakis, M.A., McNaughton, N. & Whitehead, C. (2014) Medical Education … Meet Michel Foucault. *Medical Education*, **48**, 551–645., June 2014 (published ahead of print May, 2014)

29 Martimianakis, M.A. & Hafferty, F. (2013) The world as the new local clinic: A critical analysis of three discourses of global medical competency. *Social Science and Medicine*, **87**, 31–38.

30 McNaughton, N. (2013) Discourse(s) of emotion within medical education: the ever-present absence. *Medical Education*, **47**, 71–79.

31 Razack, S., Lessard, D., Hodges, B.D., Maguire, M.H. & Steinert, Y. (2014) The more it changes; the more it remains the same: a Foucauldian analysis of Canadian policy documents relevant to student selection for medical school. *Advances in Health Sciences Education*, **19**, 161–181.

32 Whitehead, C., Kuper, A., Freeman, R., Grundland, B. & Webster, F. (2014) Compassionate care? A critical discourse analysis of accreditation standards. *Medical Education*, **48**, 632–643.

**PART 3**

# Developing your practice as an educational researcher

# 22 How to tell compelling scientific stories: tips for artful use of the research manuscript and presentation genres

*Lorelei Lingard and Erik Driessen*

'It's none of their business that you have to learn to write.
Let them think you were born that way.'
Ernest Hemingway

## Introduction

Why do researchers communicate their work to others? Certainly there are the pressures of academia, which demand peer-reviewed presentations and publications as symbolic evidence of scholarship. But more importantly, researchers communicate their work because knowledge-building is a social and rhetorical act: that is, an act of sharing ideas, of argument and persuasion to come to agreement about what is known. In order to move our field of knowledge forward, we need to talk with one another about what we have learned: we need to report our insights, question one another's methods, argue the relevance and application of emerging ideas, and extend our insights by building on one another's efforts. Scientific knowledge advances not only through systematic procedures, careful analysis and thoughtful contemplation of results, but also through social – and rhetorical – acts of knowledge creation. This is why researchers communicate their work to others. And, therefore, no researcher can afford to treat lightly the issues of effective research writing and presentation.

In framing dissemination as a social and rhetorical act, we draw attention to the role of genres in research writing and presentation[1]. Following rhetorical genre theory, we use the term 'genre' to mean more than mere structure[2,3]. While structure is important, it is shaped by three other dimensions of genre: purpose, audience and occasion. To communicate effectively, a researcher needs to understand all four aspects of the genre in which

she is participating: What is the required structure? Who is the intended audience, and what are their shared values and generic expectations? What is the genre's purpose? And what is the occasion in which this genre is an appropriate communication strategy? In summary, genre is how we recognise and construct types of communication actions within types of communicative situations. It is how we create a shared sense of order, and accomplish shared goals[2,4].

Writers and presenters tend to focus almost exclusively on the structural dimensions of genre. They worry about which sections/headings are required in their power point presentation, or about the word limit for their paper. However, a simple comparative example will serve to illustrate why all four dimensions of genre are necessary for effective communication. Imagine that you want to communicate about your last research study to your colleagues in a national conference presentation, your extended family at Thanksgiving dinner, and your vice-dean in the elevator. In the occasion of the conference presentation, your purpose is to offer, in the allotted time, a detailed explanation of the means and outcomes of your research for the purpose of incremental knowledge-building with an audience of disciplinary peers. In the occasion of Thanksgiving dinner, your purpose is to tell an anecdote in conversational language that your family (who, we will imagine, does not share your disciplinary expertise) will find engaging and relevant, and to tell it in a manner that will not last until dessert (and, in our family cultures, that isn't too self-aggrandising). In the third occasion, your purpose is to report a research highlight in accessible but still formal language that will signal your work's importance and recognition before the elevator door opens. The first occasion demands the generic structure of introduction, methods, results and discussion to satisfy the expectations of the audience; in the other two occasions, this generic

* Arnold Samuelson (1984) *With Hemingway: a year in Key West and Cuba*. New York: Random House

structure would be a serious rhetorical faux pas. What this example illustrates is that, notwithstanding our tendency to privilege structure when we are writing papers or preparing talks, structure is only one part of effective dissemination, and it is dictated by purpose, occasion and audience. Therefore, this chapter offers tips that will keep you attuned to all four features of written and oral research dissemination genres. The chapter will also briefly discuss the possibilities that social media offer for communicating science.

## Writing Up

This section provides advice about five key aspects of research writing: Entering the conversation, Mapping the gap, Telling the story and Crafting the language (see Box 22.1).

> **BOX 22.1   Key principles for approaching research writing as a social & rhetorical act**
>
> Join a conversation
> Identify a problem
> Map the gap
> Have a hook
> Tell a story
> Craft the language with care

### Entering the conversation

The first thing to remember about writing up is that you are not writing up a *study*. You are writing up a *story* that emerges from the results of a study. This is a critical rhetorical shift: it turns the act of writing a paper from being a descriptive report of something *you did* as a researcher, to being a persuasive story about something in the reader's world. Remember: nobody cares about your research study *per se* (sad, but true). But they may care about your story *if* you can convince them that it is relevant to a salient problem in their world, and enter the scholarly conversation that is currently going on about that problem. For this reason, the first question a writer should ask herself is 'what problem in the world is this paper about?'

The second question a writer should ask herself is 'where is the scholarly conversation about this problem taking place?' These questions guide your selection of journal audience, your situation of the work within the literature, and your organisation of results and discussion. It is very useful to start thinking about journals not as bound collections of papers but as social contexts for scholarly conversations about shared problems. From this perspective, getting your paper accepted is at least in part a matter of signalling that you offer a relevant and logical 'conversational turn' in an ongoing discussion about a shared problem. And so, you need to select a journal not (only) for its impact factor, but (also) for alignment between the problem you are writing about and the problems its community cares about.

Once you have selected the conversation you are joining, and found journals in which this conversation is taking place, positioning your conversational turn as relevant requires an understanding of the journal's values. Do they value work with international dimensions? Do they privilege work that engages in theory-building? Do they prefer work with relevance to more than one educational context, or work that addresses the policy dimensions of a problem? Exploring the values of the journal can help you articulate the problem your story explores in ways that will resonate with its audience. In the example in Figure 22.1, the authors gathered information about the journal's values by communicating with the editor and reading papers the journal had published on similar topics, and then set up their introduction to reflect these values of: relevance to patient outcomes, newsworthiness, scientific top quality and journalistic style.

The conversation metaphor can also usefully guide your sense of the purpose of the literature

---

Whether or not 'experience' means 'making the same mistakes with increasing confidence over an impressive number of years'[1] depends on how self-analytical and critical you are. When you speak of your students needing to be 'more reflective' you mean that they should let their future behaviour be guided by systematic and critical evaluation and analysis of actions and beliefs and the assumptions that underlie them.[2] All UK doctors are now expected to make reflection a critical foundation of their lifelong learning[3] on the assumption that patients will benefit.[4] This emphasis on reflective learning in medical education is relatively new, and certainly no hard evidence exists yet that patients benefit directly from doctors' reflective learning.[5] However, evidence suggests that reflection could help students to learn from their experiences.

Excerpted from: Driessen, E.W., Tartwijk, J. & Dornan, T. (2008) The self-critical doctor: helping students become more reflective. *British Medical Journal*, 336, 827–830.

*Figure 22.1* Signalling the journal's values.

Many have characterised the clinical activities related to non-acute patients as possessing limited educational value, naming these activities 'clinical service' or, more pejoratively, 'scutwork'[1–7] . These terms refer to tasks that are necessary for patient care but are not educationally valuable, or are repeated more often than necessary for education purposes. In a published commentary, one internal medicine resident labelled clinical service tasks as 'non-educational, non-physician level scut'[4] (p. 13). Residents spend a significant amount of their time (approximately 25 %) on service activities[1,2,9]. If these activities are truly non-educational, this is time which may be reallocated to improve education[3,7]. However, there is disagreement over whether or not particular tasks have educational value[5,6], with experienced physicians arguing that this service or 'scut' work is essential to developing clinical acumen and practising the art of healing[10]. For instance, activities such as talking to families, often considered non-educational by residents, provide an opportunity for teaching 'patient care, professionalism, and communication skills'[9] (p. s17). Disagreements over whether an activity is perceived as educational or non-educational[5,6] suggest that there may be opportunities to realise different types of learning from these tasks, depending on the environment in which they are encountered.

Excerpted from: Vanstone, M., Goldszmidt, M., Weijer, C., Watling, C. & Lingard, L. (2013) Resigned Professionalism? Non-acute inpatients and resident education. *Advances in Health Sciences Education*, 17(4), 247–255.

*Figure 22.2* Literature review as a portrayal of conversational turns.

review that often opens a paper. You are not aiming for an exhaustive romp through all that has been said on a topic; you are mapping the highpoints of the conversation before your contribution, and arranging them so that your contribution is a natural next step. Think of your literature review not as a dry list of citations, but rather as a means of creating a sort of gravitational pull – the reader should experience a powerful and explicit logic that leads, inescapably, to the point that your paper is poised to share. And search the literature to find actual conversations: commentaries on published papers, editorials, podcasts, often cited papers that get taken up in variable ways in other's work. As much as possible, view the literature as being a record of conversational turns expressing the views of scholars in the field – not *just* as references. As the following second paragraph of an introduction illustrates, you want to signal that people are actively building knowledge in your field, and you are joining them. (Figure 22.2)

Many of us are good conversationalists but our wits seem to desert us on the page. Thus, it can be helpful for a writer to imagine herself as part of a social conversation, because it allows him/her to draw on intuitive communication etiquette. In spite of academic writing's unique rhetorical occasion, the basics often still apply. For instance, imagine yourself at a cocktail party with senior researchers in your field. If you wish to join a small group enthusiastically engaged in conversation,

you must first eavesdrop, catch the thread of the argument, and then position your contribution to be relevant and timely. You have to choose the right moment and judge your tone, so that your entry is smooth and engaging rather than abrupt and impertinent. You do not want to be that dreaded person whose interruption drags lively conversations off course, or who evangelically holds forth with utter disregard for other positions in the debate. The same is true for research papers submitted to journals, so treat your writing as a conversational turn.

**Mapping the gap**

We have established that your paper is a conversational turn, telling a story which contributes to the audience's evolving understanding of a problem that matters in their world. To be a compelling conversational turn, then, the paper must establish three things before the introduction ends (and preferably in the first few paragraphs): (a) Identify a problem in the world, (b) Establish a gap in current knowledge or thinking about the problem and (c) Articulate a hook that convinces readers that this gap is of consequence. Consider the example in Figure 22.3, which quickly lays out the problem, the gap and the hook in the first paragraph:

You might have heard that an introduction must include a 'clear research question' or a 'purpose statement': in fact, these may be two of the 'golden rules' of introductions that you are familiar with.

With the advent of interprofessional care[1,2], new questions about leadership and teamwork have arisen. How should responsibility be shared and power differentials mitigated? How has the physician's role changed?[3] How do healthcare teams view these dimensions of their work? Without insight into these issues, we cannot know how best to educate physicians and other clinicians regarding their responsibilities on collaborative teams.

Excerpted from: Lingard, L., Vanstone, M., Durrant, M., Fleming-Carroll, B., Lowe, M., Rashotte, J., Sinclair, L. & Tallett, S. (2012) Conflicting messages: examining the dynamics of leadership on interprofessional teams. *Academic Medicine*, 87(12), 1762–1767.

*Figure 22.3* Laying out the problem, the gap and the hook.

And while of course it might be helpful to do either or both of these things, neither has the rhetorical weight and prominence of the problem, the gap and the hook. You could have a lovely research question about something your audience does not recognise as a problem that matters. Or you can have a clear purpose statement that sends the work off into directions where there is no gap in knowledge. Do not put your faith in a clear research question or purpose statement to compel the reader's attention. The problem, the gap and the hook are necessary components to establish your story as one that matters.

The three steps of problem, gap and hook are most useful if you remember the premise laid out at the beginning of this chapter: research dissemination is a social and rhetorical act. Your audience will have evolving impressions of what constitutes a problem that matters in the world, and you need to have your finger on the pulse of this evolving social context as you do your literature review. Are you writing about a problem that is inarguably novel (a rare event), one that is actively being worked on, or one that might be perceived by some readers to be already solved? As an example of the latter case, consider the problem of 'professionalism' in medicine. In the late 1990s in medical education research journals, this was a fairly novel problem; today, a researcher with a professionalism story to tell enters a crowded landscape in which much has been said and editors and readers may have developed a sense of ennui, a belief that surely we have figured this problem out by now. As Figure 22.4 shows, the establishment of the gap is a particularly critical step in such a case:

This example acknowledges that much progress has been made exploring professionalism as behaviours and competencies, and that context has been recognised as important, while focusing in on the problem of 'translation of abstracted principles into action' as the gap remaining to be filled.

Similarly, you might identify a problem that resonates with your readers and clearly claim for yourself a gap in current knowledge. However, if the reader does not believe that this gap matters – that is, that filling the gap will change anything – then your story has no 'hook' to draw them in. For instance, I may assert that poor staff communication in nursing homes is a problem that matters in the world, and I may illustrate a gap in our understanding of how shift work contributes to that problem. But if I do not have a hook – such as an argument that the causal relationship between communication breakdowns and medical errors in other settings centres on information handover between shifts – then readers may not see the gap as one worth filling. If that happens, it does not matter how elegantly my study was designed or how robust my results were; without a hook, which I would define as a claim to the significance or relevance of the gap, which draws on our shared values (here, the value of patient safety and error reduction), the story will lack vigour.

### Telling the story

As we have said, the best academic papers tell a story, rather than reporting a study. Among the features shared by good stories, recognisable characters and a cohesive plot are critical. A common problem for writers of research stories is that the text can get crowded with an ever growing list of characters – concepts, theories and keywords. This problem may emerge because many healthcare professional education problems are complex phenomena, requiring the writer to position them

---

Evaluating professionalism has become an important issue for medical educators, with the current trend focusing on observed behaviours and competencies to maximise reliability and validity.[1,2] Although direct observation is clearly important, assessing behaviours in isolation is insufficient—evaluators must also consider the context in which behaviours occur, any values conflicts that may be present, and the resolution of the situation.[3,4] It is clear that behaviours themselves are not always transparent indicators of 'professionalism' and that the translation of abstracted principles into action is complex.[4,5]

Medical students' professionalism is primarily evaluated by faculty attendings, but little is known about how they think students should act. In a recent study, we found that attending physicians often disagree about what students should or should not do in challenging situations. Significant inconsistency existed between and even within individual faculty about what they considered to be appropriate medical student behaviour in a given scenario.[4] In an effort to move beyond the simple analysis of behaviours, some of our other work has examined students' reasoning in the face of professional dilemmas. This research demonstrated that when faced with challenging professional situations, students are motivated to act based not only on the principles of professionalism, but also on the basis of affect (or 'self') issues, or potential implications of their actions.[6] Knowing how students reason through these dilemmas provides important insights into how they make decisions about how to act when faced with these sorts of challenges. However, it is still not clear how faculty would reason through such dilemmas when considering how students should behave.

Excerpted from: Ginsburg, S., Lingard, L., Regehr, G.R. & Underwood, K. (2008) Know when to rock the boat: How faculty rationalize students' behaviours. *Journal of General Internal Medicine*, 23(7), 942–947.

*Figure 22.4* Establishing the gap in a well-studied field.

## Introduction

Research suggests that inadequate communication is a primary cause of medical errors and that communication among the professions in the operating room (OR) is essential to patient safety[1–4]. In research on nurse–physician communication in settings such as ORs or ward rounds, nurses persistently report that they are perceived as a passive audience for others, and that they are constrained in what and when they are able to communicate[5,6]. The communicative constraints on nurses have been analysed in terms of the ways that knowledge and competence are displayed in the 'theatre' of the OR[7,8], the continued dominance of biomedical discourse over other types of healthcare discourse[9,10], and the disempowered or 'oppressed group' status of nurses[11,12]. Nurses also report seeing themselves as 'keepers of the peace' whose role is to maintain a calm environment for surgeons to focus on their work, sometimes described as a gendered role or a 'female thing'[7].

Survey research on team communication in the OR indicates that nurses and anaesthesiologists have less positive perceptions of the effectiveness of their communication compared with surgeons, and are less likely to respond positively to the statement 'I am comfortable intervening in a procedure if I have concerns about what is occurring'[13]. In our own ethnography, leaders of the different professions spoke to us about occasions when something of concern took place in the OR and 'nobody said anything'. Because of their central role in patient safety and advocacy, nurses are often the subject denoted in questions about why no one spoke up.

To date, there has been no research directly examining the speech practices, including silence, that are identified as constrained or problematic. This is understandable given the difficulty of documenting silences in communication and the traditionally marginal role of silence in qualitative research[14]. Using observational data from a multi-year study of interprofessional communication in three hospital ORs, our objective in this paper is to directly examine instances of silence and constraint in communicative exchanges in the OR using a critical ethnography approach.

Excerpted from: Gardezi, F., Lingard, L., Espin, S., Whyte, S., Orser, B., & Baker G.R. (2009) "Why didn't anybody say anything" Silence, power, and communication in the operating room. *Journal of Advanced Nursing*, 65(7), 1390–1399.

*Figure 22.5* Keywords as characters in your story.

within an interdisciplinary set of literatures. When keywords pile up, however, incoherence can set in; that is, readers simply cannot follow the plot because there are too many characters on stage, coming and going, and their relations to one another are not entirely clear. As this explanation suggests, one heuristic for ensuring coherence in your story is the metaphor of a drama. Treat keywords and ideas as actors in a play. Ask yourself, among all these actors, which has the lead role? Which have supporting roles? In the sample introduction that follows, although there are numbers of keywords – 'communication', 'patient safety', 'operating room teams', 'gender', 'nurses' and 'silence' – the organisation signals that the main character of this story is 'silence', and the other ideas are in service to that. (Figure 22.5)

As you write the paper, the lead role(s) should not change; the main character from the introduction should still be featured in the discussion, although you may add new characters as necessary as long as relationships are evident. New characters joining the discussion can productively complicate the plot line, if it is clear to the reader why these characters have appeared. At any time in the text, it should be clear to the reader which ideas are in the front-stage of the unfolding drama, and which are in the backstage.

The discussion may be the most difficult part of your research story to write. Why? Because the story's plot line needs a dramatic 'arc' – it needs to go somewhere, to climax, before resolving the questions or tensions and concluding. Many writers resolve without any climax: their discussions summarise, review design limitations, point to future research – but do not take the story of the results anywhere interesting. Writers who overlook the 'so what?' altogether may have falsely assumed that having done a study is reason enough to write a paper. Not so, because, as we have argued, study and story are not the same thing.

Many commentaries on academic writing have argued for the critical importance of the 'so what?' in academic research papers[5]. Why do the results matter? How do they reframe the problem, challenge common assumptions, advance the conversation you are joining? Your results are only part of your contribution to the conversation; your discussion of 'so what?' is the other part. You are telling a story that contributes important insights about a problem in the world that an audience is having a conversation about. One key to explicating the 'so what?' is to think of it as the piece that readers not precisely interested in your study details may still care about. For instance, in the work of one the authors of this chapter (LL), that could mean imagining what someone not interested in operating rooms or team communication practices might find valuable in his/her study of how surgical residents participate in operating room banter. The 'so what?' in such an instance could be that language is the central force in the hidden curriculum; if so, the introduction and discussion of his/her paper will need to engage the conversation about hidden curriculum to propose the central role of language and illustrate *why it matters* that we recognise this role in medical education. As this example suggests, the 'so what?' often reaches past the setting of the particular study you conducted. This is achieved through a process of abstracting, linking and extending – but there is a fine line! Beware of arm-waving or broad overgeneralisations that are inappropriate given the nature of your data.

## Crafting the language

So far, our advice has been largely conceptual: think of your research paper as joining a scholarly conversation in the field; articulate a problem, gap and hook to gain entry to that conversation; and tell a story with clear characters, a strong plot and an explicit 'so what?'. Unfortunately, a writer can follow all of this advice and still produce a weak paper. Why? Because writing is only partly conceptual; it also involves careful attention to the crafting of the language itself.

As Helen Sword has recently pointed out, academic writing is, unfortunately, not often stylish and compelling; more often it is ensnarled in labyrinthine logic and weighed down by what she calls 'soggy syntax'[6]. This chapter does not aim to provide a fulsome guide to the craft of writing; we highly recommend Sword's book, which crosses disciplines, draws on empirical evidence, and entertains with its own stylish, humorous prose. We will, however, briefly consider the main causes of and solutions for these main problems.

The first problem we have called labyrinthine logic, to reflect the experience of the reader who gets lost in the twists and turns of your argument. This problem is usually related to the problem of too many main characters that get introduced, seemingly at random, throughout the paper without signalling their relationship. This situation can be helped a great deal with effective use of the first sentence of each paragraph, the topic sentence, which signals the paragraph's main idea and links it to the idea immediately preceding. To check whether your topic sentences are doing this job properly, try cutting and pasting your topic sentences into a list. When you read the list, it should lead you through the logical steps of the story. Or, to use another metaphor, you can think of topic sentences as 'signposts', telling the reader where we are going next in the paper, and how that destination relates to where we have been.

The second problem, 'soggy syntax', refers to sentence constructions that bog the reader down rather than carrying him/her swiftly along[6]. Writers often create soggy syntax through their use of the subject position (the agent of the main verb) or the main verb (the source of the action) in simple sentences, or their handling of multiple subject positions and verbs in complex sentences.

The subject position of the sentence is the agent of the action; to use our drama metaphor, it is where you place your main characters. Academic writing loses vigour when the subject position is a nominalisation, otherwise known as an abstraction embodied in a noun phrase. Consider this example: *In the face of both globalisation and inter-professionalism, the conceptualisation of competence in medical education is changing.* Grammatically, there is nothing wrong with this sentence. But it lacks vigour because the noun phrase in the subject position – *the conceptualisation of competence in medical education* – is an abstract idea. Ideas do not make clear, vigorous agents of a verb's action. Of course, academic research writing is full of ideas, so writers need to learn how to handle them without creating cognitive burden for the reader. The sentence could express the same idea more vigorously by editing to: *Globalisation and inter-professionalism change how medical educators conceptualise competence.* The main change here is that the noun phrases are simplified by removing layers of prepositional phrases, *of competence* and *in medical education*. Ideas are still in the subject position – *globalisation and inter-professionalism* – but they are not elaborated with such layers, so they are less likely to bog down the reader.

The revision – *Globalisation and inter-professionalism change how medical educators conceptualise competence* – also addresses the second problem underlying soggy syntax: passive verb constructions. Passive verbs remove the agent of the action so that no one is actually doing anything in a sentence. To illustrate: 'The researchers interviewed medical students' is an active verb construction and it is clear who did the interviewing, whereas 'Medical students were interviewed' is a passive verb construction, which removes the agent of the interviewing (researchers). In the first version of our aforementioned example sentence, the verb phrase *is changing* removes the agent from the subject position and puts it into a prepositional phrase at the end of the sentence: *in the face of both globalisation and inter-professionalism.* The revision puts the agent into the subject position, customarily placed before the verb, which gives the sentence more energy. Now the agents, *Globalisation and inter-professionalism,* are clearly doing the action of *change.*

As a related tip, writers should watch out for iterations of the verb 'to be', which can signal passive constructions: *The study was conducted; Findings were identified.* Passive constructions make readers labour to sort out 'who's kicking whom?'[7] Even when used actively –*Globalisation is an important movement* – 'is' does not have much expressive power, nor do other favourites such as 'makes', 'shows' and 'does'. Verbs are where you create action in your prose, so use verbs that act! Usually the sentence that needs revision already includes, in noun form, the word that would create action if you put it into the verb position, as illustrated by our revision, which changed the noun *conceptualisation* to the verb *conceptualise.*

Finally, soggy syntax can be caused when sentences present the reader with multiple candidates for the main idea – that is, multiple nominalisations. In our original example – *In the face of both globalisation and inter-professionalism, the conceptualisation of competence in medical education is changing* – the prepositional phrase, *In the face of both globalisation and inter-professionalism,* introduces two nominalisations or abstract ideas (globalisation and inter-professionalism) before the reader gets to the main character of the sentence. Remember, the main character is housed in the subject position of the main clause: in this case, it is *the conceptualisation of competence in medical education.* In this case, the poor reader is already faced with three big ideas before the main verb has appeared, and she may be understandably confused about which of these she should focus on as the story's main character. The problem worsens in complex sentences with subordinate clauses, which have two subjects and two verbs, only one of which is the 'main' subject and verb of the sentence. Consider this example: *Although globalisation and inter-professionalism are relatively new concerns, the conceptualisation of competence is changing in the face of them.* In this example, the subordinate clause is the one starting with the subordinate adverb, *Although.* This clause has a subject position slot, filled by *globalisation and inter-professionalism,* and the main clause (the one without a subordinating adverb) has a subject position slot too, which is *the conceptualisation of competence.* The reader may understandably be overwhelmed by the presence of two elaborate nominalisations in the subject position slots of these two clauses. Lessening the sentence's vigour even further, both clauses use a limp 'to be' construction for the verb. Our point here is not that subordination should be avoided in academic writing; it is necessary to establish complex relations between ideas. But writers should consider how subordination can affect the reader's appreciation of the main idea and the main action in the sentence, and use such sentence structure strategically.

## Presenting your work

Try to remember the last presentation that you attended as a spectator. The odds are good that this presentation was tedious, and that your thoughts wandered away as the presenter, positioned with his/her back to you, read from PowerPoint slides filled with text and raced the clock through the final batch of slides. Stroll through any convention centre during an international meeting and this, sadly, is the bulk of what you will see.

Why do scientists persist in delivering boring presentations? Because we think that this is what is expected from a scientist. After all, this is how our supervisors delivered their presentations and it is what we see when we go to meetings. 'Rhetorically weak' appears to be how we signal 'scientifically credible'. We are afraid that a more simple and entertaining presentation will contaminate our scientific ethos with an aura of shallowness. And, of course, this fear is compounded by a general human fear of speaking before a group; in fact, it is 'the number one fear among American adults – ranking above the fear of snakes, heights, disease, financial problems or even death'[8]. Most of us stand with leaden feet in front of an audience, abandoning any good intentions to engage the audience the moment we mount the stage. Scientific knowledge, however, is built through publically sharing our insights so that they can be refined, challenged and elaborated. Therefore, as scientists, we must learn to handle this fear of presenting.

Most of the advice we gave for writing up science, also holds true for presenting science. Our central message – you are not presenting a study, but a story arising from your study – is even more important in case of an oral presentation. The concentration span of audiences is limited and often your presentation will be one in a row of many during a long conference day. It is, therefore, essential to grab the audience at the outset of your presentation and to sustain their interest for the duration. The start of your presentation should observe our problem-gap-hook structure: make clear to the audience what problem you are focusing on, what conversation is happening regarding it, and why your contribution today matters to them. Centred on this structure, this section offers a selection of recommendations for both short and long presentations based on our own experiences as presenters and spectators.

### Story telling

Besides interesting study data, stories, anecdotes and examples are the basic ingredients of your

---

**The power of stories**

One of the authors of this chapter (ED) was invited to deliver a presentation about – in that time – a fairly new topic: portfolios. Arriving in the meeting room, he experienced a hostile atmosphere and from remarks of the meetings' chair he discovered that the audience – teachers with an interest in medical education – had already decided to disagree with him before he had even said a word. In their view, portfolios sucked, and from their questions and comments it was quite clear that they had no confidence whatsoever in the main messages of the presentation. Completely frustrated with the fact that he had failed to make the presentation about this new topic a success, he thought about how to prevent a disaster to happen on a next occasion. How to persuade a strongly opposed audience to have faith in lessons from the literature? He found the answer in making explicit effort to connect himself as a presenter and the topic (portfolios) with the world of the audience (doctoring and medical education). He would open his next presentation with a personal story about a paediatric surgeon who had performed a complicated operation on his son. The story would on a content-level make tangible the complexity of the profession of doctors and at the same time explain how portfolios can be used to learn and assess this complexity. At a relational level, moreover, the story would connect the presenter with the audience. It was an emotional story with a happy ending, which directly appeals to the audience: most of them would be doctors and many would be parents too. The next time he had the chance to present about portfolios, the presentation was unexpectedly powerful. The story helped to tear down the wall between him and the already disagreeing audience and to gain trust in his words. From that day stories, narratives, examples and anecdotes have become the essential ingredients for his presentations ever since.

*Figure 22.6* Story telling during presentations.

presentation[9]. Stories help you to connect with your audience. This can be very important, as the story in Figure 22.6 makes clear.

Stories have to reflect your core message and should not be irrelevant to the rest of your abstract messages. Only then can they bring to life the abstractions in your presentations. Most presentations of science are highly abstract, dwelling on new, abstract theories and data. Listeners require time and effort to digest abstract messages, and wrapping them up in stories makes them both more palatable and more memorable. Stories place your abstract message in a context and we know that context plays a very influential role in the construction of knowledge[10].

**Kill your darlings**

It is easy to understand why most presenters feel that they have too much to tell in too little time. For over a year, you have been working hard on your study, and now you are anxious to share the lessons you learned from the literature review, account for methodological choices you made, explain the results, present your conclusions and offer important recommendations. The trick is to cook all this work down into a 10-minute talk that will not be used for email catch-up time by your audience. Our drama metaphor for writing is equally valid for presenting. In a 10-minute drama, there is only room for the main characters; therefore, in your short presentation, you must discipline yourself to stick to one, and possibly two, main messages. This means that, besides storytelling, selection is the second main ingredient of an engaging and effective talk. As one of our colleagues puts it, to engage people

in your presentation, you should keep it *simple* and keep it *short*; to increase their engagement, you should keep it even *simpler*, and keep it even *shorter*.

This is a difficult thing to accomplish. You want to share what you know, to dazzle with your ideas and insights – in short, to show off your darlings. Instead, though, the adage should be: *kill your darlings*. Include only those messages that help to communicate your main message to your audience, leaving out anything else that does not directly help to convey this main message, regardless of how much you love it. The principles that we discussed in the 'Writing Up'-section, together with what you know about the prior knowledge of the audience, should guide your selection.

**Using visuals**

For most of us, preparing a presentation comes down to drafting a PowerPoint presentation. This likely explains why, for most of us, delivering a presentation comes down to reading out the text on the PowerPoint slides. Whether or not visual aids such as PowerPoint slides help to convey your message depends on the occasion and the generic expectations that occasion sets up in the audience. However, it is safe to say that when PowerPoint produces reading, rather than presenting, it has not helped you engage the audience. So dispense with the slides-as-crutch approach and consider what the slides do for the audience, not what they do for you.

When your audience is relatively small, it may be helpful if you provide handouts that contain, for instance, a summary of the data, which you then discuss during the presentation instead of using a PowerPoint presentation. If you do use visual aids such as PowerPoint slides, then the first thing you need to do is to make sure that these aids visually support your story and messages. For several reasons, slides full of bulleted text, instead of supporting them, merely obstruct your story and messages. First of all, the structure disembowels a good story, because bullet points lead to abstract overviews instead of detailed narratives. Secondly, a presentation predicated on text-heavy PowerPoint requires an audience listen and read simultaneously, which can generate extraneous cognitive load (see the chapter by Lippink et al. in this book for more on cognitive load). This is exacerbated by the fact that your spectators may read your slides more quickly than you talk, impacting your ability to control the timing of the story. Timing is central to a speaker being able to effectively construct a dramatic arc in their story. Good storytellers build climaxes, weave in complications, insert surprises and achieve resolutions, all of which is threatened if the reader jumps ahead.

So use your PowerPoint slides wisely, as aids rather than as spoilers or crutches. We recommend slides with relevant pictures or drawings and with minimal text. And we do not recommend distributing handout versions of your slides before your talk: that is just tempting people to see how the story ends before you have even started. If you intend to give a handout to the audience, it should be something different from a mere printed version of your slides. For instance, it could include a full study synopsis and methodological details that would weigh down your oral story but might be of interest to some listeners. Garr Reynolds book on the design of PowerPoint presentations is a good guide for making your PowerPoint less text-rich and more visual[11].

While we would not argue that speakers should have their talks memorised, having the first few slides memorised helps with presentation jitters, which tend to be worse at the start of the talk. And you should have a memorised script for the closing lines as well; a good talk can be easily ruined when the speaker ends with a limp closer such as 'That's it.' or 'I'll take questions now.' The last line should be something memorable and reflective of the main thrust of the story. Similarly, speakers should be familiar enough with their presentation that they can maintain regular eye contact with the audience in order to judge their reactions to the presentation as it unfolds. This means paying attention to how your body is oriented at the podium: make sure that you look at the audience and not at the screen. Before you present, ask if you will have a laptop at the podium. If you do, there is no need to turn your back on the audience. If you do not, then you will need to rehearse your talk until you know where each slide comes in the story, and you can advance without having to look each time and present without reading the text. Think too, about transitions between slides: ideally, the presenter starts talking about what is coming next before the slide appears, helping the listener to make the logical transitions in the story easily.

## Communicating science on social media

When thinking about possibilities for communicating their work, most scientists think about writing up their work into journal articles or (chapters of) books and presenting their work at conferences, symposia or other meetings. The use of social media for communicating their work is less common but becoming increasingly important. This could be attributed to the unfamiliarity with the medium, in combination with the fear to make highly visible mistakes on the new medium. Another factor that could make scientists reluctant to use social media is the assumption that most communication on social media is superficial and uncontrollable and therefore unsuitable for the communication of something as serious as your scientific work. In spite of this, more and more scientists are discovering the possibilities that social media offer for discussing science and communicating their work[12]. Blogs, Twitter and Facebook can help to improve the visibility of the scientific work and the researcher. For example, on Twitter articles are recommended and discussed and picked up by a potentially broad audience. These media offer possibilities to bring your paper to the attention of a broader audience than the readers of the journal in which your article was published.

Social media not only provide the opportunity to increase the impact of your work, they also offer new possibilities that traditional scientific journals do not have. Communicating about science does not have to wait until the study has been finished and has been published. During the design of the study, for instance, researchers can tweet a question or dilemma that they have and use the discussion on Twitter to shape their understanding of the subject matter. Such possibilities to communicate and discuss with other researchers can boost the development of knowledge and spark scientific debate in your domain. Researchers who do not have the support of a research group that organises journal clubs or other scholarly activities can participate in online journal clubs and discussions on social media.

## Conclusion

We have used a rhetorical approach to dissemination in this chapter, to get writers and speakers thinking about how to tell a compelling story from their research work. The tips we have laid out arise from our own experience and from the role models we have both sought throughout our scientific careers as writers and presenters. We recommend 'following' the writing and presenting of people whose communication practices you find effective. Be analytical when you read or hear their work: How did they structure their paper? What makes their style so effective? What separates them from other presenters? If you need help finding speaker role models to follow, a good source of excellent presenters in action is the TED (Technology, Education and Design) website (www.ted.com/talks). We also suggest looking for role models outside your research community: scientists from other disciplines, or authors writing in non-research genres can also inspire your academic communication.

---

**Practice points**

- Think of your paper or presentation as a contribution to a scholarly conversation.

- In your opening, aim to identify the problem, map the gap, and articulate the hook.

- Tell a story with clear characters and compelling plot arc.

- Craft the written language attention for carrying the reader smoothly through the story.

- Keep the story simple for brief presentations, and use visuals strategically.

---

## Further reading

Writing up
1  Sword, H. (2012) *Stylish Academic Writing*. Harvard UP, Cambridge, MASS.

2  Glasman-deal, H. (2010) *Science Research Writing for Non-Native Speakers of English*. Imperial college press, London.

Presenting
3  www.ted.com/talks
4  Heath, C. & Heath, D. (2007) *Made to Stick: Why Some Ideas Survive and Others Die*. Randomhouse, New York.
5  Reynolds, G. (2012) *Presentation Zen: Simple Ideas on Presentation Design and Delivery*, 2nd edn. New Riders, Berkeley.

Social media
6  http://socialnetworkingforscientists.wikispaces .com/General
7  http://superfund.oregonstate.edu/apha-round table-communication-strategies#.U6vzNI1_sRV

## References

1  Devitt, A.J. (2004) *Writing Genres*. Southern Illinois University Press, Carbondale.
2  Miller, C.R. (1984) Genre as social action. *Quarterly Journal of Speech*, **70**, 151–167.
3  Lingard, L. & Haber, R.J. (1999) Teaching and learning communication in medicine: A rhetorical approach. *Academic Medicine*, **74**, 507–510.
4  Bazerman, C. (1988) *Shaping Written Knowledge: The Genre and Activity of the Experimental Article in Science*. University of Wisconsin Press, Madison.
5  Taylor, R.B. (2005) *The Clinician's Guide to Medical Writing*. Spring, New York, pp. 23.
6  Sword, H. (2012) *Stylish Academic Writing*. Harvard UP, Cambridge MASS, pp. 6.
7  Lanham, R.A. (1992) *Revising Prose*, 3rd edn. Macmillan P, New York.
8  Motley, M.T. (1997) *Overcoming Your Fear of Public Speaking-A Proven Method*. Houghton Mifflin, New York, pp. 3.
9  Heath, C. & Heath, D. (2007) *Made to Stick: Why Some Ideas Survive and Others Die*. Randomhouse, New York.
10  Brown, J.S., Collins, A. & Duguid, P. (1999) Situated cognition and the culture of learning. *Educational Researcher*, **18**, 32–42.
11  Reynolds, G. (2012) *Presentation Zen: Simple Ideas on Presentation Design and Delivery*, 2nd edn. New Riders, Berkeley.
12  Bik, H.M. & Goldstein, M.C. (2013) An Introduction to Social Media for Scientists. *PLoS Biology*, **11**, e1001535. doi:10.1371/journal.pbio.1001535)

# 23 Leadership, management and mentoring: applying theory to practice

*Judy McKimm and Helen O'Sullivan*

*You have a mixed portfolio of clinical, teaching, management and education research activities. You are really interested in the work-based assessment area of healthcare education research and have published a few papers over the years on this topic, mostly using student interns and internal funds to facilitate the data collection and analysis. You cannot do any more by yourself, and have just been asked to act as the project manager for a new national project looking at work-based assessment from an inter-professional perspective. How do you lead and manage this new inter-professional research team given your other commitments, and how do you make sure that you fulfil the conditions of the funding in terms of project delivery?*

## Introduction

Whether you are a new researcher about to start on your first project or an experienced researcher with a large team, it can be helpful to understand more about how leadership and management theory can help your (and others') research run more smoothly. Throughout the chapter, we will consider some relevant theories, models and ideas and how these might be applied at three levels:

- The intrapersonal – understanding yourself and your motivations, strengths and limitations;
- The interpersonal – working with other researchers, study participants and sponsors;
- The organisational or system – locating your research in organisations and complex systems[1].

By the end of this chapter, you should be able to describe:

- Key concepts, theories and models of leadership and their application to healthcare professions education research
- The differences between leadership and management and how to use both sets of skills appropriately
- Principles of project management
- Your own role as a research leader
- How to develop and mentor healthcare education researchers
- Build organisational research capacity.

## Leadership and management theories

Many leadership and management theories exist and are described more fully in the following sections. Whereas 'management' is often described as providing stability and order, concerned with planning and problem-solving, leadership tends to be associated with change, movement, direction setting and vision. In reality, of course, both are needed in the research setting. There is no point having a vision of running a large-scale national study if do you do not manage the resource to do this effectively. Studies also need to fit with education and health service directions so as to inform future policy and practice and they need to be well managed so researchers gain, or maintain, their own and the organisation's reputation.

As with most aspects of education, these approaches are subject to cultural influences, events and trends. At any one time, while various theories and approaches may dominate, what tends to happen is that multiple paradigms exist with people holding varying perspectives about what leaders should (or should not) be doing and how they should behave (akin to the concept of worldview in research presented earlier in this book). In the interests of space, this chapter will not describe the many theories in depth but instead select related approaches that might be helpful in different situations and contexts, which are relevant to healthcare education research.

An influential set of concepts are the context and contingency theories, including situational leadership[2,3]. From this perspective, leaders need to learn adapt their behaviour and style to fit the situation or context: leadership is, therefore, contingent on the situation. This may seem very obvious, but one reason that leaders struggle or fail is that they do not change their ways of working quickly enough appropriate to a given situation, especially in times of rapid change. For example, your style of leadership would probably be very different when working with new researchers than with a

*Researching Medical Education*, First Edition. Edited by Jennifer Cleland and Steven J. Durning.
© 2015 John Wiley & Sons, Ltd. Published 2015 by John Wiley & Sons, Ltd.

very experienced, senior researcher who can be left much more to develop and run projects themselves.

Early explanations of leadership focussed heavily on the personal qualities or personality traits of individual leaders: the hero leader who was expected to lead 'from the front' and by example. We still see echoes of this today (for example, when a surgeon dominates an operating theatre while the team is hesitant to challenge) and one of the tensions in leading and managing research activities is to achieve a balance between what individuals do versus a team or group approach. University practices can exacerbate tensions between individual and group activity in that they often measure and reward individual effort (e.g. by promotion or tenure) rather than collaborative, team achievements[4]. This contrasts with the shift in healthcare leadership, which is (at the time of writing) moving towards more collaborative or distributed[5] leadership approaches: leadership activities are thus highly devolved throughout the organisation and responsibilities and accountability are shared. 'Collective leadership'[6] is currently being promulgated as a way of improving health services from the bottom up as well as top down. These concepts fit closely with core values in health and education, which often embody ideas from servant leadership[7] – sustainability, facilitation,

stewardship, making a difference, work as vocation – or eco-leadership, where leadership is engaged with the environment, aiming for sustainability and works within interrelated systems. This highlights, first, that health education research is carried out in a complex, rapidly changing world. Second, that researchers need to use adaptive leadership[8], that is the process of understanding the meaningful steps that need to be taken to improve an organisation. Adaptive leaders help move organisations and individuals towards this goal through gradual evolution, they have insight into and understanding of this complexity so as to ensure their research 'fits' with professional, disciplinary, organisational, systems or service directions or needs – all of which will be different, and indeed sometimes competing[9]. This understanding is important, not only for your own satisfaction and motivation – most of us want to feel that our research is 'making a difference' somewhere - but also when seeking funding or support and when disseminating the outputs of research.

Table 23.1 summarises some of the leadership and management approaches that have dominated at various times. Please note this is broadly chronological but not comprehensive (see Further Reading for more detailed descriptions).

*Table 23.1* Key features and assumptions of predominant leadership approaches

| Leadership approach | Key features | Key assumptions |
| --- | --- | --- |
| Trait theories | Personality based, heroic leader, 'great man', resides in individual leaders' qualities | Leaders are born, not made |
| Task versus team, styles | Managing is a balance between task, team and individual | Leaders are managers, others' behaviours can be modified |
| Contingency theories Situational leadership | Leaders' styles and behaviours are contingent on the situation | Leaders' behaviours can be modified |
| 'New paradigms' – transformational, charismatic | Leaders can transform people/organisations through a mix of personality and 'people work' | The individual leader is essential to organisational success Leaders can 'learn leadership' |
| Followership | Followers are as important as leaders | Followers and leaders together co-create what leadership entails |
| Servant leadership | The leader wants to serve first and make a difference | That leaders' values are aligned with the organisation |
| Authentic, value-based, moral leadership | Followers value leaders who are consistent and authentic | Leaders own values are important |
| Adaptive leadership | Leaders need to adapt to and be comfortable working in complex situations in order to drive organisational change | Leaders work within complex, organic systems Those in the system have 'agency' |
| Distributed or dispersed leadership | Leadership is at 'all levels' of an organisation | Leadership is a process, building social capital important |
| Collaborative, collective, shared leadership | Leadership is about working together to achieve shared goals and outcomes | The more power we share, the more power we have |
| Eco-leadership | Leadership needs to be carried out in relation to the wider environment | Sustainability and social accountability important |

For researchers working at the interface of health services and academic institutions, understanding predominant leadership approaches and prevailing cultural norms and values is vital. This is particularly important when working at the 'evaluation' or 'improvement' end of the research continuum. It is one thing for a laboratory-based researcher to spend a lot of time working on a discrete project or part of a project alone or in a small team, but very different skills and approaches are needed when working, for example, on a large scale, multi-agency research study aiming to improve and standardise undergraduate or postgraduate assessments This is where project planning, stakeholder analysis, risk management and managing expectations are essential – discussed further in the subsequent sections.

An influential paradigm found in both education and healthcare organisations is that of 'transformational leadership'[10,11]. Transformational leadership combines the personal qualities of an effective leader (being inspiring, motivating, charismatic) with those of being able to take a visionary, strategic, direction-setting approach to transform services, organisations and ways of thinking. Whilst transformational leadership has been critiqued for its possible overemphasis on individual qualities (how does one learn 'charisma' for example?), promoting narcissistic leaders[12], emphasising more masculine characteristics and being 'Western' in its orientation, it is still the case that 'followers' expect something from a leader and that includes being inspired, motivated and attended to as individuals. Leaders, therefore, need to draw on their personal strengths and qualities in the primary role of building and maintaining relationships with other people. This is why understanding yourself and what makes you 'tick' is so important as you move into leadership roles. The very qualities that might be essential in your day-to-day research activities (such attention to detail, high conscientiousness, setting high personal standards) may hinder relationships with others who do not work in the same way and may feel you are being critical or over-demanding.

## Followership

As described in the previous section, much research focuses on leaders' qualities, behaviours and styles and, more recently on leaders' interaction with and influence on organisations, teams and systems. In studies that focus more on leaders, followers are either not considered or seen as fairly passive. However, a large body of work exists on followership and many researchers believe that more attention needs to be paid to the way those working to or

with the leader behave[13]. The relationship between leader and follower involves some dominance and some deference, but it is not always one-way. Leaders and followers can be described as passive followers, active followers, little 'l' leaders and big 'L' leaders[14]. This is a useful way of conceptualising where you and others fit in the leader–follower relationship or activity. You can provide lots of opportunities for students and early career researchers to engage in active followership or little 'l' leadership through small projects, taking a lead on research activities or working alongside more experienced researchers while they learn their 'craft'[15].

From a more detailed perspective, which helps explain why leaders have difficulties with some followers (and vice versa), Kelley's (1998) model suggests that five types of followers exist:

1 *Sheep*: passive, require external motivation and strong direction and supervision from the leader.
2 *Yes-people*: committed to working with the leader to achieve goals and tasks. They are conformists, tend to be unquestioning of the leader and very loyal.
3 *Pragmatics*: stay 'on the fence' and in the background and will not commit to innovation or major change until this is fully agreed.
4 *Alienated*: can be very negative, confrontational and disruptive of a team through questioning the leaders' (and others') decisions and actions. They often see themselves as the rightful leader of the team/organisation/project.
5 *Star followers*: positive, active and independent thinkers who do not accept the leaders' decisions or actions of a leader until they have evaluated them completely. Their independence and intelligence means that they can succeed without the leader being present[16].

Thus, contemporary research focuses on the active role of followers, how followers shape the behaviour of leaders and how power, dependence and social influence need to be considered.[17] In terms of Kelley's model, a leader needs to be aware of how each follower may perceive situations and thus how they may behave, which in turn will influence how a leader acts. For example, if your research group has a number of projects on the go with competing deadlines, you will consider your 'followers' skills, perceptions of the studies and previous performance when allocating tasks. Sheep and yes-people might be best working on the more innovative projects under the direction of a star follower, whereas more work and support will need to be done with the alienated or pragmatics, who may be best working on more routine, less critical projects, at least until you can get them on side and motivated. Depending on how your followers responded (for example if a pragmatic became fully on board with a study), again your leadership style may have to be modified and you may give this person more responsibility – this is how the relationships are co-created.

Power depends on many factors including control or influence over resources (e.g. funding, space, equipment or people with the right skills), access to people who have those resources and the position in the organisation. Leaders depend on followers to support them in decision making (and sometimes to challenge), to provide information, to meet personal needs and to behave in certain ways. Thus, a mutually beneficial contract (implicit or explicit) occurs between leaders and followers. It is important that followers learn to know their leader so that they can exert social influence safely. 'Diehards' or 'whistle-blowers', or followers who challenge leaders may find themselves at risk. Oc and Bashshur suggest that followers should be aware of the leaders' needs (have you got something they need such as expertise or skills?), build strength and power (through resources, information) accordingly, reduce social distance (get 'near' to the leader) and find safety in numbers (build coalitions)[17].

## Yourself as a research leader

### Personality type and leadership
Are leaders born or made? Can anyone become a leader or do you need an immutable set of personality traits and characteristics before you can become a successful leader? This question has been the subject of much debate in the management and leadership literature over many years. Judge et al. (2002) carried out a large scale research project looking at various personality traits and correlating them with successful leadership[18]. They also reviewed a number of other studies by colleagues who had looked at a whole range of personality traits to see if there was strong evidence that leadership was trait dependent. Many studies indicated that that successful leadership was linked to a variety of personality traits such as emotional maturity, adaptability and sociability but the only two traits where a robust correlation has been demonstrated are self-confidence and extraversion[18,19]. Although the term extraversion has a popular understanding, in psychology it is defined in terms of obtaining energy from interactions that take place outside of the self. So extraverts gain energy, drive, and motivation from working with people.

## Identifying your skills, strengths and motivations
Given the lack of real evidence linking substantial numbers of personality traits to successful leadership, this 'trait theory' of leadership has been heavily criticised and has given way to theories of leadership such as contingency leadership (where the leaders uses the most appropriate style for the context), transformational leadership (where a leaders uses his or her vision to motivate followers to change their expectation and perceptions to move the organisation towards a common goal), distributed (where boundaries of leadership are open and negotiable and where all members of the team share responsibility for the leadership) and collaborative leadership (where the leader's role is to build collaborations and cross-boundary leadership teams as discussed earlier[20]. However, whichever theory or theories of leadership you think most relevant to your personal context, personal development as you engage with your leadership journey will enable you to reflect on your leadership styles and performance and help you to develop and grow as a leader. The best foundation for this personal development journey is a thorough insight into your existing skills, strengths and motivations. This can be challenging and even difficult, especially if you are already established in a professional career and have never really reflected on your strengths and weaknesses. However, it can be enormously powerful and can help explain difficult relationships and areas of work that you have found frustrating. It can also give insight into the areas of work and leadership that you may have natural preference for and may indicate some limitations in terms of your current skill set.

### Analytical tools and leadership inventories
Entering 'leadership inventory' into an online search engine yields over 55 million results! There is no shortage of analytical tools and inventories to help you with self-analysis and insight. Some organisations may have a development unit that runs a variety of inventories, helps with analysis and reflection and can facilitate or recommend courses. Other organisations run local or regional courses or workshops at conferences, which you may wish to undertake.

Two popular approaches to development are worth engaging with:
- Inventories based on Myers Briggs Personality Type Indicator™ – these are powerful because there is no right or wrong type and it will help you to understand not only your own preferences and

behaviour but also how other colleagues think and behave[21,22].

- Inventories based on 360 degree feedback – these are especially useful when they can be administered online and your colleagues can give feedback anonymously.

However, all of these inventories should be approached with healthy scepticism! All the most commonly used inventories have criticisms associated with them and none of them explains every aspect of your potential leadership style. Their use is at its most powerful when used in collaboration with a well-supported personal development plan – either in an institutional programme of organisational development or working with an experienced and supportive mentor or coach. It is also natural to focus on the weakness or shortcomings of your leadership style. However, it is just as important to look at your strengths as you will often take these for granted. Being very clear about your strengths, preferences and motivations can help you develop your career in a way that plays to these strengths.

## The leadership journey

Whether you are an established leader who is taking on research leadership or whether research leadership is your first taste of leading others, you are on a leadership journey that will be characterised by challenges and setback, frustrations and successes. Many people can help to provide support and you will find yourself playing different support roles for others. In addition to formal line management, supervision, mentoring and coaching are also useful skills to develop. At different points in your career or in different situations you may wish to take advantage of them yourself.

Broad definitions are as follows:

- *Mentoring*: providing guidance, support and sometimes advice for the benefit of the mentee to help make transitions or changes or to assist professional development.
- *Coaching*: developing individual capabilities and potential to unlock performance and achieve personal and/or organisational goals.
- *Supervision*: overseeing performance, giving feedback and supporting professional development.

Finding an experienced and supportive mentor can help you navigate what can be a difficult journey. Your organisation may run a formal mentoring system and this can be helpful in brokering the mentoring relationship and providing a formal structure for the mentoring to take place. If not, it is advisable to find a mentor through your own efforts. Think about colleagues who are successful in your area; you should be sufficiently familiar with their work that you admire what they have achieved. They can be in your own organisation or outside it but for practical reasons they should be close enough geographically to enable reasonable access. You could ask your line manager for recommendations. When you approach your potential mentor, make it clear that the first meeting will be to establish if there is a basis for a mentoring relationship. You need to be very clear about what support you want to get out of the relationship (e.g. around promotion, large grant application process, managing a research team or raising your profile) and make a mentorship agreement that will specify how often you will meet, how long the relationship will last and so on. It is possible to have several mentors through a career, so having a time limit of, say, two years helps to prevent a mentoring relationship limping along for years when it is no longer effective. Coaching can be useful if you find yourself at a career crossroads, find personal life events are impacting on your work and career plans or if you want to consider career and lifestyle choices and options. It can also be useful to help you identify and develop strengths and strategies for getting the best out of yourself and others.

## Authenticity, integrity and resilience

A prominent leadership theory, which has application to research leadership, is that of 'authentic leadership'[23]. Authentic leaders are deemed to possess (or can acquire) a set of qualities and behaviours. These include the following:

- *Insight*: more than just having a vision of the future, insight means that the leader can cut through complexity and decide the best course of action.
- *Initiative*: they take the lead and do not ask followers to do something they would not do themselves.
- *Influence*: the leader draws people to their vision and values and has good personal networks in order to effect change.
- *Impact*: they make a difference, and (like servant leadership) it is the wanting to make a difference that drives them to make sustainable change.
- *Integrity*: value-driven, open and honest in transactions and communications – a 'moral compass' that is in tune with society's norms and values.

A large-scale research project conducted by Beverly Alimo-Metcalfe and colleagues into leadership concluded that 13 attributes of leaders have a significant impact on the effectiveness and success of the team that they lead. Of these, a leader's personal integrity and genuine concern for their team members can explain much of that effectiveness[24].

Developing personal integrity as a leader is crucial to gaining and keeping respect and credibility with those who you lead. The first step to leading with integrity is to examine your own moral and ethical codes and your own value systems and work out the extent to which you already follow those values. For example, as a healthcare practitioners, respect for patients' confidentiality and dignity is second nature, but if your research fails to safeguard your students' confidentiality or dignity, you will have failed to transfer your own values and ethics systems and this will be uncomfortable for you. Develop a culture of open communication and be generous in recognising and rewarding achievements and success in others. Keeping to your own values can be a challenge, especially in organisations that are undergoing significant change or at a time of resource constraints, but ultimately, only you can decide whether the organisation that you work for can support you in maintaining that integrity. If not, you may have some big decisions to make!

All leaders will come upon difficult situations and difficult colleagues. Leading education research can be punctuated by failed grant applications, rejected papers, studies that go wrong and colleagues who do not behave as expected. A good leader has the ability to bounce back from these setbacks, learn from them and carry on. This ability, or resilience, can be developed and having a supportive objective colleague such as a mentor or critical friend whom you can talk over difficulties with, and who can offer you an objective perspective, can help. Part of developing resilience is to develop an approach to work-life balance that is appropriate for you – make time for activities that revitalise you physically, emotionally, spiritually and intellectually.

## Leading change

Leaders need to be comfortable with managing and leading change. Researchers by their nature are inherently curious (I wonder why? I wonder how? I wonder if?) and this curiosity is allied closely to a positive leadership trait of being open to new experiences. What needs to be borne in mind is that different people or groups may have different psychological responses to change and various ways of viewing change. One of your roles as a leader is to convey your vision to other people and groups, and this requires knowing their position so you can present your pitch accordingly. For example, presenting the evaluation evidence for

reforming part of a healthcare curriculum may be received very positively by one group of colleagues but another group, who may feel that their role is being threatened by the change or who feel that the change is aimed at forcing them to change a long entrenched practice, may become defensive and obstructive. They will need more careful handling, lots of discussion and communication and need to trust that the change will have positive impact on them and their practice. Any change involves loss and anxiety, even if the change is positive (such as winning a large amount of funding for a study or centre or being promoted to a new job) some loss is incurred in working out what you will have to give up as a consequence and self-doubt may set in about whether you are up to the new challenges. Thinking of change in terms of the loss-grief cycle, Change curve[25] or Transition curve[26,27] helps to explain your own or others' responses. Most of these cycles identify common responses and stages of adapting to change:

- early immobilisation or denial;
- a dip in competence or productivity;
- frustration, resentment or anger;
- a move towards accepting the new reality and letting go;
- starting to make sense of the new way of working and behaving;
- finally, integrating the change into everyday life.

So, as part of developing the research culture in your organisation, you may decide to change the way that research students are managed from an ad hoc system where each supervisor does their own thing to a more collaborative process where research student training is done collectively and where processes for reviewing progress are more systematic. A starting point would be to work out who is going to be affected by the change and who might see it as a threat to their autonomy and potentially, even their competence. It would also set out the benefits of the change such as improved student experience, improved efficiency of the process and therefore saving time in duplicating effort, as well as support and guidance for new supervisors. If possible, engage a colleague who is very positive about the change and who can see the benefits and provide lots of opportunities for consultation and for colleagues to voice their concerns. Engaging senior colleagues, students and the correct committees can give you a mandate for change and help with issues of authority.

Managing change by understanding and reducing negative consequences (real or perceived) can help individuals work through this cycle by planning well, providing time and support to adapt to change, allowing grieving for what has gone to occur and expecting a (hopefully temporary) loss of competence or productivity.

Aside from the intrapersonal or intrapersonal aspects of leading change processes, other change models or approaches, which focus more on the system organisational aspects, can be useful, particularly when planning or when things go wrong or stall.

## Using a project management approach

Leaders need to keep sight of the wider aspects of change management as described earlier and managing multiple priorities may seem like second nature for those experienced in healthcare practice or managing education programmes. However, the success of a research project depends on the researcher's ability to plan, carry out, analyse and then write up their research. A formal project management process will help you anticipate problems and hence contain stress. This section does not advocate highly formal project management procedures but suggests that using the principles of project management will make your research more productive and enjoyable.

### Defining success
It is often helpful to start by working out what you want to get out of the project. If your project is externally funded, you will probably have already set this out in a grant application. The end points of a research project can be divided into two categories:
- *Outputs*: are tangible, usually physical things such as a journal paper or a conference presentation. They could also be a product, such as an assessment tool or some online learning material.
- *Outcomes*: is what happens as a result of the outputs; for example 'undergraduate medical students will perform better in their clinical exam'

Defining these very clearly at the outset enables you to evaluate the project against these at the end. See further reading for examples.

### Stakeholder analysis
Healthcare education research usually involves a number of different groups of people with potentially conflicting interests. Research in a university or other educational setting will probably involve healthcare students, faculty and professional services' colleagues and may involve other student groups. Where the research is situated in a healthcare setting (such as examining the process of

workplace based assessments in postgraduate medical training), you can add in the involvement of healthcare colleagues and patients. By working out who the stakeholders are for your project, you can plan how to involve them and communicate with them appropriately. Getting key stakeholders 'on side' from the very beginning can make a real contribution to the success of your project. For bigger projects, stakeholders (or their representatives) are often included as part of a steering or governance group. You will also need to ensure your research plan is reviewed and approved by governance bodies such as research ethics committees, if applicable to your setting/country.

### High-level time line
Once you know what you are trying to achieve and who you need to involve, you can produce a high level timeline for your project. The end date for your project may be defined by the terms of a grant application or by the fixed nature of a temporary position. So, for example, a high level timescale for a 1-year MPhil studentship may look like this.

| | |
|---|---|
| August/September | Research ethics application |
| August | Start literature review |
| September | Organise focus groups |
| October/November | Write up focus groups, plan questionnaire |
| December | Pilot and validate questionnaire |
| January–March | Distribute questionnaire and follow-up |
| March–April | Analyse questionnaire data |
| May–June | Write up thesis |
| August | Viva |

Healthcare education researchers are often juggling service delivery and teaching responsibilities, so the timeline needs to be realistic and take into account other significant tasks as well as life events and holidays. For example, if you know that your researcher is a doctor doing a part-time masters' project, for which they have been released from clinical duties for two days per week, it is sensible to estimate the work plan bearing that in mind. The work plan for someone doing full-time research would be very different.

### Work breakdown
The next stage of the planning process is to break down each of the main tasks into the small steps that make up the bigger task. A common approach

to this stage is to write down all of the small stages on post-it notes and then group or arrange them on a whiteboard or flip chart paper spread over a table. This has the advantage that you can rearrange the post-it notes and experiment with different ways of organising the project before settling on a final project plan. Other people find that using a mind map approach at this stage is more useful. However you do this part of the project plan, it is very useful to ask an experienced researcher to review your plan at this stage. They will be able to point out places where you have underestimated the time something will take, or missed out a crucial stage. Once you have got your post-it notes/flip chart paper/mind maps into a format that you are happy with, it is useful to photograph your detailed plan. If you are lucky enough to have a budget for your research project, you need to include costings to the various parts of the project so that you can keep track of expenditure during the project.

Once you have your work breakdown you can experiment with different ways of scheduling your project through relatively simple tools such as spreadsheets or Gantt Charts or more sophisticated software if your project is much larger or more complex. These are a matter of personal preference and are out of the scope of this chapter but there are plenty of books, websites and courses that describe and advise on different approaches and techniques.

### Identifying and managing risks

During the planning stage, you should identify some of the main risks for your project and work out how to minimise the risk in advance or plan what you might do in the event of one of the potential risks actually happening. For example, risks in healthcare education research might include the following:

- Very low numbers of students volunteering to take part in project;
- Data is poor quality and does not really show anything;
- Someone publishes the exact same study a week before you finish;
- You lose your laptop with all of your data on.

Once you have thought through and listed all possible risks to your work (even if some of them seem a little over dramatic!) you can prioritise your risks by giving them a value of 1–5 depending upon how serious the impact on your project would be and then again 1–5 depending on how likely the scenario is (probability). Each risk will then have a score from 1–25 and you can plan a mitigation strategy for each one that scores over 10.

So your mitigation strategy for the aforementioned risks might look like this:

| Risk | Mitigation |
|---|---|
| Very low numbers of students volunteering to take part in project; | • Communicate with students in advance about the benefits of the research;<br>• Identify advocates from the student body who can mobilise support;<br>• Provide appropriate incentives for taking part in the research. |
| Data is poor quality and does not really show anything; | • Pilot the study;<br>• Regularly review the data as it is collected. |
| Someone publishes the exact same study a week before you finish; | • Attend conferences and network;<br>• Consult with leaders in the area;<br>• Present pilot studies and ideas at conferences and get feedback. |
| You lose your laptop with all of your data on. | • Store data in more than one location. |

### Managing the project

Once your project is up and running, it is essential to manage and monitor your project so that you can deal with any unexpected issues or just get the project back on track if deadlines start to slip. This is particularly important if there is a team involved in the carrying out the research. Monitoring can be achieved through regular structured team meetings where each member of the team report on their progress. A simple report form can be developed by adapting the following headings

- Progress this month;
- Targets for next month;
- Any issues/barriers to progress/items for discussion.

It is also crucial to track your expenditure and manage the budget. Your own organisation will have a financial reporting mechanism but it is also useful to keep your own income and expenditure accounts to make sure that your budget is properly accounted for.

## Take time to finish off

Perhaps the part of a project that receives the least attention is the end of the project. All projects should have a formal end point and often this is a natural stage – the paper is published, the PhD is submitted, the research assistant's contract finishes. There are some obvious steps at the end of project such as completing a report for the grant awarding body or writing a final report for a research ethics committee. It is also really important that you conduct an evaluation of the project even if this is not formally required by anyone else. There are valuable lessons that can be learned during this period of reflection and it does not have to be very long or over complicated. Kirkpatrick's model for evaluating training programmes can usefully be adapted for evaluating educational research projects.[28,29] A quick note of the lessons learned can help you in planning your next project.

## Developing and sustaining research capacity in organisations

### The challenges of building research capacity in education

Healthcare education research is usually carried out in a university, a healthcare setting or jointly between the two types of institutions. For these organisations, education research is often subjugated in priority to service delivery, teaching and biomedical sciences research. Part of your role as a leader of healthcare education research is, therefore, to build research capacity in your organisation. Building capacity can refer to two major areas:

- Building skills and expertise in yourself and colleagues who wish to carry out educational research.
- Securing resources – both tangible resources in terms of equipment, financial resources for consumables, travel and so on and human resources; in other words, time!

Research leaders can also achieve results through seeking ways to enhance scholarship and improve education; putting faculty into positions of influence within their communities; gaining a reputation for the place that sets the research agenda and facilitating translational and applied research[30].

### Leveraging financial resources

It is very difficult to secure large grants for new programmes of education research. Funders will usually need to see a successful track record of completed projects and publications so that the risk of funding your project is minimised. However, this leads to the question; how can I get started if I cannot get a grant? Your own institution may offer small sums of money to pump prime new educational research areas and lots of external organisations offer small grant schemes. These are for relatively small sums of money but they enable you to get started and to demonstrate that you are capable of delivering an externally funded project.

### Developing human resources

As a research leader, the amount of hands-on research that you can carry out will be limited by the amount of time that you have available. Even if you have no other professional responsibilities, this time will be finite and the only way to expand this capacity is by taking on PhD students and/or research assistants. As stated earlier, the opportunities to bid for externally funded research studentships are rare but there may be institutionally funded studentships that you can bid for or part time self-funded students that will be interested in your work.

You may have more senior colleagues who are established healthcare professionals who have very little experience of conducting research projects. You may even have colleagues who are very experienced in one area of research (for example biomedical sciences) but who aspire to conduct educational research. If these colleagues are without a PhD then encouraging them to study for a PhD on a part time basis is an excellent way for them to develop the necessary research skills. However, this needs to be taken on with realistic notion of the time involved. Other possibilities include them taking an MPhil or MRes, an MA in Medical/Healthcare Education or intense courses in research methods.

Even if your research team is just you and a part-time PhD student, it is worth engendering a 'research group' ethos from the start. By setting up a seminar series, workshops and a journal club and encouraging colleagues to present their work at national and international conferences, you can prevent feelings of isolation and encourage an open and evaluative culture in your research. This has the added benefit of raising your profile internally and externally. The ability to network is important when setting up your research group and successful networking will lead to opportunities to collaborate and, therefore, expand your capacity to carry out research, write and publish.

## Interdisciplinary working and working across institutions

One way of expanding your capacity and extending your work is through interdisciplinary and multi-disciplinary work. A simple way to start is to apply the methodology from a completed research project to another professional group, preferably one that you have easy access to through a personal connection and geographical location. So, for example, if you have just conducted a study on peer assisted learning in medical undergraduates, it may be possible to extend that project to nursing students in the same organisation. Another way of doing this might be to bid for a grant to look at peer assisted learning in medical, dental, nursing, physiotherapy and veterinary medicine students. Organisations are often more likely to fund bids where they can see that the impact is in more than one professional area or setting. It is possible to build institutional capacity by collaborating with other institutions and this can be especially powerful when collaborating internationally.

## The planned opportunist

In order to develop and accomplish a successful body of research and outputs, you need to be very clear about the programme of research that you wish to pursue. However, calls for funding and invitations to collaborate may not align perfectly with this programme and your plans or vision. Sometimes you need to be opportunistic and modify your research to fit in with a particular priority of a funding body or organisation. Being open to changing your research area slightly to fit in with an opportunity will give your research career sustainability. Linked to this is horizon scanning (which helps develop insight) – keeping up to date with national and international policy and issues, understanding local and national priorities in healthcare education and understanding the potential consequences of critical incidents on national policy. There are news alerts and email groups that you can sign up for to help with this and membership of professional groups can provide an opportunity to discuss these issues with colleagues.

## Conclusion

In summary, the leadership literature can provide helpful perspectives, models and explanatory frameworks on how both leaders and followers can work more successfully in healthcare education research. Developing self-knowledge and insight into your strengths, motivators and preferences is key to working more effectively and interacting with others to get the best out of them. The role of research leaders as change agents and as capacity builders is also vital. Research is often carried out in teams and the role of a research leader is to support, develop and grow the capacity of students, colleagues and the organisation in learning and applying the evidence from research. Getting to know the systems and organisations (both formal and informal) in which you work and with which you interact will also help you develop longer term vision, a power base and enable you to seize opportunities when they arise. Finally, it is reassuring to remember that leadership is a process: it is a journey that lasts a lifetime that no one ever gets perfect.

---

**Practice points**

- Leadership and management are different, but both are needed in healthcare education research

- Leadership can be thought of at the interpersonal, the intrapersonal and the organisation or system level – essentially, leadership is about knowing yourself, relationships, conversations and change

- Understanding some leadership theories and approaches can help you lead more effectively

- A project management approach can help avoid pitfalls and failure in healthcare educational research

- Coaching and mentoring can be useful for you and for your team but individual development needs to be coupled with organisational capacity building

---

## Further reading

Bolman, L.G. & Gallos, J.V. (2010) *Reframing Academic Leadership*. John Wiley and Sons Inc, New York.

Goffee, R. & Jones, G. (2006) *Why Should Anyone be Led by You? What it Takes to be an Authentic Leader*. Harvard Business Review Press, Boston, MA.

Leadership Quarterly Yearly Review e.g. 2013 *issue 'Advances in traditional leadership theory and research', guest editor Chester A Schriesheim – these annual reviews provide excellent summaries of the latest in general leadership research and development.*

McKimm, J., Cotton, P., Garden, A. & Needham, G. (2013) Educational leadership. In: Walsh, K. (ed), *Oxford Textbook of Medical Education*. Oxford University Press, Oxford.

Obolensky, N. (2010) *Complex Adaptive Leadership: Embracing Paradox and Uncertainty*. Gower/Ashgate Publishing Ltd, Farnham.

Preedy, M., Bennett, N. & Wise, C. (2012) *Educational Leadership: Context, Strategy and Collaboration*. Open University/Sage, Milton Keynes.

Swanwick, T. & McKimm, J. (2014) Educational leadership. In: Swanwick, T. (ed), *Understanding Medical Education: Evidence, Theory and Practice*. Wiley Blackwell ASME, Chichester.

Many web resources exist which provide information and examples of useful management tools which can be used in research projects (e.g. strategic management; SWOT, PESTLE, risk analysis; options appraisal, stakeholder analysis), including:

The JISC site has many resources openly available for researchers, especially in universities

www.jiscinfonet.ac.uk/infokits

Mindtools – lots of resources on leading and managing yourself and teams, career and professional development, Free weekly newsletter with lots of hints and tips and a club

www.mindtools.com

Businessballs - career and personal development as well as more explanation of some of the models and frameworks described in the chapter

www.businessballs.com

## References

1 Swanwick, T. & McKimm, J. (2014) Faculty development for leadership and management. In: Steinert, Y. (ed), *Faculty Development in the Health Professions: A Focus on Research and Practice*. Springer, Dordrecht.

2 Fiedler, F. (1964) A contingency model of leadership effectiveness. In: Berkowitz, L. (ed), *Advances in Experimental Social Psychology*. Academic Press, New York, pp. 149–190.

3 Hersey, P. & Blanchard, K. (1988) *Management of Organizational Behaviour*. Englewood Cliffs, NJ, Prentice Hall.

4 Leiff, S. & Albert, M. (2010) The mindsets of educational leaders: how do they conceive of their work? *Academic Medicine*, **85**, 57–62.

5 Bolden, R. (2010) Leadership, management and organisational development. In: Thorpe, R., Gold, J. & Mumford, A. (eds), *Gower Handbook of Leadership and Management Development* (5e). Gower, Farnham, pp. 117–132.

6 Eckert, R., West, M., Altman, D., Steward, K. & Pasmore, B. (2014) *Delivering a Collective Leadership Strategy for Health Care*. The King's Fund, London.

7 Greenleaf, R.K. (1977) *Servant Leadership: A Journey into the Nature of Legitimate Power and Greatness*. Paulist Press, Mahwah, NJ.

8 Heifetz, R.A. & Linsky, M. (2004) When leadership spells danger. *Education Leader*, **61**, 33–37.

9 Randall, L. & Coackley, L. (2007) Applying adaptive leadership to successful change initiatives in academia. *Leadership and Organization Development Journal*, **28**, 325–335.

10 Bass, B.M. & Avolio, B.J. (1996) 'Postscript' In *Improving Organisational Effectiveness Through Transformational Leadership*. Sage, London.

11 Leithwood, K., Jantzi, D. & Steinbach, R. (1999) *Changing Leadership for Changing Times*. Open University Press, Buckingham.

12 Maccoby, M. (2007) *The Leaders We Need and What Makes us Follow*. Harvard Business School Press, Boston.

13 Kellerman, B. (2008) *Followership: How Followers are Creating Change and Changing Leaders*. Harvard Business Press, Boston, MA.

14 Kelley, R.E. (1988) In praise of followers. *Harvard Business Review*, **66**, 142–148.

15 Bohmer, R. (2010) Leadership with a small 'l'. *BMJ*, **340**, c483.

16 Kelley, R.E. (1998) Followership in a Leadership world. In: Spears, L.C. (ed), *Insights on Leadership Service, Stewardship, Spirit and Servant Leadership*. John Wiley and Sons, Inc, New York, pp. 170–184.

17 Oc, B. & Bashshur, M.R. (2013) Followership, leadership and social influence. *Leadership Quarterly*, **24**, 19–934.

18 Judge, T.A., Bono, J.E., Ilies, R. & Gerhardt, M. (2002) Personality and leadership: a qualitative and quantitative review. *Journal of Applied Psychology*, **87**, 765–780.

19 Siebert, S.E. & Kraimer, M.L. (2001) The five factor model of personality and career success. *Journal of Vocational Behavior*, **158**, 1–21.

20 Storey, J. (2004) Changing theories of leadership and leadership development. In: Storey, J. (ed), *Leadership in Organisations: Current Issues and Key Trends*. Routledge, Abingdon.

21 Myers, I.B. & Myers, P.B. (1995) *Gifts Differing: Understanding personality type*. Mountain View, CA, Davies-Black/CPP Inc.

22 Quenk, N.L. (2002) *Was That Really Me? How Everyday Stress Brings Out Our Hidden Personality*. Mountain View, CA, Davies-Black/CPP Inc.

23 George, B. (2007) *True North: Discover Your Authentic Leadership*. John Wiley and Sons, New York.

24 Alimo-Metcalfe, B., Alban-Metcalfe, J., Bradley, M., Mariathasan, J. & Samele, C. (2008) The impact of engaging leadership on performance, attitudes to work and wellbeing at work: a longitudinal study. *Journal of Health, Organisation and Management*, **22**, 586–598.

25 Kübler-Ross, E. & Kessler, D. (2005) *On Grief and Grieving: Finding the Meaning of Grief Through the Five Stages of Loss.* Simon & Schuster Ltd, New York.

26 Fisher, J.M. (2005) A Time for change. *Human Resource Development International*, **8**, 257–264.

27 Parker, C. & Lewis, R. (1981) Beyond the peter principle: managing successful transitions. *Journal of European Industrial Training*, **5**, 17–21.

28 Kirkpatrick, D.L. (2009) *Evaluating Training Programs: The Four Levels*, 3rd edn. Berrett-Koehler, San Francisco.

29 Kirkpatrick, D.L. & Kirkpatrick, J.D. (2007) *Implementing the Four Levels.* Berrett-Koehler Publishers.

30 Cross SE. 2013 *A leadership model for the research university. 3rd International Conference on Leadership, technology and innovation management, Procedia - Social and Behavioural Sciences; 000-000, Elsevier Ltd. table*

# 24 Programmatic research: building and sustaining capacity

*David Taylor and Trevor Gibbs*

*After your appraisal, you return to your office and reflect on the discussion. Due to external pressures, the focus of your work is becoming more and more to do with education, and it is getting harder and harder to keep the momentum up in all of the strands of your busy life. You need to drop some commitments and consider where to focus your time and enthusiasm. The things that have been interesting you most recently have been the conversations you have had with students, and you find yourself wondering where they have got their ideas from? You reflect on this for a few days and realise that the most obvious, and the most interesting, path to develop further in your career portfolio is healthcare education research. You are not starting from scratch: you have already published a few articles in the medical education literature, presented at national conferences and have the beginnings of a network of research-interested colleagues. But how best to use your limited time effectively? Would it be better to join forces with research-active colleagues who have similar interests as you, go it alone or start the process of setting up a new research group?*

## Introduction

Research is stimulating, even fun, and most of us who get involved in it are highly motivated to understand more about the things that interest us and the things that matter. Our belief is that motivation- and enquiry-based approach to our everyday working lives is now the norm. However, it is all too easy to slip into being involved in a *'bit of research'*, often squeezed in and around clinical and/or teaching commitments, rather than working in ways that create long-term sustainable research programmes, which will build knowledge and understanding of a topic. This habit can be further compounded by spending too much time and energy in repeating the studies that have already been carried out by other people. This chapter sets out guidance to help readers consider how to move on from 'doing' a study as an individual to leading

or collaborating in a team-based, sustainable programme of educational research. We write from the viewpoint of being UK-based researchers, but the messages of this chapter are transferable to all contexts.

## Developing a research idea: the initial steps

An important starting point in developing any project is to verbalise the issue, problem or gap. An example of this would be: *'My students never appear to read the material associated with my lectures in advance. Why is this? I wonder if not doing so means they don't understand what I am saying in the lecture?'* The research question could then focus on exploring student attitudes towards preparatory reading, or in identifying barriers to preparation, or in considering if there are other, more effective, ways of teaching the topic in question.

From here, the process of research has already begun, but even at this early stage, challenges can arise. By looking through the literature for evidence on your topic or idea, you may discover that your question has already been answered. More likely, the existing evidence may have partially answered your research question and identified the need for further research. Even before you embark on your investigation(s), this step is influencing your work – your research is taking shape, you are asking questions, seeking and finding answers or even gaps in knowledge. It is at this point that you need to think if this is something that still interests you. Do the gaps in the literature fit with your research interests, knowledge and skills? Indeed, is it something that you would like to develop further? Is it something that is within your academic capabilities and time constraints? Can you do it alone or will you need help? If it is the latter, then who would you like to work with who has the necessary knowledge and skills? This period of

*Researching Medical Education*, First Edition. Edited by Jennifer Cleland and Steven J. Durning.
© 2015 John Wiley & Sons, Ltd. Published 2015 by John Wiley & Sons, Ltd.

personal constructive reflection is an essential first step in research. Whichever route you decide on, you are going to need to feel committed to, and positive about, the project.

A meaningful programme of research takes time; it needs time and energy, perseverance and resilience. Remember that even the most successful researchers are not always successful in grant applications, nor do they have their papers accepted without revisions. Sound decisions based upon realistic expectations, even at this early stage, can help ensure long-term sustainability of a research programme.

If you find that your question or idea has not been addressed, and/or there are other questions of interest still to be asked, and you are still confident that this is what you wish to pursue, then it is time to start a process of refinement. This involves developing some structure around your aims – what you want to find out – and objectives – how you will find it out. This is discussed in detail in Chapter 3. At this stage, you may also wish to discuss your research question with your colleagues – several heads are typically better than one – to ask if they feel that your ideas are relevant, logical, appropriate and feasible. You may also wish to communicate with individuals or groups working elsewhere, who have a track record of research on the topic under consideration.

Contacting others can be useful for many reasons, not the least of which is finding out about work in submission or preparation, the existence of which influences your choice of research question. Just as there is no point in repeating a study that is published, there is no point in starting a study that has already been done but is not quite yet available in the public domain. More positively, sometimes contacting an established research team can lead to collaborations, to 'win-win' situations where there is synergy across those working in the same area.

At this point, you should also reflect on your worldview (see McMillan, Chapter 2) and your preferred ways of working in terms of philosophical approach and the aligned methodologies and tools (see Cleland, Chapter 1). It is crucial to consider both of these carefully, and not, for example, launch down the pathway of using one particular data collection method merely because you have experience of using it before rather than it being fit for purpose[1].

This stage of research, identifying a problem and then a question and thinking through the process of developing a research focus and question, is often a lengthy and creative process, but an important one. A logical approach at this early stage provides a strong basis for your research, as well as gives an indication of how much work may be involved to achieve your research aims and objectives.[2].

Carefully choosing your research questions has three additional advantages:

- Through careful thought and discussion, you will probably end up concentrating on a more refined and narrow range of activities, where there is an increased and reasonable chance of gaining a real understanding of what is going on.
- You will foster the development of your own personal expertise.
- Careful planning and discussion usually means that you explore the 'so what' value of your research, which then has an ability to transform or change the present state of knowledge.

Moving from a single research question and study to a research programme, there are four overlapping elements that underpin a successful and sustainable programmatic approach to research. These are: topic focus, support from others, resource, and education and training of team members.

## Focus

One of the things that matters most in our current research environment is impact; the 'so what' factor; a concept of transferability or translation to the real world. One way of ensuring impact or transferability is to be sure that there is a common theme underpinning the research programme(s). This can be made more likely when a programme of research is based upon the needs of individuals, a community or a region – it becomes purposeful, has meaning and its outcome is likely to be effective. For example, with reference to other chapters in this book, many different programmes have evolved on the basis of need – for example, how best to discriminate between applicants at the point of selection into medicine or how best to understand learning processes (see a number of chapters in this book, including those of Torre and Durning, and Leppinck et al.).

Embedding individualistic research questions under a common umbrella of research on a specific subject frequently increases the chances of success in the area, increased publications, increased probability of research grants, and, hence, increased long-term sustainability. In an article written to mark his receipt of a Karolinska Institute Prize for research in medical education, Cees van der Vleuten gives a vivid description of the importance of a focused programme of research, in his case into assessment, which flourished because of focus, as well as good collaborative relationships across relevant disciplines (see later)[3].

Indeed, most institutions now concentrate their research on a small number of themes. In this way, the institution, not just the individual, develops the reputation of leading the way in a particular field. This protects a research programme against collapsing if any one individual leaves, and attracts others who are interested in working on the same programme in the institution. Having 'a track record' or a solid reputation in a field is important to funders, who usually need evidence of both expertise and ability to deliver on time, and to budget. Note that the size of any research group is not fixed: this is likely to be dictated by the local circumstances and success of the team in attracting funding to pay for dedicated research staff. The size of any group may fluctuate over time depending on the amount of ongoing research activity in progress.

Choosing the theme and focusing on the programme is essential. At Liverpool University Medical School, Liverpool, UK (www.liverpool.ac.uk/medicine), for example, members of the Medical Education Research Unit were interested in epistemology, widening participation, applying best evidence in medical education and professionalism. Through discussion, they decided to align all of their research interests under the umbrella of 'communities of practice' (CoPs: see Torre and Durning in this volume for more discussion of CoPs) in relation to how students 'become' doctors[4-10]. There are numerous examples of programmatic research in medical education: Jeroen van Merrienboer's programme of work on learning and instruction, Maastricht University, The Netherlands; Jennifer Cleland's work on selection and assessment, University of Aberdeen, UK; Kevin Eva's work on mini-multiple interviews (MMIs), University of British Columbia, Canada, to name but a few.

## Support

The research environment itself is fundamental[11]: it must encourage thinking and debate, and support research activity.

Support mechanisms tend to fall into two categories: formal structures and personal support. In terms of formal structures, in many institutions, researchers are required to discuss their projects with others before they apply for ethics review and grant funding. These systems of internal peer review can benefit both parties. The individual researcher is challenged to articulate clearly what he/she wants to do and why. The end product of, for example, an application for external funding is better articulated and more likely to be successful as a result.

At the more formal end of the continuum of support, it is important to have a mentor. A mentor is someone with sufficient experience and wisdom to be able to guide and advise a researcher. There is strong evidence that mentoring is both important and effective[12], provided that there is a good relationship between the mentor and the mentee and that they share similar outlooks. A strong mentorship programme has the potential to sustain a strong learning community[13]. See Chapter 23 by McKimm and O'Sullivan for further discussion on mentoring in education research.

It is also important to invest in people and encourage those involved in education research to acquire the appropriate qualifications[3]. Although, previously, many of those working in medical and healthcare education research developed their skills and knowledge 'on-the-job', the current climate encourages formal learning and recognised qualifications. This is partly for the benefit of the individual and for the benefit of professionalising the community[14].

Less formal support systems also exist. It can be very helpful to present ideas at research group meetings, journal clubs, at internal research days or at academic meetings and conferences. Questions and responses from the audience can shed light on weak points in the research and give pointers as to how to progress.

Other strategies for support at a personal level include the following:

- There is tremendous advantage in finding a critical friend[15], who is someone with whom one can talk honestly and openly and share ideas. You may be lucky enough to find this person in your own organisation, or you may have to look outside. It does not need to be anyone particularly senior, just someone who can understand what you are aiming at and why.
- The second strategy is to get into the habit of regular writing[16]. It can be a painful business but, particularly if you are the one who has to be putting the grant proposals and the papers together for the team, it is a very useful habit. One of us (DT) has just completed a Doctorate in Education (EdD), which required around 3000 words a week to be submitted every week over a two-year period. This regular activity became habit forming[17]. Since for most of us, the act of writing a paper is effectively 'writing up the study', there is considerable benefit in writing things as you go along[18]. Other ideas will occur to you as you write, and you will be encouraged to check and re-check sources. You will also then have a record that you can reflect upon to

help develop your understanding[19]. Being able to share the writing within the team, promoting active discussion and using each other as reviewers help solidify the quality of the written material.

The third element required for success is collaboration or adopting a collaborative approach. There may be some individuals who can go it alone, but most of us find it helpful to work with colleagues, librarians, psychometricians, psychologists, sociologists or those who work in education research but are not immersed in the world of healthcare education. As mentioned earlier, it is the team, not the individual, that builds a programmatic research[20]. Moreover, by working across disciplines, you see things from others' perspectives, which can be helpful in terms of holistic understanding[21]. This can help improve the quality of research in numerous ways, including in reaching the appropriate balance between what is theoretically important and what is pragmatically possible[22,23]. The second reason is that it encourages people to see things from other theoretical perspectives and, therefore, leads to a more holistic understanding of the issue under scrutiny[21].

Last, but not least, keeping up to date of publications in the field helps in planning future studies. Attending conferences or research seminars is a really good way of widening one's horizons and challenging one's ideas. One caveat: although it is fun to travel far and wide and a good way of building your own networks, it is important to remember that there may be someone in the next corridor or building who is thinking about the same sort of things as you[24]. Moreover, there are also countless, helpful online resources, from TED Talks® to Med-EdWorld (www.mededworld.org).

## Resources

Ultimately, building research capacity and maintaining sustainability requires resources. Resources encompass IT systems; library and online access to journals and other sources of information; equipment; staff time; as well as the less tangible resource of an organisational ethos, which encourages research (see earlier).

Staff time is arguably the most important, and the most expensive, resource in medical and healthcare education research. In the preliminary stages of a programme of research, realistically, projects may depend on internal resources such as interns, students wishing research experience and/or small funds. These are very useful means of developing ideas into proposals, carrying out feasibility or pilot studies (e.g. small amounts of funding can fund

interview transcription, or some statistician time) or even releasing some of your time from other commitments so that you can write an application for funding. Where the wider institution has a clear research mission, aligning one's own programme with that mission is strategic. Doing so can enable access to (re)sources of internal funding, training and professional development opportunities, and other support from within the organisation (e.g. your department head assigning some of your teaching to a new staff member to free you to write up a paper).

However, these days, it is essential to attract external grant funding. This is not easy – research is under-funded and hence opportunities to win funding are highly competitive. You also need a track record of attracting external funding (and delivering externally funded projects on time and to the budget) to be seriously considered for larger grants. It is, therefore, sensible to start small – as a collaborator rather than a lead applicant on a grant, then as a lead applicant on a small grant, then on a larger grant, then as a co-applicant on a large supranational research grant, and so on. Small grants may not look worth the effort of slaving over the application form and pulling together a team, but success in obtaining a small grant signifies to others that your work is of sufficient quality and importance to attract external interest and investment. Remember, everyone has to start somewhere!

## Training

The final major element in building research capacity is education and training. The best time to start learning about research is as an undergraduate – this was one of the striking elements of the consensus that came out of the MEDINE 2 project funded by the European Union[25]. However, vocational degree programmes such as medicine, which have to fulfil the demanding regulator standards and requirements, have long struggled with finding time for significant research training within the formal curricula. While bearing this in mind, it is important to create opportunities and expose students to research processes (how did we find out that drug A is better than drug B in treating the later stages of chronic obstructive pulmonary disease), as well as outcomes (drug B is recommended by the guidelines) in stimulating ways, at every opportunity. One approach to doing so is that of 'student-selected components', used in the United Kingdom for various purposes, including to give medical students the opportunity to explore research and equip them with at least the basic skills and knowledge (e.g. how to search the literature)[26].

The attractor for the student is that engaging in the research process may lead to presentations and even publications, as well as generic skills development[27]. (Our experience is that students are really very motivated to engage in research for these reasons.) Moreover, encouraging research activity early on can contribute to sustained activity and hence capacity building: Thirty percent of Liverpool Medical School students, all of whom carry out a structured programme of research training, go on to complete Masters programmes within 5 years of graduation.

Interestingly, Van der Vleuten[3] compared research training with the concept of CoPs in that research can be nourished by a group activity that involves all levels of researchers, from undergraduates, faculty who have developed an interest in research, to those involved in full time research. A research CoP encompasses the values of inclusiveness, openness, supportiveness, nurture and mentorship and, by maintaining a close proximity to a themed research programme, extends corporate knowledge about a given area.

Training also implies formal educational programmes. In medical education, these range from programmes such as the series of Essential Skills in Medical Education courses that are run by the Association for Medical Education in Europe (AMEE) (http://www.amee.org/amee-initiatives#esme) through to Masters and Doctoral programmes of which there are a now a multitude[28]. The need for postgraduate candidates to perform a real piece of research provides an incentive to plan opportunities within a programme, resulting in 'win-win' situations where the student gains a good project within a research team and the research team gains the resource of a keen and motivated student.

There is a place for running local training programmes, since these make it easier for busy trainees to attend and have the advantage of situated cognition (see Chapter by Torre and Durning in this volume). Such programmes can help align practice with current research in the very specific local context[16,29]. They also help people over the threshold of the local research environment[30], making it more likely that they will recognise and identify with the local landscape of practice[24] and may even choose to join the programme.

The range of opportunities for using faculty development to build research capacity has recently been covered in some detail by Hodges[31]. The essential element is to help people develop their way of thinking about things, rather than simply providing them with a set of skills. In planning training, it is important to recognise that even

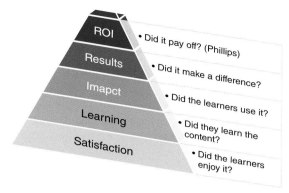

**Figure 24.1** A modified version of the Kirkpatrick[33] model of evaluation.

within a well-functioning team, there are different levels of understanding and confidence about theoretical issues. The research environment should empower people to articulate their understandings and recognise when their colleagues understand something differently[3,32].

It is up to the institution to determine whether the investment in training for research and in the research itself has had an impact. There are several potential avenues to explore[33], but at some stage, the Kirkpatrick model ([34,35]; see Fig. 24.1) needs to be extended to include a consideration of a return on investment[36].

Given the focus of our intention in this chapter, one of the returns on investment may be the implementation or sustaining of some change in medical or healthcare education, which ultimately benefits patient outcomes. For example, there is a growing literature on shared decision making and how it can lead to improved healthcare outcomes[37] and how training on communication skills can improve patient satisfaction and outcomes[38,39]. This endpoint may not be appropriate for all educational research, but where it is, it should not be neglected.

## Conclusion

Most people who get involved in research are highly motivated to understand more about the things that interest them and the things that matter. However, no matter how good the intentions and how keen the individuals are, some research fails to achieve its outcomes, not because of its ideas or content but because of its failure to be planned in a way that ensures long-term effectiveness. Sustainability and long-term effectiveness can be achieved by moving research from an individual activity to a group process. There are some fascinating and inspiring vignettes of those who have faced these challenges, and there is a growing research literature about the research process. We outlined the importance of building a team-based research programme around four action terms: focus, support, resource planning and training and education. This approach can facilitate success, helping to ensure that research achieves its goals.

---

### Practice points

- Early and in-depth, shared discussion about the research question can go a long way in ensuring sustainability of a research programme.

- A team approach to research is usually more successful than an individual approach.

- An effective research team typically encapsulates diversity of expertise and experience.

- Formal and 'on-the-job' training is critical to ensure a sound knowledge base and continue professional development for all researchers.

- Transferability of the research outcome to real life practice (impact) is important in terms of recognition and hence for long-term success.

---

## References

1 Crites, G.E. *et al.* (2014) *Medical education scholarship: An introductory guide: AMEE Guide No. 89. Medical Teacher*, **36**, 657–674.

2 Donnon, T. (2013) Quantitative research methods in medical education. In: Walsh, K. (ed), *Oxford Textbook of Medical Education*. Oxford University Press, Oxford, pp. 626–637.

3 van der Vleuten, C.P.M. (2014) *Medical education research: a vibrant community of research and education practice. Medical Education*, **48**, 761–767.

4 Wenger, E. (1998) *Communities of Practice: Learning, Meaning, and Identity*. Cambridge University Press, Cambridge, New York, Melbourne, Madrid, Cape Town, Singapore, Sao Paulo, Delhi.

5 Kadushin, C. (2012) *Understanding Social Networks: Theories, Concepts and Findings*. Oxford University Press, Oxford, New York.

6 Maudsley, G. & Strivens, J. (2000) 'Science', 'critical thinking' and 'competence' for tomorrow's doctors. A review of terms and concepts. *Medical Education*, **34**, 53–60.

7 Maudsley, G., Williams, E.M. & Taylor, D.C. (2008) Problem-based learning at the receiving end: a 'mixed methods' study of junior medical students' perspectives. *Advances in Health Sciences Education: Theory and Practice*, **13**, 435–51.

8 Maudsley, G. & Taylor, D.C.M. (2009) Learning professionalism in a Problem-based curriculum. In: Creuss, R.L., Creuss, S.R. & Steinert, Y. (eds), *Teaching Medical Professionalism*. Cambridge University Press, New York, pp. 211–224.

9 Watmough, S.D., O'Sullivan, H. & Taylor, D.C.M. (2010) Graduates from a reformed undergraduate medical curriculum based on Tomorrow's Doctors evaluate the effectiveness of their curriculum 6 years after graduation through interviews. *BMC Medical Education*, **10**, 65.

10 Garner, J. *et al.* (2010) Undergraduate medical student attitudes to the peer assessment of professional behaviours in two medical schools. *Education for Primary Care*, **21**, 32–37.

11 Arnold, L. (2004) Preface: Case studies of medical education research groups. *Academic Medicine*, **79**, 966–968.

12 Eby, L.T. *et al.* (2008) Does mentoring matter? A multidisciplinary meta-analysis comparing mentored and non-mentored individuals. *Journal of Vocational Behavior*, **72**, 254–267.

13 Stewart, R.W. *et al.* (2007) The new and improved learning community at Johns Hopkins University School of Medicine resembles that at Hogwarts School of Witchcraft and Wizardry. *Medical Teacher*, **29**, 353–357.

14 Reznick, R.K. (2014) Lessons learned in the pursuit of a dream. *Medical Education*, **48**, 768–775.

15 Baskerville, D. & Goldblatt, H. (2009) Learning to be a critical friend: from professional indifference through challenge to unguarded conversations. *Cambridge Journal of Education*, **39**, 205–221.

16 Zerubavel, E. (1999) *The Clockwork Muse: a Practical Guide to Writing Theses, Dissertations, and Books*. Harvard University Press, Cambridge, Massachusetts and London.

17 Lally, P. *et al.* (2010) How are habits formed: Modelling habit formation in the real world. *European Journal of Social Psychology*, **40**, 998–1009.

18 Badley, G. (2009) Academic writing as shaping and re-shaping. *Teaching in Higher Education*, **14**, 209–219.

19 Archer, M.S. (2012) *The Reflexive Imperative in Late Modernity*. Cambridge University Press, Cambridge.

20 Eva, K.W. & Lingard, L. (2008) What's next? A guiding question for educators engaged in educational research. *Medical Education*, **42**, 752–754.

21 Eva, K.W. (2009) Broadening the debate about quality in medical education research. *Medical Education*, **43**, 294–296.

22 Albert, M. (2004) Understanding the debate on medical education research: A sociological perspective. *Academic Medicine*, **79**, 948–954.

23 Albert, M., Hodges, B. & Regehr, G. (2007) Research in Medical Education: Balancing Service and Science. *Advances in Health Sciences Education*, **12**, 103–115.

24 Wenger-Trayner, E. *et al.* (2015) *Learning in landscapes of practice: Boundaries, identity and knowledgability*

*in practice-based learning*. Routledge, Abingdon, New York.

25 Maerz, R., Dekker, F.W., van Schravendijk, C., O'Flynn, S. and Ross, M.T. (2013) Tuning research competencies for Bologna three cycles in medicine: report of a MEDINE2 European consensus survey. *Perspectives on Medical Education*, **2**, 181–195.

26 Riley, S. (2009) Student selected components (SSCs): AMME Guide No. 46. *Medical Teacher*, **31**, 885–894.

27 Bate, E., Hommes, J., Duvivier, R. and Taylor, D.C. (2013) Problem-based learning (PBL): Getting the most out of your students-Their roles and responsibilities: AMEE Guide No. 84. *Medical Teacher*, **36**, 1–12.

28 Tekian, A. & Artino, A. (2013) AM Last Page: Master's Degree in Health Professions Education Programs. *Academic Medicine*, **88**, 1399.

29 Irby, D.M. (2014) Excellence in clinical teaching: knowledge transformation and development required. *Medical Education*, **48**, 776–784.

30 Land, R., Cousin, G., Meyer, J.H.F. and Davies, P. (2005) Threshold concepts and troublesome knowledge (3): implications for course design and evaluation. In: Rust, C. (ed), *Improving Student Learning–equality and diversity*. Oxford Centre for Staff and Learning Development, Oxford.

31 Hodges, B. (2014) Faculty development for research capacity building. In: Steinert, Y. (ed), *Faculty Development in the Health Professions: A Focus on Research and Practice*. Springer-Science+Business Media, Dordrecht, pp. 79–96.

32 Taylor, D. & Hamdy, H. (2013) Adult learning theories: Implications for learning and teaching in medical education: AMEE Guide No. 83. *Medical Teacher*, **35**, e1561–e1572.

33 Spencer, J., Faculty development research: the "State of the Art" and future trends, In: *Faculty Development in the Health Professions: A focus on Research and Practice*, Y. Steinert, (ed) 2014, Springer Science+Business: Dordecht. p. 353-374.

34 Kirkpatrick, D.L. (1967). In: Craig, R. & Mittlel, I. (eds), *Evaluation of Training, in Training and Development Handbook*. McGraw-Hill, New York, pp. 87–112.

35 Steinert, Y., Mann, K., Centen, A., *et al.* (2006) A systematic review of faculty development initiatives designed to improve teaching effectiveness in medical education: BEME Guide No. 8. *Medical Teacher*, **28**, 497–526.

36 Phillips, J.J. (1996) ROI: The search for best practices. *Training and Development*, **50**, 42–47.

37 Leader, A., Desblabis, C., Braddock, C.H. 3rd, *et al.* (2012) Measuring informed decision making about prostrate cancer in primary care. *Medical Decision Making*, **32**, 327–36.

38 Clark, N.M., Gong, M., Schork, M.A. *et al.* (1998) Impact of education for physicians on patient outcomes. *Pediatrics*, **101**, 831–836.

39 Clark, N.M., Gong, M., Schork, M.A. *et al.* (2000) Long-term effects of asthma education for physicians on patient satisfaction and use of health services. *European Respiratory Journal*, **16**, 15–21.

# 25 Conclusion

*Jennifer Cleland and Steven J. Durning*

The intent of *Researching Medical Education* was to provide an authoritative guide to promote excellence in educational research in the healthcare professions, including medicine, nursing and dentistry, thereby progressing knowledge and understanding in these fields. This book has sought to help provide a bridge between theory and practice, which ultimately could improve the care of patients.

The chapters in this book have been drawn from the contemporary education literature on healthcare professions, and from several other fields including education, expertise, psychology and sociology, to name a few. Our objectives were to introduce a breadth of conceptual frameworks, theories, research designs, methodologies and methods relevant to our field and to illustrate their application in the educational settings across the international healthcare professions. By explicitly linking these areas, we believe that the book you are reading fosters quality improvement, capacity building and knowledge generation. It is timely here to extend our gratitude to the *Researching Medical Education* International Editorial Board members for their guidance based on which theories, models and methods were included in this book. We also thank them for their help during the process of reviewing submissions and guidance on the final product.

Given our broad target audience, which includes Masters and PhD students in healthcare profession education and their supervisors; those who are new to the field, generally inexperienced in research or new to the field of educational research but with prior research experience in the clinical or biomedical domains; and the experienced researchers seeking to explore new ways of thinking and working, the book was divided into three sections. The first was a primer. This section introduced the initial steps in the research process including considering your research philosophy, worldview, ontology and epistemology; carrying out a literature review; writing a research question and considering the number of participants required in your study. The next section of Researching Medical Education introduced a broad array of theories, methodologies and methods relevant to education and research in healthcare professions today. We emphasised the practical aspects of the theory, methodology and/or method through a sample vignette, multiple examples, practice points and key references in each chapter. Finally, the last section of the book provides guidance on developing your practice as a healthcare educational researcher, looking forward from 'doing a study' to disseminating your work and developing leadership in your field.

We cross-referenced chapters as appropriate to highlight to the reader about the common terms and understanding. We believe that this cross-referencing and merging between related fields is a key to advancing our understanding, and thus we highlight some key connections here. Firstly, there is a commonality across the chapters in terms of the overarching framework, or the unifying 'grand' theory. A number of chapters explicitly refer to social constructivism, whereas a post-positivist stance underpins the research reported in other chapters. The importance of workplace teaching and learning in healthcare education practice is reflected by its centrality in a number of quite diverse chapters. Other chapters clearly illustrate the application of theories imported or borrowed from other discipline areas, such as mathematics, education, a number of different branches of psychology and human communication. The introduction to such a wide range of topics in one volume helps the reader understand the key differences and similarities between the topics in terms of their use of theory – for example, what are the commonalities across those chapters focusing on the 'social' or those where the focus is on the 'individual', and how do these approaches differ in their assumptions about the meaning of knowledge and reality?

All the chapters bring not just a topic area but also a number of different ways of studying that topic to the reader, thus illustrating that there is more than one way to build a programme of

*Researching Medical Education*, First Edition. Edited by Jennifer Cleland and Steven J. Durning.
© 2015 John Wiley & Sons, Ltd. Published 2015 by John Wiley & Sons, Ltd.

research. Importantly, several chapters emphasise the importance of aligning and considering the critical foundations of worldview or philosophy, ontology and epistemology, design and methods, no matter what the research topic is. The importance of this basic foundation is also illustrated by the chapters in the book which show how different theoretical lens or methodological approaches can be used to inform understanding and the subsequent action of a given phenomenon.

We must stress here that no one volume can cover all the theories and approaches that are applicable to healthcare profession education. For example, there is little about the philosophy of education in this book; yet, this is critical to questioning the very foundations of healthcare education. For example, the relationship between power and knowledge and how these are used as a form of social control are not covered in depth, although the theories of Foucault and other philosophers[1] are gaining popularity in educational research in healthcare professions. Nor does the book examine in detail the influence of historical, social and cultural factors on what is (currently) seen as legitimate and valued in healthcare education and its associated research.[2] In terms of theory, the emerging work from the neuroscience literature, which is providing important biological insights into our understanding of learning and performance,[3] is neglected by us. Equally, there is little in this book in terms of how theory from organisational psychology and management science can be applied to healthcare profession education.[4]

Many different data collection approaches are illustrated in this book, but again, these examples are not all encompassing. We urge the readers with an interest in qualitative approaches to also explore methods such as the guided walk[5] and creative methods, which employ art, drama, poetry and so on to engage participants in a more holistic way.[6] Those with a more quantitative worldview may have noticed that reliability and generalisability theories are not covered. Nor is there an example of a case-control study although these are not uncommon in studies of healthcare professional training.[7]

Although the book covers a range of topics, from selection to workplace-based learning, motivation to communication, as with theories and methods, we have not been able to include all the topics that are considered legitimate areas of study in healthcare profession research. The (enormous) research topic of formal assessment would require a volume of its own. Research on curriculum change is not introduced. In addition, we are also extremely

aware of our neglect of e-learning and e-research methods.

In short, please do not think if a theory, methodology or a method is not mentioned in *Researching Medical Education*, then is not potentially useful. Moreover, given that our field has always drawn from others and will continue to do so, it is important to be aware of theoretical and methodological developments in other disciplines. An approach that is considered relatively mainstream in, for example, sociology may be appropriate, novel and original in educational research in healthcare professions.

This brings us to an issue, which is very pertinent to the last section of the book on disseminating and developing your research. There is a need for collaborative research into educational research in healthcare professions. Many of the problems and questions that need to be explored are not unique to any one area. Indeed, many are 'grand challenges' (such as widening participation) that require the bringing together of resources and knowledge from different fields and disciplines to understand and perhaps even solve complex, real-life problems.[8,9] It is important to stress the need for interdisciplinary in addition to than multidisciplinary research. In the latter, research problems are investigated from different disciplines, while in the former, theories, insights and methods from different disciplines are integrated to investigate a jointly defined problem. Interdisciplinary collaboration has the potential to forge new research fields.[10] Collaboration of this type is, however, not always easy – different disciplines have different assumptions, language, methods and viewpoints, as well as different journals, publication norms and standards.[10–12] Both of us have had the personal experience of working with colleagues from education where, after talking at apparent cross-purposes for sometime, we often realise that we are actually saying the same thing, but using a very different language to do so. O'Sullivan *et al.*[12] provide a thoughtful overview of the gains and potential pitfalls of collaborative research in medical education, which is essential reading if one is considering embarking on an interdisciplinary project or programme of research. Finally, and on a practical note, funders often like – and look for – multidisciplinary collaborations. Indeed, the right team is a core feature of a successful grant application. Given that educational research in healthcare professions is inherently interdisciplinary – this book provides a number of examples of collaborative working across scientists, social scientists and clinicians from around the globe – the time is right to further diversify the perspectives brought to research questions in our field.

Finally, this book would not have been possible without the support and efforts of the International Editorial Board members, the chapter reviewers and the chapter authors. The book represents a truly global achievement, drawing on intellectual contributions from colleagues working across Africa, Asia, Australasia, Europe and North and South America.

We hope *Researching Medical Education* stimulates fresh thinking and new ideas, stretching the readers' understanding and encouraging them to engage further with new theories, models, methodologies and analysis approaches introduced here for purposes of improving the work that we do.

## References

1 Oakeshott, M. (2000) *The Voice of Liberal Learning*. Liberty Fund, Indianapolis, IN, pp. 69.

2 Kuper, A. & D'Eon, M. (2011) Rethinking the basis of medical knowledge. *Medical Education*, **45**, 36–43.

3 Mareschal, D., Tolmie, A. & Butterworth, B. (2013) *Educational Neuroscience*. John Wiley and Sons Ltd., London, UK.

4 Venance, S.L., LaDonna, K.A. & Watling, C.J. (2014) Exploring frontline faculty perspectives after a curriculum change. *Medical Education*, **48**, 998–1007.

5 Moles, K. (2008) A walk in thirdspace: place, methods and walking. *Sociology Research Online*, **13**, 2.

6 Wiles R, Pain H, Crow G (2011) Innovation in qualitative research methods: a narrative review. *Qualitative Research*, **11**, 587–604.

7 Wayne, D.B., Didwania, A., Feinglass, J., Fudala, M.J., Barsuck, J.H. & McGaghie, W.C. (2008) Simulation-based education improves quality of care during cardiac arrest team responses at an academic teaching hospital. *Chest*, **133**, 56–61.

8 Committee on Facilitating Interdisciplinary Research, Committee on Science, Engineering, and Public Policy. National Academy of Sciences, National Academy of Engineering, and Institute of Medicine of the National Academies (2005) *Facilitating Interdisciplinary Research*. National Academies Press, Washington, DC. http://dels.nas.edu/resources/static-assets/bls/miscellaneous/NRCInterdisciplinaryResearch-Summary.pdf [accessed on 7 August 2014].

9 European Commission (2011). *Commission Staff Working Paper: Horizon 2020 – The Framework Programme for Research and Innovation: Impact Assessment*. SEC (2011) 1427 final.

10 Visholm A, Grosen L, Nom MT, Jensen RL. (2012) *Interdisciplinary research is key to solving society's problems*. Copenhagen, DEA. http://dea.nu/sites/dea.nu/files/Resume_Interdisciplinary%20Research.pdf [accessed 7 August 2014]

11 Gill, D. & Griffin, A.E. (2009) Reframing medical education research: let's make the publishable meaningful and the meaningful publishable. *Medical Education*, **43**, 933–935.

12 O'Sullivan, P.S., Stoddard, H.A. & Kalishman, S. (2010) Collaborative research in medical education: a discussion of theory and practice. *Medical Education*, **44**, 1175–1184.

# Index

Note: Page numbers in *italics* represent figures, those in **bold** represent tables.

*Researching Medical Education*, First Edition. Edited by Jennifer Cleland and Steven J. Durning.
© 2015 John Wiley & Sons, Ltd. Published 2015 by John Wiley & Sons, Ltd.